Robotic Surgery Devices in Surgical Specialties

João Pádua Manzano • Lydia Masako Ferreira

Editors

Rafael Silva de Araújo

Associate Editor

Robotic Surgery Devices in Surgical Specialties

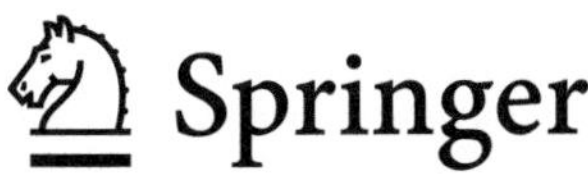 Springer

Editors
João Pádua Manzano
Department of Surgery
Universidade Federal de São Paulo
São Paulo, Brazil

Lydia Masako Ferreira
Plastic Surgery Department
Universidade Federal de São Paulo
São Paulo, Brazil

ISBN 978-3-031-35104-4   ISBN 978-3-031-35102-0   (eBook)
https://doi.org/10.1007/978-3-031-35102-0

This Springer imprint is published by the registered company Springer Nature Switzerland AG
The registered company address is: Gewerbestrasse 11, 6330 Cham, Switzerland

Preface

In the last few decades, surgical procedures have seen remarkable advancements through disruptive technologies. The introduction of minimally invasive techniques in surgery has revolutionized the way surgical procedures are performed, allowing for faster recovery times, less pain, and fewer complications for patients. The next step in this evolution is robotic-assisted surgery, which is expanding rapidly and has the potential to be the most significant advance in surgery for generations to come.

The current robotic platform, the Da Vinci system, is the product of an evolution that began with the US Department of Defense's efforts to provide advanced surgical care to frontline soldiers from remote locations. The system's enhanced dexterity, based on an anthropomorphic model that mimics the human hand's range and freedom of movements, has allowed both average and skilled surgeons to push the envelope in the complexity of minimally invasive procedures. The robotic approach has now permeated essentially every specialty in surgery.

The true potential of robotic surgery lies in two new dynamics between patient and surgeon. The master-slave relationship, where the surgeon is remote from the patient and controls a slave patient cart that is attached to the patient, enables telepresence and will have a profound impact on delivering complex care to remote locations from a command center. It will also dramatically facilitate professional education and collaborative surgery. The digital interface, which allows the collection and manipulation of data that can be used for diagnostic or interventional purposes, represents an even greater potential.

Currently, the robotic approach has permeated practically all surgical specialties. This book is the first comprehensive overview of the role of robotic surgery devices in all surgical specialties. It is intended to give a historical perspective of the evolution and applications of robotic surgery in each surgical specialty. In recognition of the importance of understanding emerging technology and future robotic platforms, this book also provides an overview of the potential impact of this technology on the future of surgery.

Each chapter in this book is written by recognized leaders in their field, examining specific applications of robotic surgery in a surgical specialty. The authors provide detailed technical aspects of each existing platform and the surgical procedures performed using this technology, as well as the results of these techniques. The editors appreciate the participation of these expert surgeons in this effort, and we hope that this comprehensive resource will advance the practice of robotic surgery.

São Paulo, Brazil	Joao Padua Manzano
São Paulo, Brazil	Rafael Silva de Araújo
São Paulo, Brazil	Lydia Masako Ferreira

Contents

History of Robotic Surgery

Lydia Masako Ferreira, Rafael Silva de Araújo,
and Catherine Maureira Oyharçabal

The first appearance of species currently described as "robots" refers to the work "Iliad" by Homer, book XVIII, from the fifth century BC. In it, it was found the activity of creating beings made of metal and gold with their own movement designed by the god of metallurgy, Hephaestus, to serve him in his tasks. In the course of history to the present day, the image of these beings has acquired different features, moving between heroes and villains in different scenarios of prosperous futures or fanciful dystopias [1].

Despite the description in the Antiquity period, the first time that the term "robot" was used comes from the Czech play "Rossum's Universal Robots," written in 1920 by Karel Capek. According to the translation of the play in the work *Rossum's Universal Robots* (Tchápek, 2010, p. 16), it is described that the word *robot* comes from the Church Slavonic term *rob*, which means *slave*, and that as a feminine noun in the Czech spelling *robota*, it translates to *forced labor* or *strenuous physical labor*. Thus, in the theatrical work, the word *robota* was used to refer to metal beings with an image similar to man and which translates to "servants" whose destiny and function was previously established: to fulfill what human beings had not had the ability or intention to perform [2, 3].

It can be seen during the play that the boring activities dedicated to the dozens of replicas allowed human beings more time to dedicate themselves to other intellectual activities, to leisure, and to idleness. In the end, Tchápek describes the awakening of the robots' consciousness in his narrative, which face their dominators with the saying: *"The human stage is outdated. A new world has begun! The government of robots!"* [3].

L. M. Ferreira (✉) · R. S. de Araújo
Plastic Surgery Department, Universidade Federal de São Paulo, São Paulo, Brazil

C. M. Oyharçabal
University of Mogi das Cruzes, São Paulo, SP, Brazil

© The Author(s), under exclusive license to Springer Nature Switzerland AG 2023
J. P. Manzano, L. M. Ferreira (eds.), *Robotic Surgery Devices in Surgical Specialties*, https://doi.org/10.1007/978-3-031-35102-0_1

1

What at first was just a science fiction dream that brought alternative realities and extraordinary battles in the field of Literature gradually brought new tools to human daily life, especially with the advancement of technologies and innovations. In the field of medicine, in the 1980s, there were already specific computer systems that guided certain procedures, such as the case of *Robodoc* for hip replacement surgeries in orthopedics or the *Programmable Universal Machine for Assembly (PUMA) 200* for performing neurosurgical biopsies. During this period, based on a proposal made by the United States Army (USA), the spark was lit for the insertion and idealization of the use of robotic machinery in surgical fields [4, 5].

The main idea of this request was based on the possibility of allowing the arrival of medical aid in military camps of difficult access, changing the previous paradigm of transferring the injured soldier to the nearest hospital and bringing the new concept of taking the operating room to the support unit. In this way, it was hoped to change the precept from "Golden Hour" to "Golden Minute," allowing for immediate intervention and improving the survival of seriously injured soldiers [5, 6].

The pioneering prototypes depended on previous studies by researchers at the *National Aeronautics and Space Administration (NASA)* and Scott Fisher, who developed a screen attached to the face through a helmet to allow a three-dimensional (3D) virtual environment. For the creation of a telepresence device, engineer Dr. Phil Green from the Stanford Research Institute (SRI), a program funded by the US government, Colonel Richard Satava, and other members of the SRI team developed what was called a "telepresence surgery system," also known as the "SRI system," consisting of a surgeon's workstation and a remote surgical unit [7].

This public initiative prototype contained a pair of instrument handlers at the surgeon's station that transmitted their movements to the remote surgical unit attached to the patient. These gauntlets did not contain an articulating wrist and therefore allowed movement in only four degrees of freedom compared to the seven possible degrees of being performed by the human hand. They were positioned below a mirror in order to give the illusion that the instrument handles in the surgeon's hand were attached to the tips projected in the image seen on a monitor. As there was a simple video system, this phase required the use of polarized light glasses to create a 3D image [7].

In the remote surgical unit, instruments could be changed through a twist lock mechanism, making it possible to use needles, intestinal forceps, scalpels, and electrocautery. A point that differentiates the SRI system from current ones is the presence of tactile feedback from force sensors in the distal portion of the instruments, which transmitted sensations to the surgeon and prohibited movements from a certain degree of resistance encountered during the intraoperative [7, 8].

Although it was initially designed for use in open surgery, in 1989, Colonel Richard Satava watched the presentation of a videotaped laparoscopic cholecystectomy performed by Dr. Jacques Perrisat at the Society of American Gastrointestinal and Endoscopic Surgeons (SAGES). This milestone made him bring to the SRI team the idea of promoting the transition from the robotic laparotomy system to a laparoscopic model. At the time, Colonel Satava argued that the robotic telepresence system offered a solution to difficulties with traditional laparoscopic tools, such as providing better-definition stereoscopic vision, improved dexterity, reduced tremor, and motion scaling, that could improve a surgeon's performance beyond their physical limitations [7].

Such action resulted in Colonel Satava's invitation to the *Advanced Research Projects Agency* in 1992 (ARPA, which became the *Defense Advanced Research Projects Agency [DARPA]* in 1993) to develop the telepresence system for potential military applications. With the aim of improving military medicine, mobile units were developed with the telepresence system coupled with tests on mannequins. Despite these initiatives, the system was never used in humans, opting for the exit strategy of patenting it between 1993 and 1994 during the performance of various tests on both live and nonliving models [7, 9].

Created in 1990 and originating from the private initiative of Dr. Yulun Wang, the *Computer Motion* Inc., from Santa Barbara, California, USA, initially aimed to develop an endoscopic support. Along with funding from *NASA*'s Small Business Innovation Research Grant, complemented by *DARPA*, in 1992, the first robotic prototype was released, approved for use in humans by the *Food and Drug Administration (FDA)* in 1994, called the *Automated Endoscopic System for Optimal Positioning* (AESOP) [9].

Its first version, AESOP 1000, was composed of a single mechanical arm coupled to a laparoscopic optic and its control could be performed by pedals. Later versions brought changes, such as the use of voice control in replacing the pedals in the AESOP 2000 and increasing degrees of freedom of movement in the AESOP 3000. In 1996, the HERMES system was announced, which incorporated voice control and haptic feedback into other operating room components, such as lighting or operating table movement, in the so-called AESOP HERMES Ready (HR) [9, 10].

When envisioned, the AESOP was designed to provide improved video image stability and eliminate the need for an auxiliary to hold the optics. Such ambitions were acquired in practice, but it was realized that the operative procedures still required the need for slight movement of the camera from time to time and the surgical team [8, 9].

In 1998, the same company that created the AESOP developed the ZEUS Robotic Surgical System®, in Goleta, California, USA. It consisted of a mechanical arm intended for optics and two independent arms with four degrees of freedom, all attached to the operating table. This system enhancement allowed the introduction of the telepresence concept of robotic surgery from a console. This surgeon's handling device consisted of a video monitor and two handles capable of controlling the instruments in a two-dimensional interface. The ZEUS system was used both in fallopian tube anastomosis and coronary artery grafting in 1998 and 1999, respectively [7].

However, the most successful milestone for this robot comes from Operation Lindbergh, the first transatlantic surgery, performed in 2001. Charles Augustus Lindbergh (1902–1974) was the American aviator who became the inspiring name for this surgery due to his heroic act of planning and performing a solo flight from New York to Paris in 1924, becoming a symbol of American freedom, pride, and daring [11].

Operation Lindbergh consisted of a cholecystectomy performed by Jacques Marescaux, a surgeon located in New York, on a patient located in Strasbourg, France. The ZEUS robot used the SOCRATES telecollaboration system, which allowed the control of robotic arms across the Atlantic Ocean. The result was the success of the operation, whose total duration was 54 min, without technical incidents [11, 12].

Concurrent with the period of development of the ZEUS system, another company created in California in 1995, called Intuitive Surgical Inc., brought its first model to the market: Lenny, an abbreviation for Leonardo. Lenny, whose prototyping continued from where the SRI system had stagnated, took a differential leap by adding a robotic pulse to handling instruments. Such action promoted the addition of the seven degrees of freedom of movement of the human hand to the robot, improving the surgeon's skill and field of action. In addition, the use of glasses with lenses synchronized with the video monitors increased vision, but the manual fixation of the three robotic arms on the operating table took a long time to prepare the room and limited the surgery. Although animal tests were performed in 1996, it was not considered mechanically reliable and still did not provide the surgeon with a very high-quality view of previous events [6, 12].

In 1997, the second generation of Intuitive, Mona, was released in honor of Leonardo da Vinci's Mona Lisa. This was the company's first robotic surgical system to be used in human trials. Unlike Lenny, Mona had an interface with four rotating ports of interchangeable instruments that could be exchanged intraoperatively in a sterile field. Mona's first procedure was a cholecystectomy, performed the same year by Jacques Himpens, a bariatric surgeon at Saint-Blasius General Hospital, Belgium [7, 8].

Despite the success of the surgery, flaws in this system were noticeable, such as the absence of an arm for the endoscopic camera, requiring an assistant to hold it, the fragile coupling of the instruments, and the difficult configuration of the equipment [6, 7].

In 1998, it was launched the robotic platform that would become the one with the greatest impact and employment today: the da Vinci® system. Different from previous robotic systems, the da Vinci obtained the differential of bringing greater ergonomics to the surgeon's movements from the increase of seven degrees of freedom, with two axes of axial rotation, and better convenience when coupling the stereoscopic viewer and the control pedal of the mono- or bipolar power to the surgeon's console. The robot consisted of three arms, two to hold the instruments and one to support the new 3D endoscopic camera, joined to only one exoskeleton, dispensing time to assemble each arm to the operating table [8, 13].

Its first iteration in human trials took place the same year as it was launched in Mexico, Germany, and France in procedures that included cholecystectomy, Nissen fundoplication, thoracoscopy mastectomy, and mitral valve repair. Its first commercial sale took place in late 1998 to the Leipzig Cardiac Center in Germany, and within a year another ten units were sold across Europe. To prove the safety of this new technology, about 300 robotic surgeries were performed on the same continent, especially cholecystectomies and fundoplications. Other registered surgeries were tubal reanastomosis, correction of inguinal hernias, intrarectal procedures, and hysterectomies [8, 14].

In the 2000s, the da Vinci system obtained approval for use in abdominal procedures by the FDA; however, by claiming the equivalence of the da Vinci technology with that of Mona, Intuitive Surgical Inc. was able to extend the authorized regions for the procedures. In 2002, based on the growing need, the company added a fourth arm to the current version to aid in the presentation of anatomical structures [6, 13].

As sales, enrollment, and employment of the new technology soared, in the following year, Computer Motion Inc. merged with Intuitive after a legal battle, halting development of the ZEUS system and migrating all efforts to the latest model [7, 9].

In 2006, Intuitive launched the da Vinci S system, in which it implemented simplifying handling of the operating system and improving quality of 3D endoscopic camera vision. In 2009, the da Vinci model was reformulated to its da Vinci Si version, the most widespread platform in the world. As a highlight, the *dual console* technology was introduced, which allows cooperation between two surgeons, either intraoperatively or in the training, and supervised simulation of surgeons. In addition to these aspects, the images presented to the surgeon obtained further improvements with the incorporation of the *Firefly* system, a technique for applying and acquiring fluorescence images in real time [6].

In 2014, the da Vinci Xi platform reached global markets with the insertion of an exoskeleton adjustable to the patient's table from any positioning angle and an integrated table motion (ITM), which allows repositioning intraoperatively, without the need to reposition the robot. Both features reduce both surgical time and the time required for equipment assembly and preparation. Likewise, the endoscopic camera has received further 3D image quality improvements with the possibility of reversing the camera angle by the surgeon at the console, eliminating the need for an assistant. Over the years, the most recent version announced by *Intuitive* is the da Vinci SP, in which a single specialized arm for minimally invasive single-port surgery features three instruments and a camera articulated to narrow spaces [6, 15].

After FDA approval in the early 2000s, the Vattikuti Institute of Detroit, Michigan, was the first to document the so-called "Vattikuti Institute prostatectomy," which become commonly recognized as one of the most performed procedures in this area: robotic-assisted prostatectomy. Nowadays, several specialties already use robotic surgery, such as gynecological surgeries for benign diseases, orthopedic surgeries for spinal procedures with lower risk of spinal cord injury, otorhinolaryngology and head and neck surgery for oncological procedures with reduced complications, and, in particular, the areas of urological surgery and surgery of the digestive system [5, 13, 15].

In 2018, the British company called *Cambridge Medical Robotics Surgical* (CMR Surgical) launched the *Versius*® robotics platform. According to Luke Hares, the company's chief technology officer, the platform was developed to address some of the limitations and needs not met by previous robotic systems. First, the system's manual controllers were ergonomically designed to optimize the surgeon's comfort, seeking to avoid neck pain and low back pain. Next, the surgeon's console has an open (i.e., non-immersive) *design* that allows the surgeon to maintain communication with his team during surgery and is height adjustable, giving you the option of sitting or standing during the procedure. Visual feedback is provided by the console surgeon's "head-up display," which displays 3D video from the endoscopic camera with an image overlay. Finally, the arms of the instruments have about eight joints, providing seven degrees of freedom of precise and stable movement during the procedure, and it is worth noting the small size of the robot, facilitating docking and transport [16, 17].

Over the years, studies have shown that the use of the robotic platform reduces blood loss and the need for blood transfusion, mean pain scores, and hospital stay compared to the open procedure. On the other hand, there are disadvantages, such as longer operating time depending on the surgery, complex installation process depending on the model used, costs, and lack of tactile feedback [4, 14].

However, perspectives indicate that robotic-associated procedures are a safe reality, superior in several patient-related elements compared to the laparotomy technique and comparable in some of these data to laparoscopy depending on the surgeon's experience and the procedure performed [14]. Despite this, it is noticeable that the history of robotic surgery is far from over, with the potential for the creation of new tools, new systems, and professionals in continuous adaptation of procedures from different specialties for use with robotics in search of excellence in the surgical results of patients.

References

1. Homero. Ilíada. Tradução Carlos Alberto Nunes. 25th ed. Rio de Janeiro: Nova fronteira; 2015.
2. Martins JO, Santos NSA. A Robótica e a Ficção Científica: Primeiras Interações. Darandina Revista Eletrônica. 2019;12:1–20.
3. Jovanovic A. Introdução. In: Tchápek K, editor. A fábrica de robôs. São Paulo: Hedra; 2010. p. 9–23.
4. Siqueira-Batista R, Souza CR, Maia PM, Siqueira SL. Cirurgia Robótica: Aspectos Bioéticos. ABCD, Arq Bras Cir Dig. 2016;29(4):287–90.
5. Gomes MTV, Costa Porto BTD, Parise Filho JP, Vasconcelos AL, Bottura BF, Marques RM. Safety model for the introduction of robotic surgery in gynecology. Rev Bras Ginecol Obstet. 2018;40(7):397–402.
6. Peters BS, Armijo PR, Krause C, et al. Review of emerging surgical robotic technology. Surg Endosc. 2018;32(4):1636–55.
7. George EI, Brand TC, LaPorta A, et al. Origins of robotic surgery: from skepticism to standard of care. JSLS. 2018;22(4):1–14.
8. Morell AL, Morell-Junior AC, Morell AG, et al. Evolução e história da cirurgia robótica: da ilusão à realidade. Rev Col Bras Cir. 2021;48:1–9.
9. Ghezzi TL, Corleta OC. 30 Years of robotic surgery. World J Surg. 2016;40(10):2550–7.
10. Matanes E, Lauterbach R, Boulus S, Amit A, Lowenstein L. Robotic laparoendoscopic single-site surgery in gynecology: a systematic review. Eur J Obstet Gynecol Reprod Biol. 2018;231:1–7.

11. Reich LS. From the spirit of St. Louis to the SST: Charles Lindbergh, technology, and environment. Technol Cult. 1995;36(2):351–93.
12. Pickover CA. The medical book: from witch doctors to robot surgeons, 250 milestones in the history of medicine. 1st ed. New York, NY: Sterling New York; 2012.
13. Li X, Wang T, Yao L, Hu L, Jin P, Guo T, et al. The safety and effectiveness of robot-assisted versus laparoscopic TME in patients with rectal cancer: a meta-analysis and systematic review. Medicine (Baltimore). 2017;96(29):e7585.
14. Oyharçabal CM, Araújo RS, Ferreira LM. Emprego De Sistemas Robóticos Em Diversas Modalidades Cirúrgicas: Revisão Sistematizada De Literatura. IJDR. 2021;11:1–10. Conclusão.
15. Intuitive Surgical. Products & services: systems. 2022. https://www.intuitive.com/en-us/products-and-services/da-vinci/systems. Accessed 25 Jan 2022.
16. Hares L, Roberts P, Marshall K, Slack M. Using end-user feedback to optimize the design of the Versius Surgical System, a new robot-assisted device for use in minimal access surgery. BMJ Surg Interv Health Technol. 2019;1(1):e000019.
17. Butterworth J, Sadry M, Julian D, Haig F. Assessment of the training program for Versius, a new innovative robotic system for use in minimal access surgery. BMJ Surg Interv Health Technol. 2021;3(1):e000057.

Robotic Devices in Aesthetic Plastic Surgery

Marco Aurélio Faria Correa

1 Introduction

We are seeing an increasing number of female and male patients presenting with small- and medium-size abdominal wall deformities coming to our clinics asking for minimally invasive and scarless procedures that can effectively improve their core muscle and the aesthetic appearance of the abdomen. In many cases the problem is not the cosmetic aspect of the skin, nor striae, nor the redundant folds of skin, nor overweight or abdominal lipodystrophy, but rectus diastasis (Figs. 1, 2, 3, 4, 5, 6, 7, 8, 9, 10, and 11). They complain that despite working hard at losing weight, having a strict and rigorous workout regime, they cannot get rid of that bulging stomach and/or the periumbilical deformity (sad belly button). The weakening of the musculoaponeurotic abdominal wall due to congenital conditions, weight variation, aging, or pregnancy is a frequent cause of rectus diastasis and/or umbilical hernia that can alter the cosmetic aspect of the abdomen [1, 2]. The rectus abdominal muscle plays an important role, not only in the cosmetic appearance of the abdomen but also in the stability of the spine. Depending of the degree of the rectus diastasis, it can lead to a vicious posture, spine problems, back pain, slipped disc, etc. Rectus plication can effectively restore function, providing a balance between the anterior and posterior muscle of the abdominal wall, and improve the cosmetic appearance of the abdomen [1, 3]. The long-term evaluation by ultrasonography and CT scan of the plication of the anterior rectus sheath [4, 5] as well as our long-term clinic follow-up (Fig. 12) has shown the efficiency of the recti plication when properly performed.

M. A. F. Correa (✉)
Singapore, Singapore
e-mail: drmarco@drmarco.com

J. P. Manzano, L. M. Ferreira (eds.), *Robotic Surgery Devices in Surgical Specialties*, https://doi.org/10.1007/978-3-031-35102-0_2

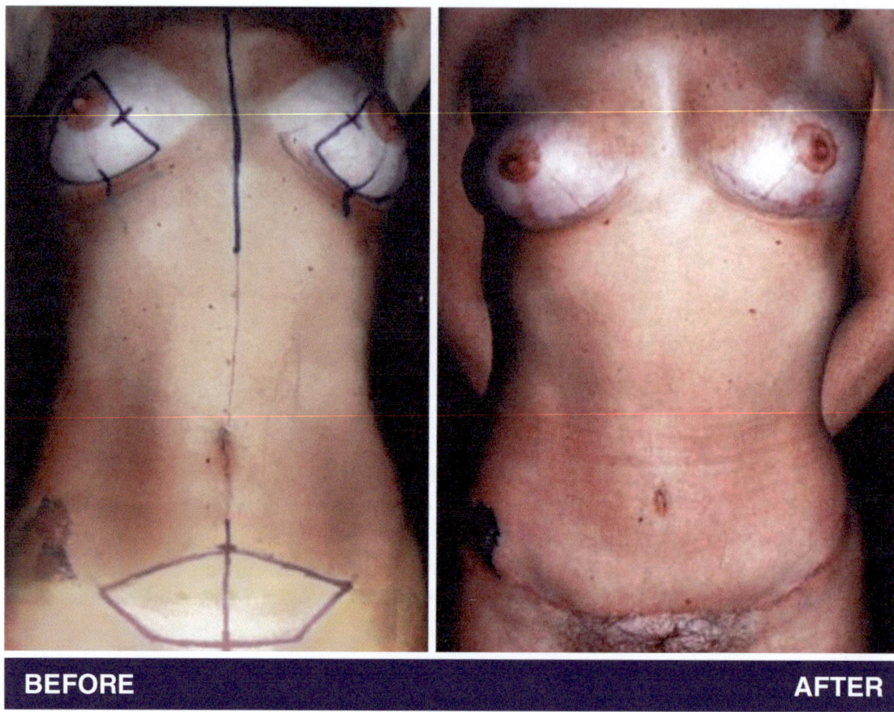

Fig. 1 Mini-abdominoplasty with mini-dermolipectomy done in 1986 caused an anatomical deformity by lowering the umbilicus position

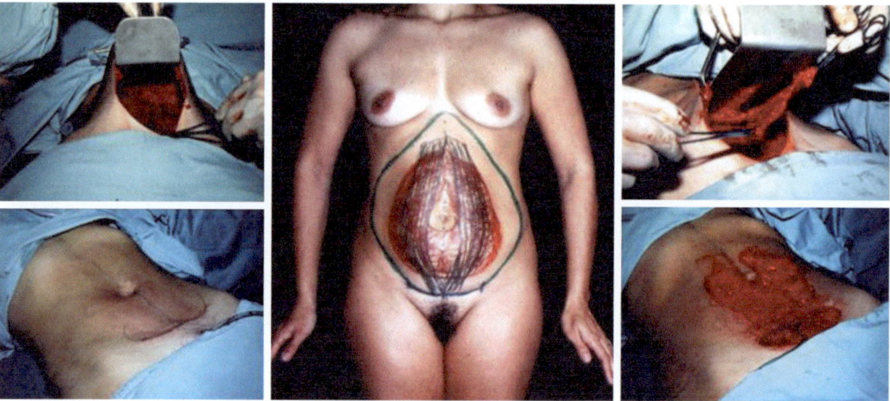

Fig. 2 Minimal scar abdominoplasty: xiphoid-pubic rectus plication, lipectomy, and no skin removal—performing the whole procedure using the previous "C-section scar" with the aid of light source retractors

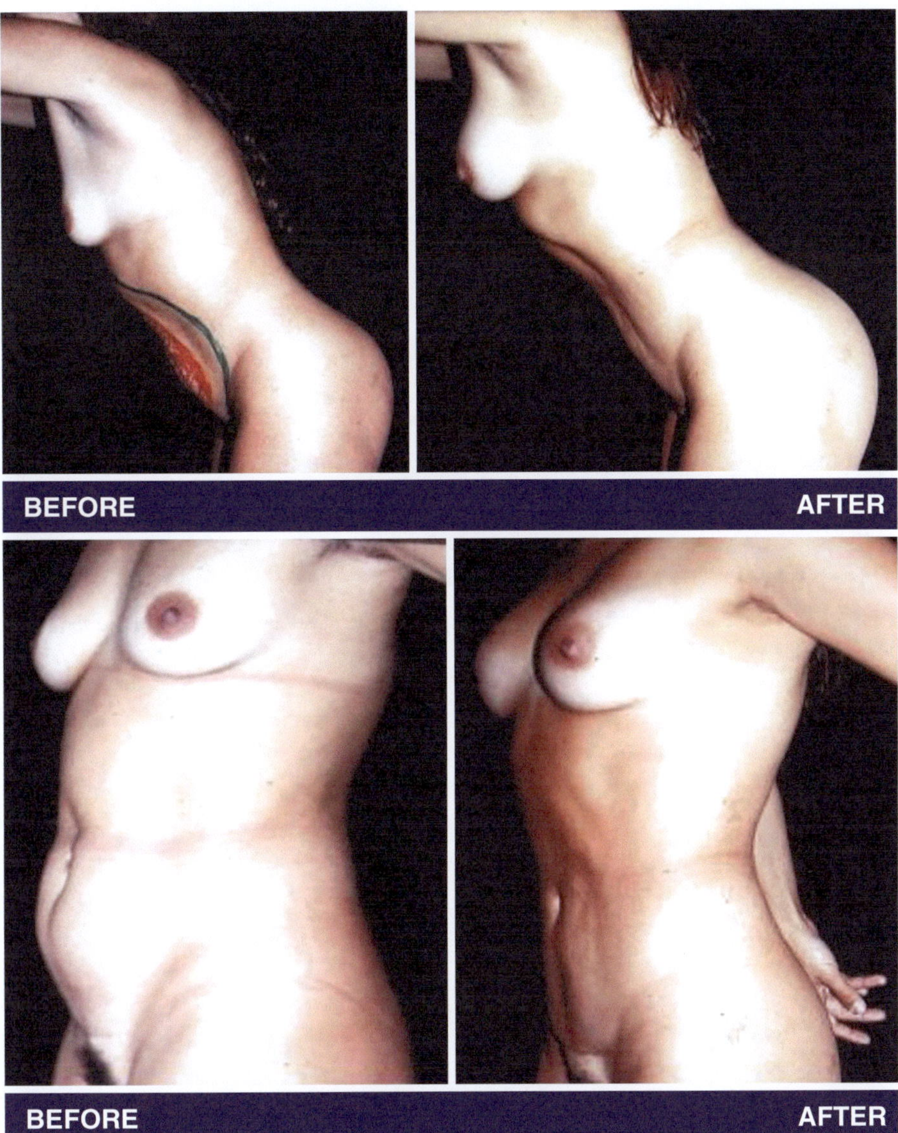

Fig. 3 Before and after minimally incision abdominoplasty

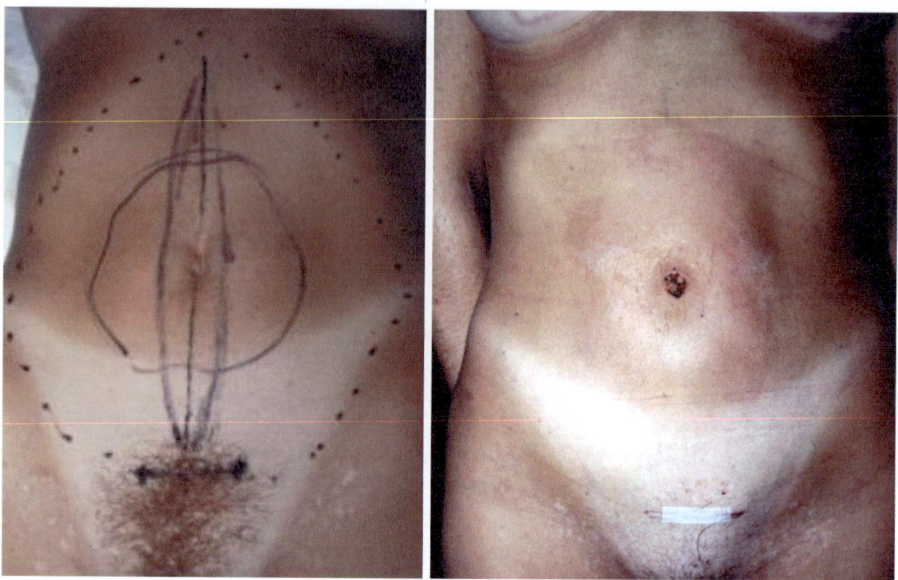

Fig. 4 Endoscopic abdominoplasty scars hidden inside the navel/umbilical and inside the pubic hair-bearing area

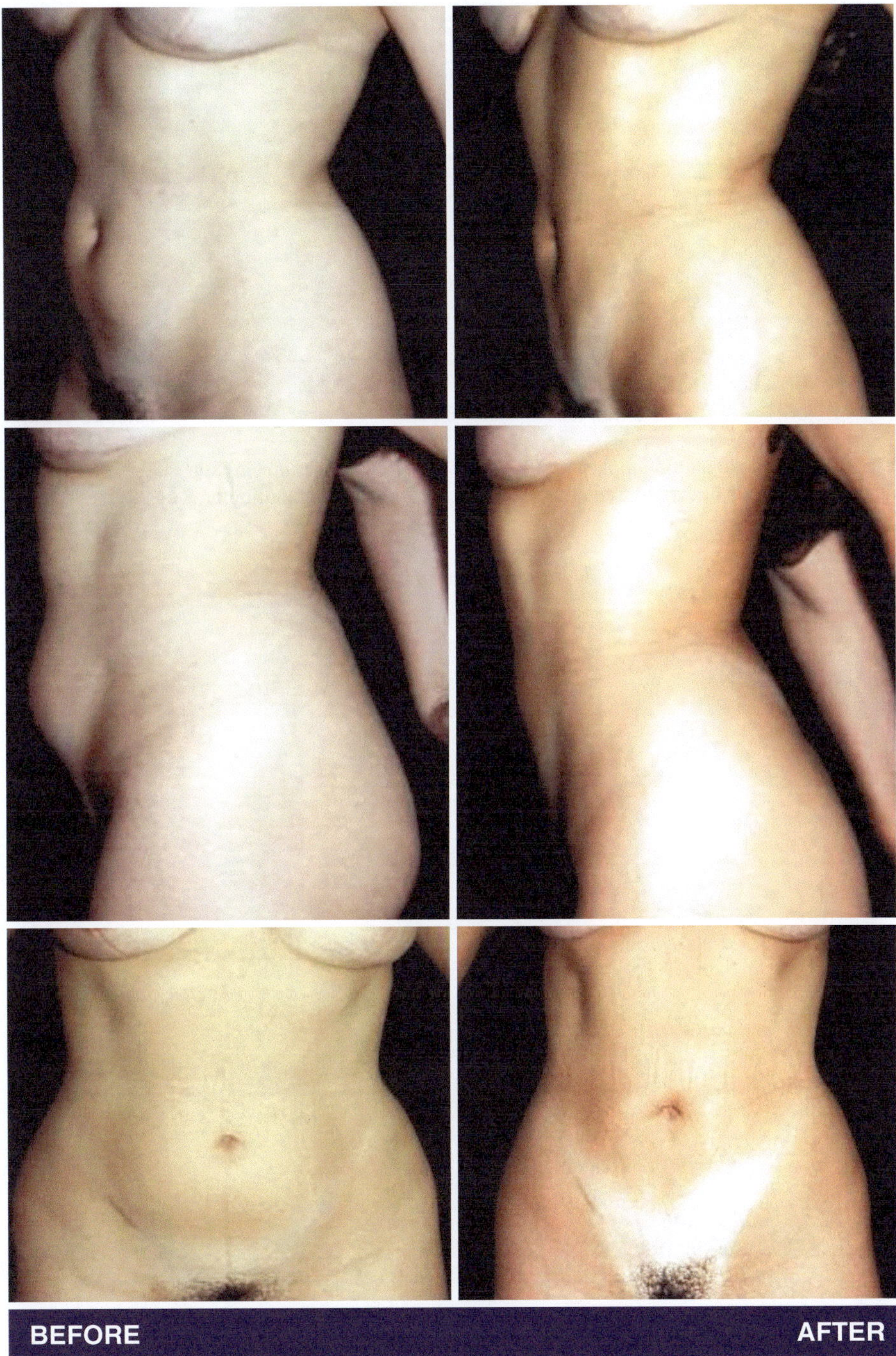

Fig. 5 Before and after endoscopic abdominoplasty

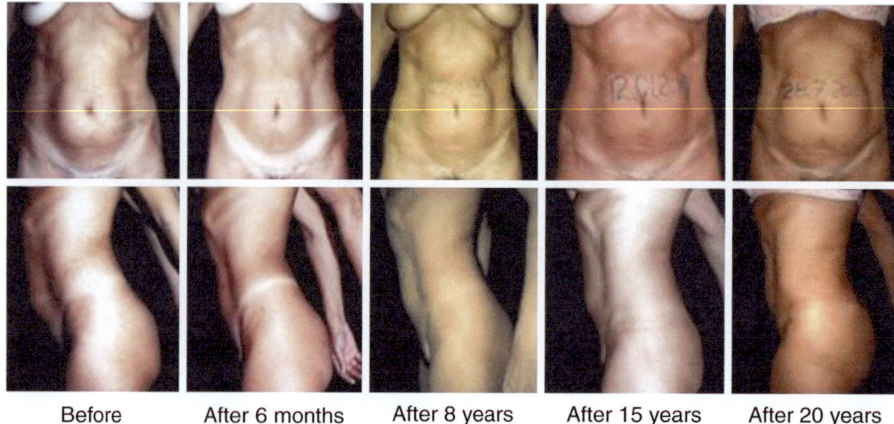

Fig. 6 Endoscopic abdominoplasty with 20 years of follow-up showing the maintenance of the result of the rectus plication even after patient aging 20 years and putting on 8 kg

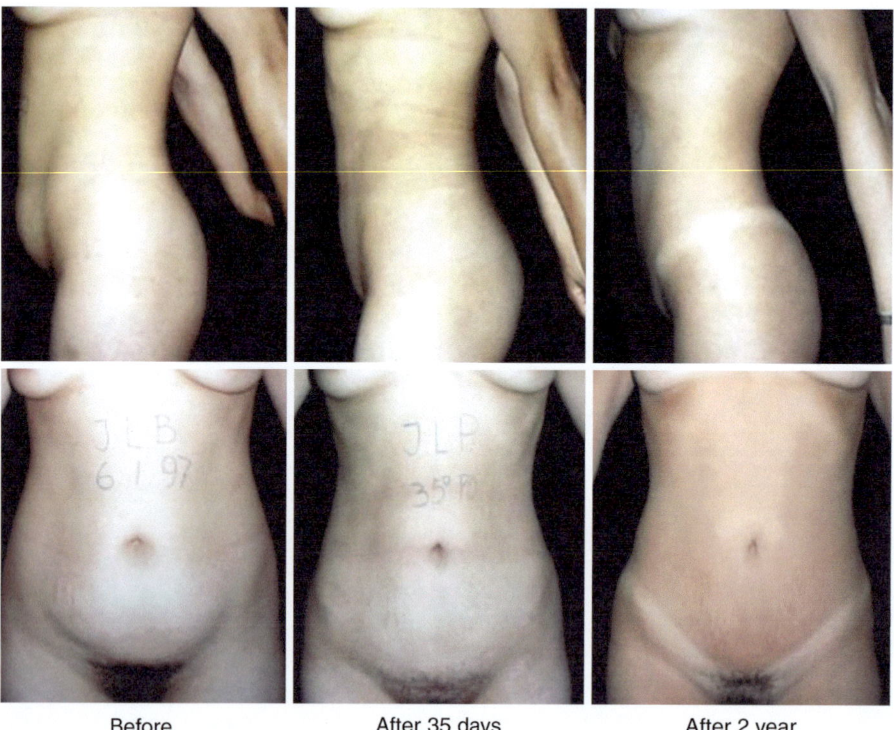

Fig. 7 Long-term follow-up of endoscopic abdominoplasty after 35 days showing a very fast recovery with minimal swelling. After 2 years showing maintenance of the result of the rectus plications and fat plication

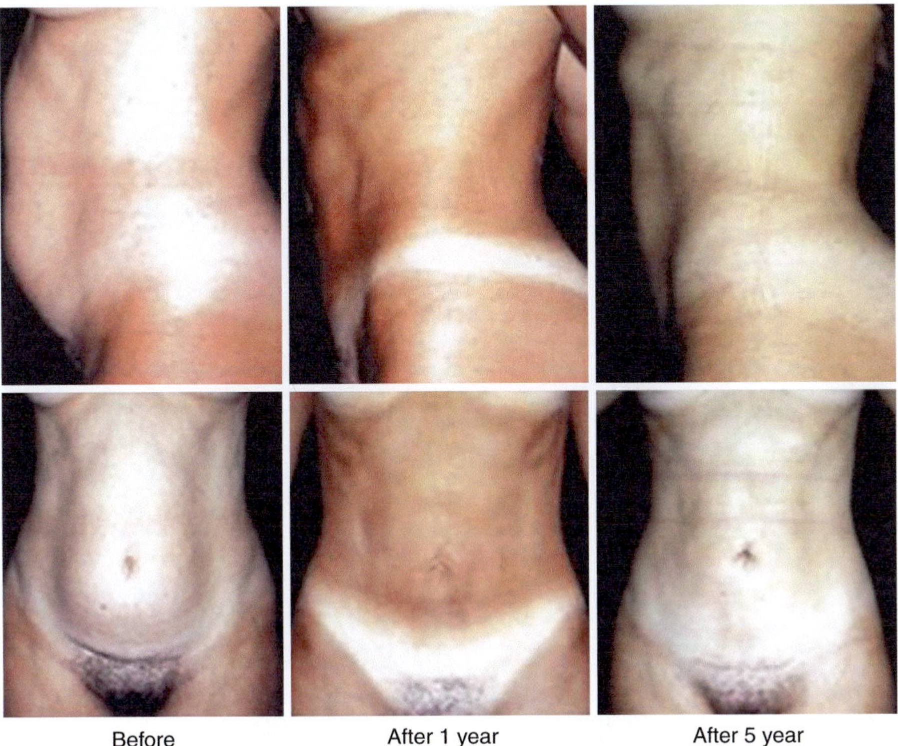

Before After 1 year After 5 year

Fig. 8 The before photo shows a patient who had abdominal deformities after the delivery of twins and was 8 kg overweight. At 1-year follow-up the patient cut down 8 kg. After 5 years post-op, the patient put back 5 kg. We observe the long-term maintenance of the result

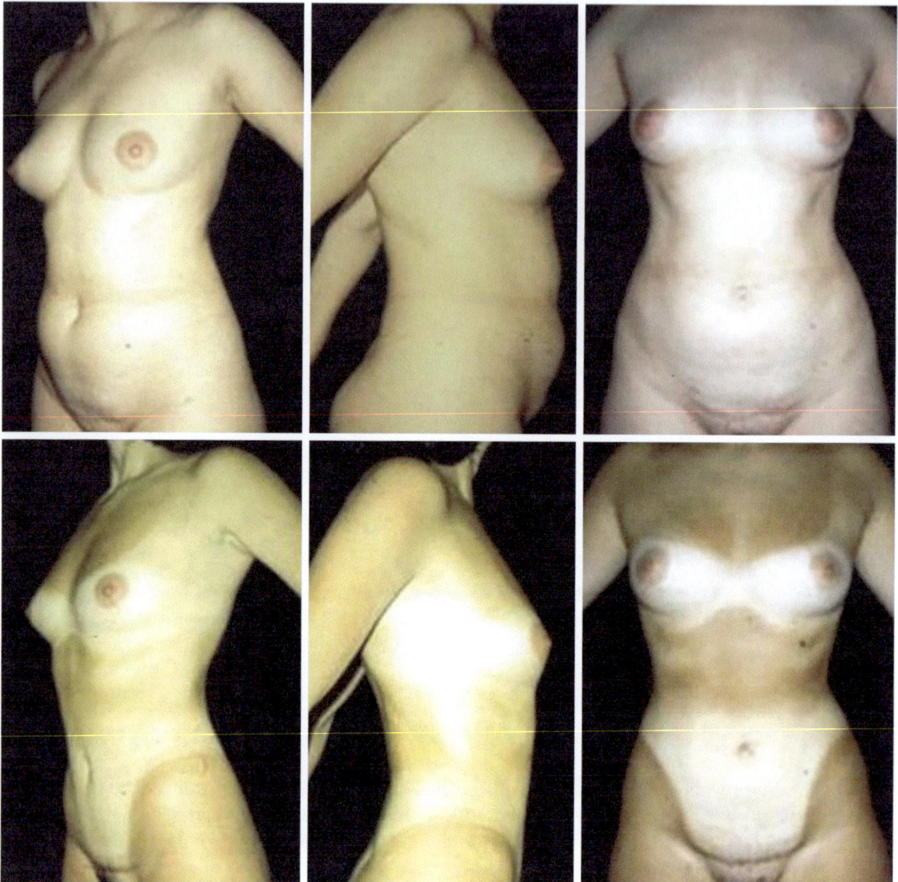

Fig. 9 Endoscopic abdominoplasty performed through C-section scar: before and after

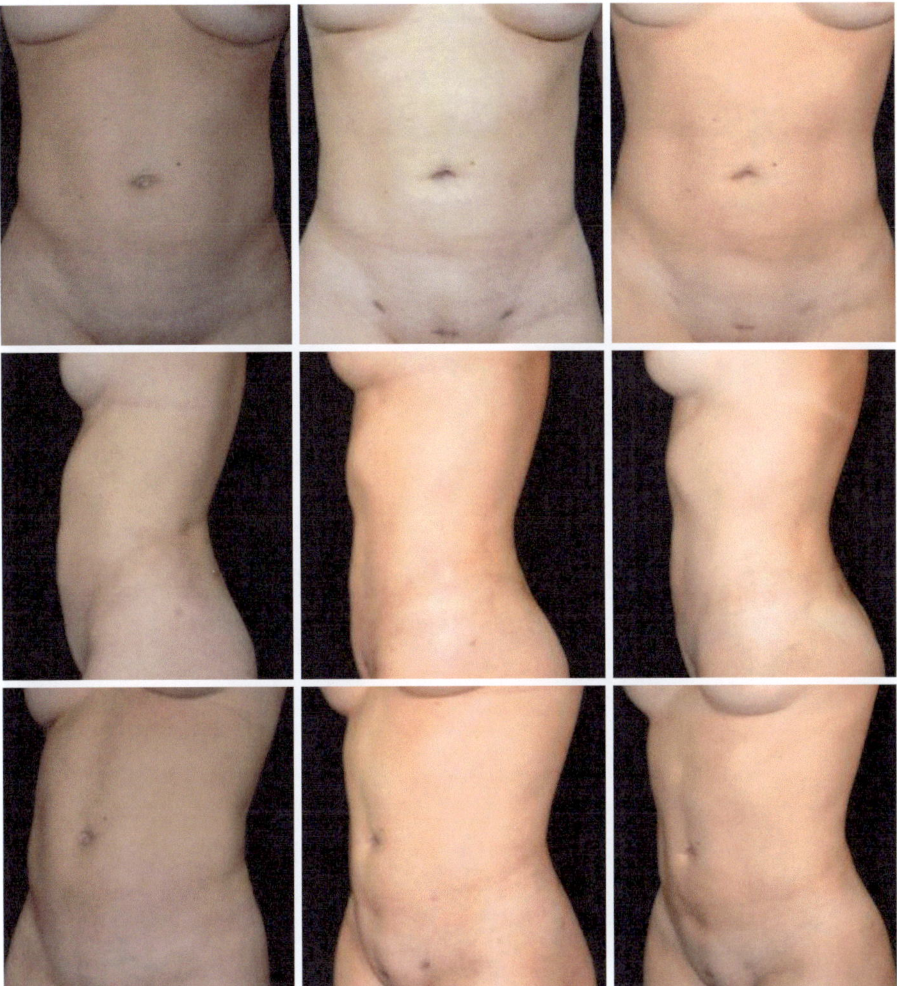

Fig. 10 Robotic abdominoplasty: before and after 3 months and 1 year. After three pregnancies a 42-year-old very fit patient started to suffer from a moderate to severe degree of rectus diastasis that was causing her back pain and urinary issues (urgency to pass urine and leaking urine when coughing and practicing sports). The patient had tremendous improvement in her spine and urinary issues after repairing rectus diastasis. We can observe in the **frontal view** the RD all along the whole abdomen before and the improvement after. In the **profile view** we observe an acute angulation of her spine and a bulging projection of her abdomen on the before view and a nice improvement after; in the **semi-profile** view we can observe a global improvement of the function of her core muscles

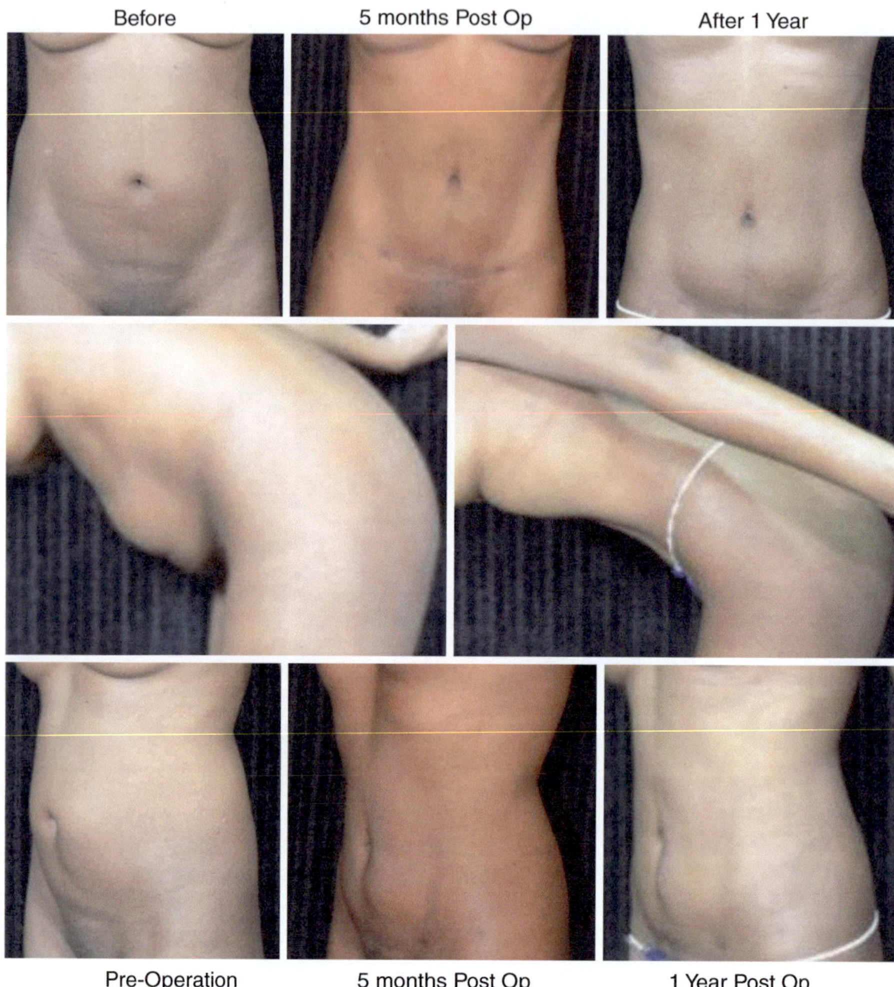

Fig. 11 Robotic abdominoplasty—before, *after* 5 months and *after* 1 year. We can observe important improvement in her posture, a new definition of her core muscle, and in the hanging abdomen before and the new capacity of holding her abdominal viscera after

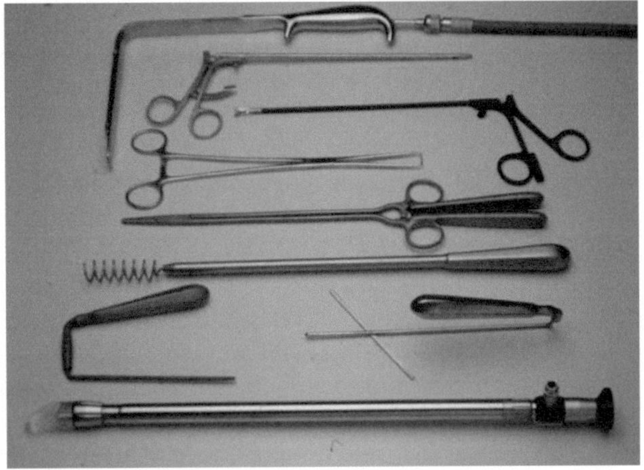

Fig. 12 Set of instrument developed by the author

2 Evolution of Thought

By analyzing the results of mini-abdominoplasty in the treatment of small- and medium-size abdominal deformities, I have drawn the following conclusions:

- Plication of the lower abdominal rectus may cause a protrusion of the upper abdomen; therefore, rectus plication from the pubis to the xiphoid process is required.
- Small skin resections in the lower abdomen will not help in the flabbiness of the abdomen and may cause dog-ears and/or long scars, so I recommend no skin resection and work through smaller incision possible in patients presenting with good skin elasticity.
- The reposition of the umbilical scar below its original position may cause a distortion of the patient's original anatomy and an unnatural and weird appearance, so I recommend reinserting it in its original site.

3 Evolution of the Method: From the Light Source Retractors to Endoscopic and to Robotic Methods

In 1989 I started performing mini-abdominoplasty without removing any skin, just using the previous C-section scar, with the aid of light source retractors freeing the umbilical scar, performing a xiphoid, pubic rectus plication, and lipectomy, and reinserting the umbilical scar in its original site (Figs. 2 and 3)—*minimal scar abdominoplasty technique.*

The beautiful results achieved by effectively treating the cosmetics and functional deformities through minimal incisions, without adding new scars, but just by using the previous scars and even improving it, gave me the enthusiasm.

In 1991 one patient came to me without previous "C-section" asking me if I could treat her using a very small scar hidden inside her pubic hair-bearing area. Attentive to the emerging video-endoscopic method, which was so promising, allowing the surgeons working through very minimal incisions, I had the idea of using endoscopic methods in plastic surgery [6–9].

Then, at the University Hospital PUC Porto Alegre, I started a research project to adapt endoscopic methods to the subcutaneous territory for treating patients presenting with rectus diastasis and no redundant skin, working through incisions as small as 4 cm hidden in the pubic hair-bearing area and inside the umbilical area [7–10] (Fig. 4). In those days there was a concept that we should not use pressured gas in the subcutaneous to develop the optical cavity, the working space, due to the risk of gas embolism when cutting perforators veins during the flap dissection and also the risk of gas dispersion causing the subcutaneous emphysema. For circumventing those risks, I developed a set of instruments to gasless, undermining the abdominal flap, tenting the flap, and stitching the muscle [6, 7, 9] (Fig. 12).

Attentive to the development of new instruments, machines, and methods in surgery that can facilitate and improve our task and result and with more than 20 years of follow-up, it shows the effectiveness of the technique and the beauty of restoring the original anatomy leaving minimal and inconspicuous scars (Fig. 4); in 2013 I started studying and training robotic surgery with the enthusiasm of going for the next level, using the da Vinci Robotic Surgery System to perform rectus plication in minimally invasive abdominoplasty [1].

Robotic surgery is the "gold standard" of minimally invasive surgery in many surgical fields. The robot high-definition three-dimensional view and the amplification of images give us a much better depth sensation of the surgical field than the 2D endoscopic view; it is even better than our naked eyes. Laparoscopic instruments have a limited range of motion; the robot EndoWrist range of movements is comparable to the human wrist. The surgeon's hand tremor is transmitted through the rigid laparoscopic instrument; this limitation makes delicate procedures more difficult [10, 11]. The superb precision and stability of the robot arms, surgical field, and instruments, all controlled by the surgeon seated at the console in a comfortable ergonomic position, without the need of coordinating camera and instrument movement with a surgical assistant makes the surgery much easier, more precise, and less stressful [1].

In urology, robotic prostatectomy is such a solid application, presenting so many advantages over the open methods as well as over the endoscopic methods [11, 12] that, if a patient has the chance to choose which methods to undergo, the best choice would be to go for robotic-assisted ones. In cardiothoracic surgery the surgical robots are also proving to be the key in transforming technically challenging open procedures like mitral valve repair and heart revascularization into technically feasible, minimally invasive procedures. In any institution where robotics "da Vinci Surgical System" is available, the tendency for laparoscopic surgery (in gynecology, colon-rectum surgery, and general surgery) is being replaced by robotic-assisted surgery due to the many advantages that robotic-assisted surgery presents over laparoscopic method [1].

In many surgical fields robots are becoming a promising technology.

In reconstructive plastic surgery it has already been used for the harvesting of latissimus dorsi in breast reconstruction, supermicrosurgery, hand surgery [10, 13, 14], and hair transplant.

So far I didn't find in the literature any report of other applications of robotics in aesthetic plastic surgery [1].

As a cosmetic plastic surgeon I feel it is very interesting that there is a fast-growing trend for the use of robot for performing trans-axillary robotic thyroidectomy and robot retro-auricular submandibular gland resection [15, 16] procedures that are improved or tweaked to minimize visible scars or even relocate the scars to other body areas that could be hidden. Yet little is done in the area of aesthetic plastic surgery, where scarring is of an important concern for patients [1].

After completing my training and certification as a robotic surgeon, I designed retractors to perform a gasless muscle—aponeurotic rectus plication in the same fashion as I do endoscopic abdominoplasty. I performed my first case in April 2015 and since then up to now 31 cases are done with no complication and very satisfactory results.

4 Surgical Robots

The equipment that I am using is the da Vinci Surgical System SI and XI. It consists of three components: the console where the surgeon sits to operate the robotic arms, a robotic cart with three or four arms on which the patient sits, and the high-definition 3D vision system.

It is the surgeon that operates. The robot system does not have autonomy to do anything on its own; every single movement is operated and controlled by the surgeon. Sitting at the console, using the joysticks, the surgeon drives the robot arms and endowrist instrument operating very precise miniaturized tools. Using the feet, the surgeon controls the camera (zoom in zoom out), monopolar and bipolar cut, and cauterization, as well as switching use of the second and the third robot-working arms, without the need of coordinating the movements with an assistant [1].

5 Surgical Technique

I use two different methods: the CO_2 method and the gasless method. In this chapter I will describe the gasless method that is the direct evolution of the minimal scar abdominoplasty. It is the method that I recommend for the beginners.

5.1 *Anesthesia*

For endoscopic abdominoplasty, epidural anesthesia or general anesthesia is used. For robotic abdominoplasty general anesthesia is my preference because after docking in the robotic arms, the patient should stay still, in a state where she could move as a reaction to pain or other stimuli. There is a so-called remote center in the trocar that must stay in place to avoid tearing the skin. All the movements of the robot arms are around a fixed rotating point.

5.2 *Infiltration*

Five hundred milliliter of saline solution and 1 mL of epinephrine (1:500,000) are infiltrated at the area to be undermined in between the fat tissue and the muscular aponeurosis to facilitate dissection and reduce bleeding as well as in the incision sites.

5.3 *Incisions*

If a patient presents with previous scars from cesarean sections or other abdominal surgery (Figs. 6, 7, 8, and 9), the surgeon assesses the need to repair the scars as well as the possibility of using them for access [6, 9].

In endoscopic abdominoplasty technique if there is no previous C-section scar, a 4 cm incision is made at the pubic hair-bearing area and another one inside the umbilical scar (Fig. 13).

In robotic abdominoplasty I use two incisions of 0.7 cm at the bikini line 20 cm far from each other to avoid instrumental collision and one incision for the camera arm at the midline of the patient's abdomen, inside the pubic hair-bearing area at the pubic bone level, 3 cm above the vaginal furcula, measuring to 2 cm, and one "Y"-shaped incision is made within the umbilical scar (Fig. 14). The umbilical port is used for the introduction of retractors for tenting the abdominal flap, for supplying sutures and gauze into the operative field, and for the surgical assistant helping with laparoscopic instruments if necessary. Liposuction can be done using the same three incisions in cases of lipo-abdominoplasty (Fig. 14).

The skin of the umbilical scar is detached from its stalk. If there is an umbilical or paraumbilical hernia to be repaired, I do it before proceeding for the rectus plication. The umbilical stalk is then transfixed using a 3-0 mononylon suture. The reinsertion of the umbilicus skin flaps is done after finishing the rectus plication, at its original site, deep inside the plication [9]. If there is redundant skin at the navel, a Y-shaped incision is made generating 3 triangular flaps [6, 9], the closure of it will leave inconspicuous converging scars, following Avelar's original idea [17]. By resecting part of these triangular flaps, we treat the redundant skin (Fig. 15) [1, 6, 9].

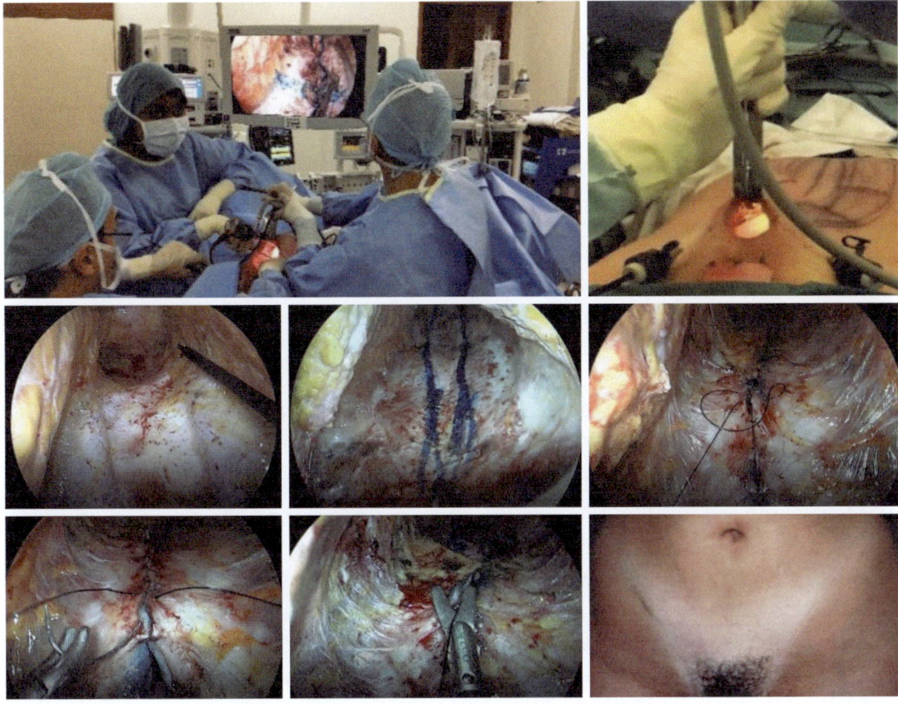

Fig. 13 Endoscopic abdominoplasty: (1) team positioning; (2) suprapubic incision; (3) dissection and identification of the diastasis recti; (4) rectus abdominis muscle inner border demarcation; (5) first layer of plication using interrupted stitches; (6) cutting tread after stitching; (7) second layer of stitching, running suture using mononylon 2-0; (8) resulting scar hidden inside the pubic hair-bearing area

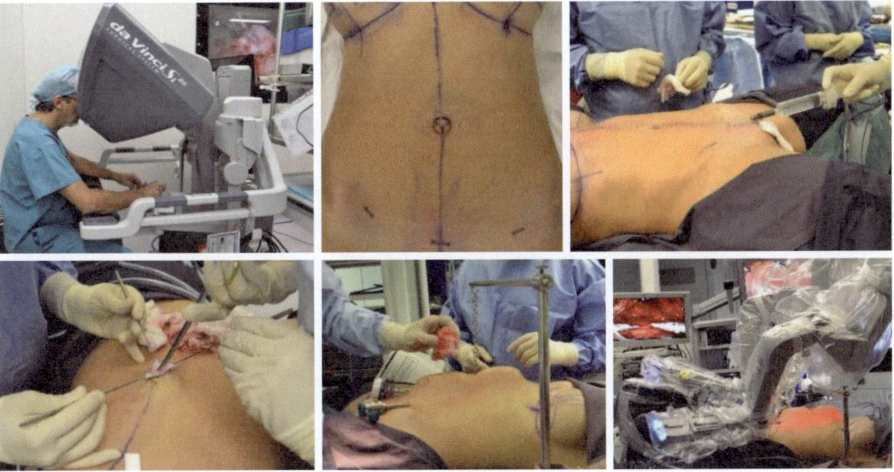

Fig. 14 Robotic abdominoplasty: (1) surgeon sitting at the console performing the rectus plication; (2) drawing the incisions; (3) infiltration of saline solution and adrenaline (1:500,000); (4) Y-shaped incision at the umbilicus; (5) Faria-Correa retractor tenting the flap to maintain the optical cavity in a gasless fashion; (6) robot arms positioned and the surgeon performing the rectus plication (1)

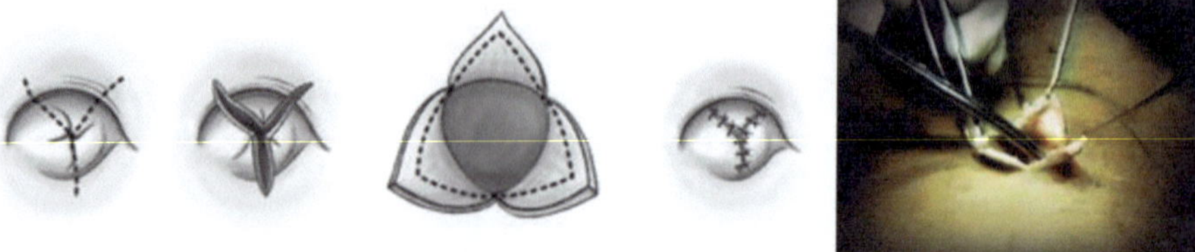

Fig. 15 The surgical sequence of umbilicoplasty technique is as follows:
• Intraumbilical Y-shaped incision
• Three triangular flaps and a wide entrance port
• Partial resection of these flaps to treat flabbiness
• Closure, leaving inconspicuous converging scars

5.4 Dissection and Elevation of the Abdominal Flap

In the gasless method the undermining starts from the umbilicus progressing downwards through the midline towards the pubis and from the pubic incision upwards, or vice versa, to meet each other. The procedure begins with the use of traditional methods with conventional instruments as far as our eyes, fingers, and instruments allow us to work safely and comfortably. With the aid of a 4 or 7 mm 30-degree endoscope, retractors, and the "subcutaneous tomoscope" [9] or electrocautery, we progress to dissecting a tunnel from the pubic bone to the xiphoid process (Figs. 6 and 13) up to the outer borders of the rectus abdominal muscles to create the optical cavity. The undermining can be done endoscopically or with the aid of the robot system. If further undermining is necessary for a proper redistribution of the abdominal flap, we do a blunt dissection, creating tunnels and preserving vessels and nerves. Tunneling preserves the sensitive innervation of the abdominal wall and provides faster recovery with earlier reduction of the edema [9] (Fig. 7).

5.5 Recti Plication

We identify the rectus diastasis (Figs. 13 and 16), and with a small cotton bud tinted with methylene blue, we demarcate the inner border of the rectus abdominal muscle aponeurosis to be plicated. Plication of the anterior rectus sheath is performed in two layers, the first layer using 2-0 or 3-0 nylon buried stitches 1.0 cm distant from each other, and the second layer of two continuous sutures using V-Loc 00 nylon: one starting from the xiphoid process running till just above the umbilical stalk, another continuous running suture starting from just below the umbilical stalk to the pubic bone.

Supra-umbilical or periumbilical flabbiness is frequent (Fig. 17). This deformity occurs during pregnancy when the abdominal muscles stretch and the subcutaneous fatty tissue attached to them is pulled away, creating a gap with skin flabbiness in the region. This subcutaneous fat gap is repaired by suturing the two edges of the fat

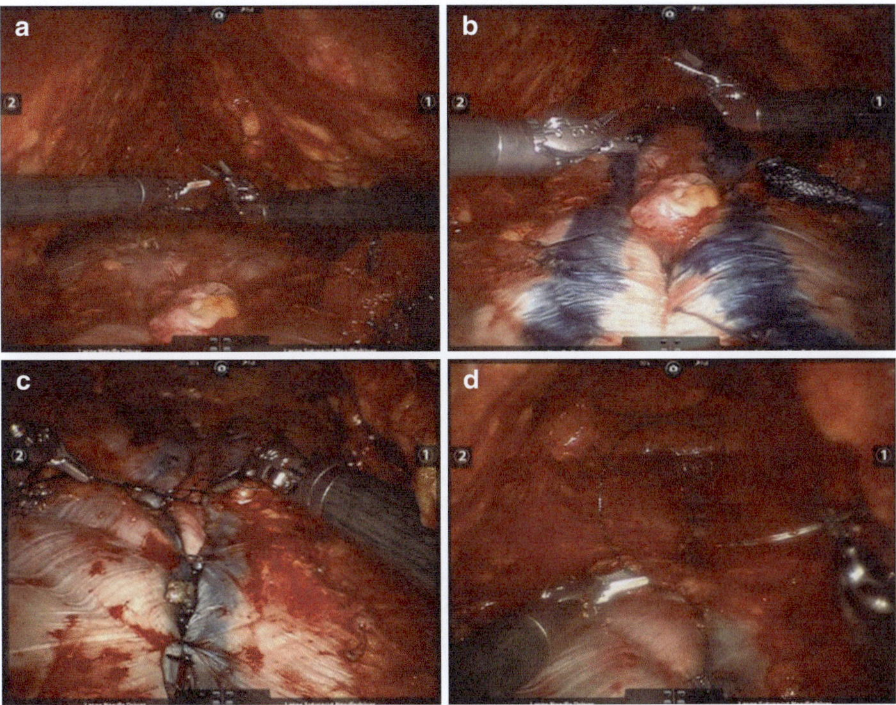

Fig. 16 Robot rectus aponeurosis plication. Surgeon's HD 3D view in the console. (**a**) Identify the rectus diastasis. (**b**) Draw the inner border of the rectus abdominis using a small cotton bud. (**c**) Plication starts using 2-0 nylon interrupted stitches 1 cm distant from each other. (**d**) Second layer of plication by using a 2-0 V-Loc nylon running suture

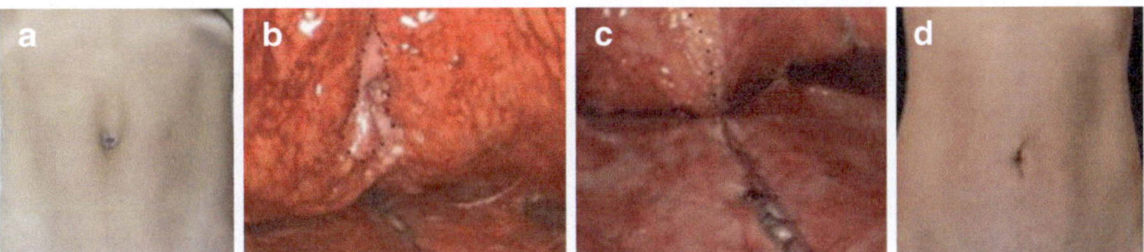

Fig. 17 (**a**) Pre-op showing the rectus and periumbilical fat diastasis. (**b**) Intra-operation, a view of the repaired rectus diastasis and the mark of the edges of the subcutaneous fat gap to be repaired. (**c**) Intra-op, a view of the rectus diastasis repaired and subcutaneous fat gap repaired. (**d**) Immediate postoperative result

tissue together with 4-0 monocryl interrupted sutures. A small hole is left between the edges to permit these small triangular umbilical skin flaps to pass through it for the reinsertion into the umbilical stalk, which was previously secured by the spare suture mentioned earlier [9].

5.6 *Liposuction*

If there is any area that requires liposuction, the liposuction will be performed after the rectus plication. We aspirate only the deep surface of the dermal-adipose flap. In the undermined areas we use the cannula with the holes facing up. In the non-undermined areas, we use the cannula with the holes facing down in the traditional way and liposuction of the deep fat tissue area, creating tunnels, preserving vessels, and creating a closed vascular system just like what was described by Avelar [18].

6 Results

I have done approximately 20 cases of minimal incision abdominoplasty from 1989 to 1992, approximately 300 cases of endoscopic abdominoplasty from 1992 to 2015, another 280 cases of endoscopic assisted abdominoplasty and endoscopic abdomino-plasty (using both the CO_2 and the gasless method) from 2015 to today, and 31 cases of robotic abdominoplasty from 2015 to today. I have many robotic abdominoplasty patients with up 5 years of long-term follow-up (Figs. 10 and 11) and endoscopic abdominoplasty cases up to 5 and 20 years of follow-up (Figs. 6, 7, and 8). We can observe an important cosmetic improvement, a much flatter abdomen, improvement in the posture, and a natural reconstitution of the patient's original anatomy leaving minimal scars, and most patients inform an important improvement in their quality of life by reducing their suffering from back pain and pelvic floor dysfunction.

The rectus plication showed effectiveness and is long-lasting in most of the cases when the plication method was done using two layers of stitching: first-layer interruptive stitches with nylon 00 and second-layer running stitches. It failed in a few patients that didn't respect the proper downtime and started exercises before 6 months.

I converted the minimally invasive abdominoplasty into a full abdominoplasty in about 20 cases. After a short period of time, because some patients had some degree of flabbiness that they did not accept, and other who were happy with the result of the endoscopic abdominoplasty for many years, after putting on weight and plus the aging process caused redundant skin, they decided to remove the redundant skin.

Overall the results are very satisfactory when it is done in the right patients with no redundant skin and with realistic expectations and that don't want long scars.

7 Complications

The complications in minimally invasive abdominoplasty, both endoscopic and robotic methods, are the same: seroma (Fig. 18) and hematoma. So far in a total number of more than 600 cases in more than 32-year experience, I never had one case of infection and skin necrosis, had some cases of skin surface irregularities due to the liposuction, and had cases of rectus diastasis failure because the patients

Fig. 18 Seroma

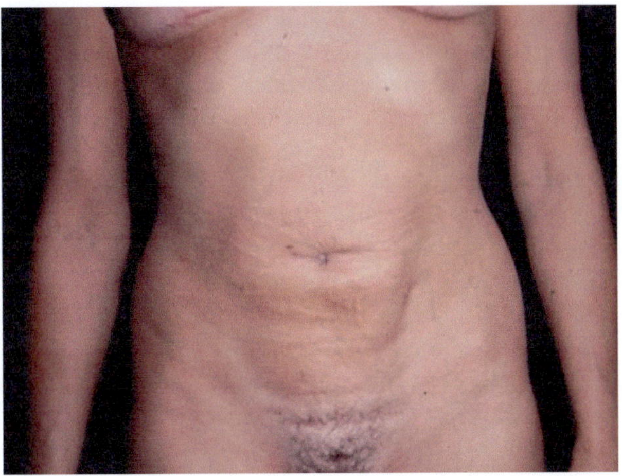

started physical activities too early, not following the recommendation of 6 months of no sports but only core muscle re-education exercises. We manage to reduce the incidence of seroma by reducing as much as possible the undermining area, creating a closed vascular system [18], and stitching the dermal-adipose flap to the muscle fascia, and suction drainage would have to be maintained minimally for 2 or 3 days or until the drainage over 24 h is less than 30 cm^3 [6, 9].

8 Discussion

A proper understanding of the patient's concern, a correct diagnosis of the issues involved, and a clear discussion with the patient about the surgical plan and the outcomes are paramount.

Treating patients with over-redundant folds of skin, flabbiness, and skin damaged by striae is an easy task. We have no doubt on what to do. Our patients will be very happy to have a long scar, that will fade as time goes by, in order to have the ugly and redundant skin removed, to get a new body contouring.

But the situation is not the same when it comes to the treatment of small- and medium-size abdominal wall deformities. They ask for scarless minimally invasive procedures that can restore their original anatomy.

Post-gestational deformities are most of the time associated with rectus diastasis and the stretching of the linea alba that causes a protrusion in the abdominal wall affecting the function of the core muscle, leading to medical and cosmetic issues. Rectus diastasis most of the time is not limited to the lower abdomen but extends towards the whole abdomen—that is why rectus plication from the pubis to the xiphoid is required for a proper functional and cosmetic result.

Many times, the skin is not the patient's concern. If the patient's skin is still presenting with good elasticity, with the capacity to retract, and is also presenting with a nice cosmetic aspect, cutting a fuse of skin in the lower abdomen will not help in treating a small degree of flabbiness, and will just create unnecessary scars, sometimes cause a lowering of the umbilicus positioning, distorting the patient's original anatomy, not contributing to the beauty of the result.

Liposuction alone will not be enough if there is a rectus diastasis. Liposuction can be associated with rectus diastasis in very selected cases of real abdominal lipodystrophy.

Pregnancies can cause an imbalance of the core muscle. After repairing and reconstructing the linea alba, a physiotherapy work may be helpful to achieve the optimal result. We recommend a postural re-education with a specialized physiotherapist to reinforce the core muscle and a proper healthy lifestyle and maintenance of the right weight.

Minimally invasive surgery presents many advantages compared to open methods, like fast recovery, less pain, lower risk of infection, and minimal scars that are our goals in cosmetic surgery. Plastic surgeons are not well trained in minimally invasive methods and it will demand a lot of time, cost, and dedication to develop skills in endoscopic surgery and robotic surgery. Robotic surgery also adds a cost to the patient and that makes it difficult for some patients to afford. In robotic surgery an initial limitation is the loss of haptic feedback (force and tactile). Conventional endoscopy presents with a 2D image view, whereas the da Vinci system presents with a high-definition precise 3D image that compensates for the loss of haptic feedback [1].

But, even if minimally invasive methods present advantages over open methods, what I consider more important in this technique is *the new concept in mini-abdominoplasty: In patients presenting with good cosmetic aspect of the abdominal skin, good elasticity, and no redundant skin, we should work using minimal incisions and do* remove any skin; plication should be performed using nonabsorbable stitches, at least one layer of interruptive stitches, and extends from the pubis to the xiphoid process; the umbilical scar should be re-inserted in its original site; and liposuction should be performed when necessary.

## 9	Conclusion

We are living a new era in plastic surgery. We have learned a lot about the skin elasticity and capacity to retract. New technologies to help the skin to retract are available. Rectus diastasis so far still needs surgical treatment. Minimally invasive methods have shown many advantages over the conventional methods, and scars are one of the most important concerns in our cosmetic patients. Robotics in aesthetic plastic surgery is still in its infancy, but it is very promising considering its many advantages in minimally invasive surgery associated with high technology that helps us work through minimal scars with incisions at remote sites, leaving inconspicuous scars that are the hallmark of plastic surgery. Over the past 30 years we are seeing an increasing number of female and male patients coming for the treatment of small- and medium-size abdominal deformities. Many of them are presenting with rectus diastasis, no redundant folds of skin, good skin elasticity, and with or without abdominal lipodystrophy. They demand for scarless procedures that can effectively correct it. Liposuction alone will not be effective enough in many cases. The long-term evaluation of midline aponeurotic rectus plication, when properly performed, has proved its efficiency. Plastic surgeons are always looking for tools and instruments that can help us to better perform our procedures with more precision, efficacy, less trauma, faster recovery for our patients, and minimal scars. Since 1991 I started using endoscopic methods for the treatment of the described deformities. The efficacy of the minimally invasive method was observed in patients with more than 20 years of follow-up, it gave me the enthusiasm of going to the next level: the "gold standard" of the minimally invasive video surgery, the use of robot "da Vinci Surgery System" for the plication of the rectus diastasis. In many areas of application like urology, gynecology, general surgery, neurosurgery, and heart surgery, robot surgery has proved to have many advantages over conventional endoscopic methods due to the robot high-definition three-dimensional surgical view and amplification of images that makes it much more accurate than the 2D view provided by the conventional endoscopic methods, the superb precision and a much larger range of motion of the robot endowrist instruments that are comparable to the human wrist, and the stability of the surgical field, camera, and instruments, all controlled by the surgeon seated at the console in a comfortable position [1]. It is time to stop creating unnecessary scars and using minimally invasive methods in body contouring plastic surgery. It is time for robotics in plastic surgery. MILA (minimally invasive lipo-abdominoplasty) is the state of art of 32 years of evolution of a new concept in mini-abdominoplasty and by the introduction of emerging technologies of endoscopy and robotic. The Endoscopic version of MILA, Endoscopic Abdominoplasty awarded by the American Society of Plastic Surgeons and Plastic Surgery Foundation in 1996 (Fig. 19a) and the Robotic Abdominoplasty awarded by six societies of cosmetic and plastic surgery in Asia in 2016 (Fig. 19b).

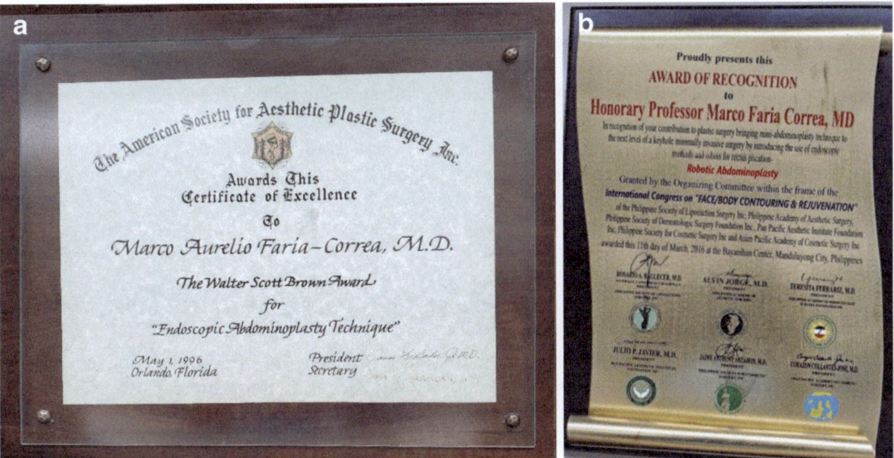

Fig. 19 (**a**) Endoscopic Abdominoplasty Technique award by the American Society of Plastic Surgeons in 1996 "*Endoscopic Abdominoplasty Technique*". (**b**) Robotic Abdominoplasty Technique received award of recognition in 2016 during the **International Congress on "FACE/BODY COUNTOURING & REJUVENATION"**—*in recognition of my contribution to plastic surgery bringing mini-abdominoplasty technique to the next level of a keyhole minimally invasive surgery by introducing the use of endoscopic methods and robots for rectus plication—robotic abdominoplasty*

References

1. Faria-Correa MA. Robotic procedure for plication of the muscle aponeurotic abdominal wall. In: New concepts on abdominoplasty and further applications, vol. 11. New York, NY: Springer; 2016. p. 161–77.
2. Nahas FX, Ferreira LM. Concepts on correction of the musculoaponeurotic layer in abdominoplasty. Clin Plast Surg. 2010;37:527–38. https://doi.org/10.1016/j.cps.2010.03.001.
3. Nahas FX, Augusto SM, Ghelfond C. Suture materials for rectus diastasis: nylon versus polydioxanone in the correction of rectus diastasis. Plast Reconstr Surg. 2001;107(3):700–6.
4. Nahas FX, Ferreira LM, Augusto SM, Ghelfond C. Correction of diastasis: long-term follow up of correction of rectus diastasis. Plast Reconstr Surg. 2005;115(6):1736–41. https://doi.org/10.1097/01.PRS.0000161675.55337.F1.
5. Nahas FX, Ferreira LM, Ely PB, Ghelfond C. Rectus diastasis corrected with absorbable suture: a long-term evaluation. Aesthet Plast Surg. 2011;35:43–8. https://doi.org/10.1007/s00266-010-9554-2.
6. Faria-Correa MA. Abdominoplasty: the South America style. In: Ramirez OM, Daniel RK, editors. Endoscopic plastic surgery. New York, NY: Springer; 1995.
7. Faria-Correa MA. Abdominoplastia videoendoscopica (subcutaneoscopica). In: Atualizacao em Cirurgia Plastica Estetica e Reconstrutiva. Sao Paulo: Robe Editorial; 1994.
8. Faria-Correa MA. Videoendoscopic abdominoplasty(subcutaneouscopy). Rev Soc Bras Cir Plast Est Reconstr. 1992;7:32–4.
9. Faria-Correa MA. Videoendoscopic subcutaneous abdominoplasty. In: Endoscopic plastic surgery, vol. IV(16). 2nd ed. St. Louis, MO: Quality Medical Publishing, Inc; 2008. p. 559–86.
10. Faria-Correa MA. Videoendoscopy in plastic surgery: brief communication. Rev Soc Bras Cir Plast Est Reconstr. 1992;7:80–2.
11. Lanfranco AR, Castellanos AE, Desai JP, Meyers WC. Robotic surgery: a current perspective. Ann Surg. 2004;239(1):14–21. https://doi.org/10.1097/01.sla.0000103020.19595.7d.
12. Lee HS, Kim D, Lee SY, Byeon HK, Kim WS, Hong HJ, Koh YW, Choi EC. Robot – assisted versus endoscopic submandibular gland resection via retroauricular approach: a prospective nonrandomized study. Br J Oral Maxillofac Surg. 2014;52(2):179–84. https://doi.org/10.1016/j.bjoms.2013.11.002.
13. Selber JC. The role of robotics in plastic surgery. St. Louis, MO: Quality Medical Publishing, Inc.; 2009. http://www.plasticsurgerypulsenews.com/12/article_dtl.php?QnCategoryID=112&QnArticleID=236.
14. Selber JC, Baumann DP, Holsinger FC. Robotic latissimus dorsi flap for breast reconstruction. Plast Reconstr Surg. 2012;129(6):1305–12. https://doi.org/10.1097/PRS.0b013e31824ecc0b.
15. Lee J, Chung WY. Robotic thyroidectomy and radical neck dissection using a gasless transaxillary approach. Robot Gen Surg. 2014;24:269–70. https://doi.org/10.1007/978-1-4614-8739-5_24.
16. Mattei TA, Rodriguez AH, Sambhara D, Ehud M. Current state-of-the-art and future perspectives of robotic technology in neurosurgery. Neurosurg Rev. 2014;37(3):357–66. https://doi.org/10.1007/s10143-014-0540-z.
17. Avelar JM. Umbilicoplastia-uma tecnica sem cicatriz externa. An do XIII Cong Bra de Cir Plast Porto Alegre; 1976, p. 81–2.
18. Avelar JM. Uma nova tecnica de abdominoplastia-sistema vascular fechado de retalho subdermico dobrado sobre si mesmo combinado com lipoaspiracao. Rev Bras Cir. 1999;88/89(1/6):3–20.

Features and Knacks of Robotic Keyhole Cardiac Surgery

Ryuta Seguchi, Norihiko Ishikawa, and Go Watanabe

1 Introduction

The da Vinci Surgical System (Intuitive Surgical, Sunnyvale, CA) has revolutionized the field of minimally invasive cardiac surgery. While it avoids sternotomy similar to conventional minimally invasive cardiac surgery via lateral thoracotomy, the robot provides clear visualization of the operation field and enables precise movements of its arms, which allows more elaborate surgery compared to those performed with human hands (Fig. 1).

Robotic cardiac surgery has mainly developed in the field of coronary artery bypass grafting (CABG) and mitral valve repair (MVR). The da Vinci Surgical System has played a key role in this development. In the year 1998, Carpentier performed the first robotic mitral valve repair using a prototypic da Vinci Surgical System. In the same year, Loulmet et al. performed the first robotic totally endoscopic coronary artery bypass (TECAB) in an arrested human heart. In the year 2000, Falk described the first off-pump robotic TECAB using an endoscopic stabilizing device. In the same year, Chitwood performed the first complete mitral valve repair using the da Vinci Surgical System [1].

In Japan, the first robotic cardiac surgery was performed by our team in 2005 [2]. In 2009, we established a method to perform robot-assisted totally endoscopic mitral valve repair using the da Vinci Surgical System [3]. We used the da Vinci S system until 2018 and then converted to using the da Vinci X system. From 2005 to October 2021, we have performed 1143 robotic cardiac surgeries. These include 191 cases of CABG, 815 cases of MVR, 98 cases of atrial septal defect (ASD) closures, 4 cases of ventricular septal defect (VSD) closures, and others.

R. Seguchi (✉) · N. Ishikawa · G. Watanabe
Department of Cardiovascular Surgery, NewHeart Watanabe Institute, Tokyo, Japan

© The Author(s), under exclusive license to Springer Nature Switzerland AG 2023
J. P. Manzano, L. M. Ferreira (eds.), *Robotic Surgery Devices in Surgical Specialties*, https://doi.org/10.1007/978-3-031-35102-0_3

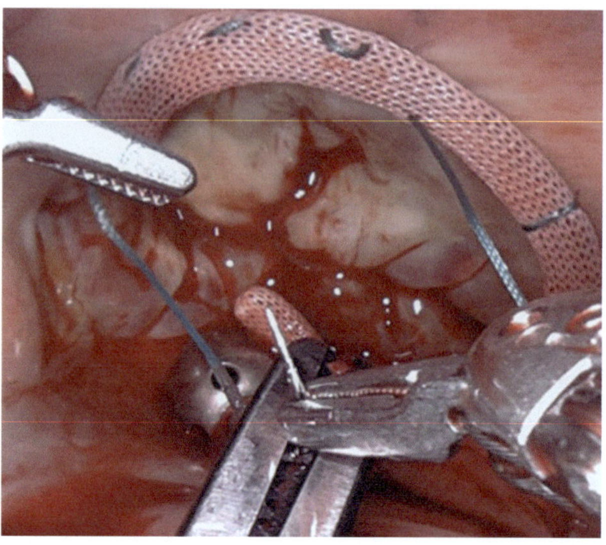

Fig. 1 Clear surgical visualization of tricuspid valve provided by the da Vinci Surgical System

In 2019 and 2020, the number of robotic cardiac cases per year in a single faculty was 212 and 178, respectively, and they were the highest in the world. We would like to introduce our basic methods and share our experiences.

2 Surgical Methods

2.1 Mitral Valve Repair

2.1.1 Patient Selection and Outcomes

Mitral regurgitation due to degenerative change or annular dilatation meets the criteria for robotic mitral valve repair. Contraindications are active endocarditis, solid mitral leaflet due to rheumatic change, and severe tethering with a severely enlarged ventricle.

Ascending aorta clamping is essential for robotic mitral valve repair. Preoperative computed tomography, preferably enhanced, is crucial for evaluating ascending aorta calcification. Patients with calcified ascending aorta should avoid undergoing robotic mitral valve repair. Other exclusion criteria are as follows: (1) severe aortic regurgitation, (2) severe lung dysfunction which cannot tolerate single-lung ventilation, and (3) preoperative history of trauma or surgery in the right pleura of the mediastinum. The third exclusion can be overcome with the use of an endoballoon, but this device is not available in Japan.

In our method, MVR is completed from four keyholes (Fig. 2). The early outcome of mitral valve repair in our faculty is described previously by Tarui et al. with an incidence of 0% mortality, 1.4% cerebrovascular complication, 1.4% reoperation

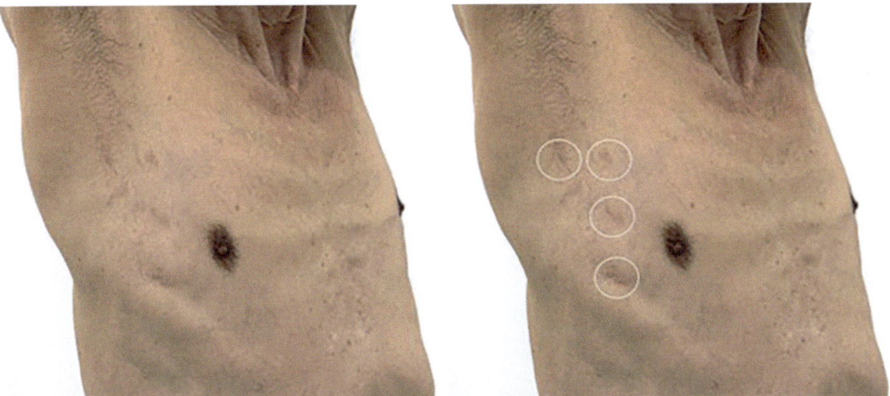

Fig. 2 Operative scars of robot-assisted mitral valve repair. The operation is completed from four keyholes

due to bleeding, 0% new-onset dialysis, 0% reoperation for mitral valve insufficiency within 30 days, and 9.4% requiring transfusion [4]. Mean operation time was 192 ± 49.8 min, cardiopulmonary bypass time was 127 ± 23.8 min, and aortic cross-clamp time was 70.1 ± 16.2 min [4].

2.1.2 Operative Method

The patient is placed in a supine position and general anesthesia is delivered through a double-lumen endotracheal tube that allows for a hemi-pulmonary collapse. A triple-lumen central venous catheter and Swan-Ganz catheter are inserted from the left jugular vein. A 16 Fr drainage tube is inserted from the right jugular vein with low-dose heparin of 3000–5000 units. Transesophageal echocardiography is performed.

Next, the patient is moved to a 30-degree decubitus position. Cardiopulmonary bypass is established following injection of full-dose heparin. A 22–24 Fr drainage tube is inserted from the right femoral vein. Combined with the jugular vein drainage, bicaval drainage is established. In cases with persistent left superior vena cava, an additional drainage tube is inserted from the left jugular vein. The first choice for the arterial line is the right femoral artery, due to its ease and safety of cannulation. In cases where there is calcification and plaques in the descending and abdominal arteries or insufficient diameter in the iliac arteries, the axillary artery is selected as an additional substitute.

Right-thoracoscopic robot-assisted procedure is performed through four ports using a surgical robot system (da Vinci X Surgical System, Intuitive Surgical, Sunnyvale, CA). Ten-millimeter ports are inserted from the third, fourth, and fifth intercostal space on the right anterior axillary line. A service port, 20 mm in diameter, is made in the fourth intercostal space on the right midaxillary line (Fig. 3). The

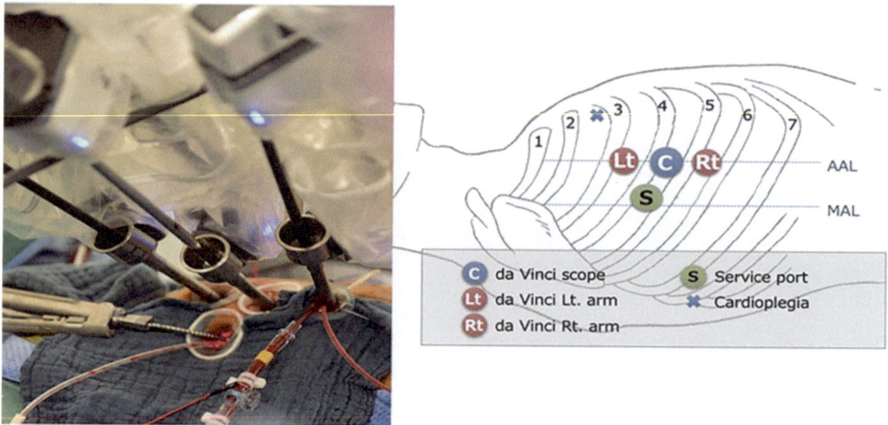

Fig. 3 Port placements in robotic totally endoscopic mitral valve repair using the da Vinci Surgical System

retractor port is added only in cases where it is required. The da Vinci Surgical System is docked to the patient. After pericardiotomy and marking of the right-side left atriotomy line, double purse-string elastic sutures are placed on the aorta around the planned site of cardioplegia cannula insertion. An antegrade cardioplegia needle is directly passed through the chest wall and then inserted through the middle of the purse-string sutures into the ascending aorta. Flexible aortic cross-clamp is endo-scopically inserted from the service port. Cardiac arrest is achieved using cold cardioplegia. Following left atriotomy, the atrial roof is lifted.

The lesion is determined by the saline test, and mitral valve repair is performed according to its etiology. Neochordae implantation, French collection, ring annuloplasty, edge-to-edge techniques, and leaflet augmentation with the pericardium are available options. The ideal leaflet mitral valve surface is confirmed by the saline test. Cryoablation with the designated probe (CryoICE, AtriCure, USA) and endocardial left atrial appendage closure with 4-0 Gore-Tex suture (CV-4; W.L. Gore & Associates, Flagstaff AZ USA) are performed in a patient with coexisting atrial fibrillation. The atriotomy is closed with 3-0 Prolene (Ethicon, Raritan, NJ) continuous suture, and a left ventricular vent tube is inserted from the incision line. The position is changed to Trendelenburg and a sufficient dose of hotshot is given. After which, the aorta is declamped. In patients with coexisting tricuspid insufficiency, tricuspid annuloplasty is performed via right arteriotomy with the superior vena cava clamped. During closure of the atriotomy, the cardia is weaned from the cardiopulmonary bypass. Following vent tube extubation, abolishment of mitral regurgitation is confirmed by transesophageal echocardiography. The cardioplegia needle is evacuated from the aorta according to the method described in Watanabe et al. [5]. Finally, the robot is undocked, cardiopulmonary bypass is disconnected from the patient, and the scar is closed.

2.2   Atrial Septal Defect Closure

2.2.1   Patient Selection

Every secundum atrial defect is a candidate for robotic closure. Exclusion criteria is the same as that for MVR.

2.2.2   Operative Method

The cardiopulmonary bypass is the same as that for mitral valve repair. Under ventricular fibrillation, the operation can be completed using only two ports (Fig. 4). Bilateral robotic arms are inserted to one scar in a cross-armed fashion (Fig. 5). The precise method is described by Ishikawa et al. [6].

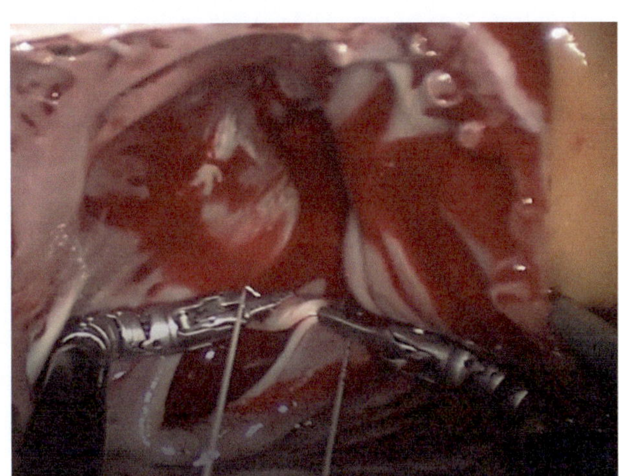

Fig. 4 Intraoperative view of robotic atrial septal defect closure [6]

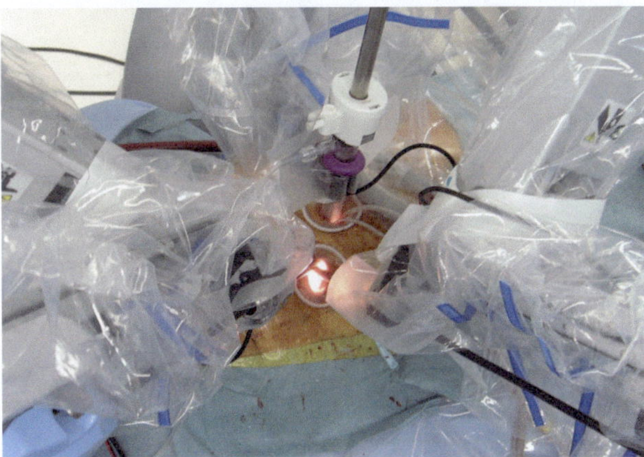

Fig. 5 Scheme and operative image of port setting in two-port robotic atrial septal defect closure. The bilateral arms of the da Vinci S system are inserted to single 20 mm port in cross-armed fashion [6]

2.3 *Coronary Artery Bypass Grafting*

The da Vinci Surgical System is tremendously useful in harvesting the left and right internal mammary arteries (IMA) for minimally invasive coronary artery bypass grafting. The scar is small, and the risk of graft damage is minimized due to its clear visualization and precise movement of the arms [7].

Regardless of the side, the port is placed in the second, fourth, and sixth intercostal space on the anterior axillary line. Single-lung ventilation and insufflation between 6 and 12 mmHg is vital to expose internal mammary arteries. The graft is harvested in a skeletonized fashion from the region between the adhesion site of the first rib to the bifurcation of the sixth rib (Fig. 6). When the IMA is covered with excessive fats and is difficult to visualize, the da Vinci Surgical System's firefly fluorescence imaging is helpful to detect the exact location of the artery [8]. In cases requiring harvesting of both the right and left mammary arteries, we usually harvest starting from the right side. In order to harvest a mammary artery, the robot should be docked from the opposing side. After peeling off the right graft from the chest wall, the robot is moved to the contralateral side. When the left graft is peeled off, heparin is injected. The peripheral portion of the left mammary artery is ligated by clips and is transected. The mediastinal pleura is then incised to visualize the right mammary artery. The peripheral portion of the right mammary artery can be transected via the left pleura with the robot.

Once the grafts are harvested, anastomosis is performed. With the use of the da Vinci S system and U-clip device (Medtronic, Minneapolis, MN, USA), totally endoscopic off-pump left internal mammary artery-left anterior descending (LIMA-LAD) anastomosis can be performed with the robotic arms. The da Vinci S system is equipped with a stabilizer and blower for totally endoscopic anastomosis [9]. In other situations, the anastomosis is performed by hand sewing from the incision made in the fourth or fifth intercostal space.

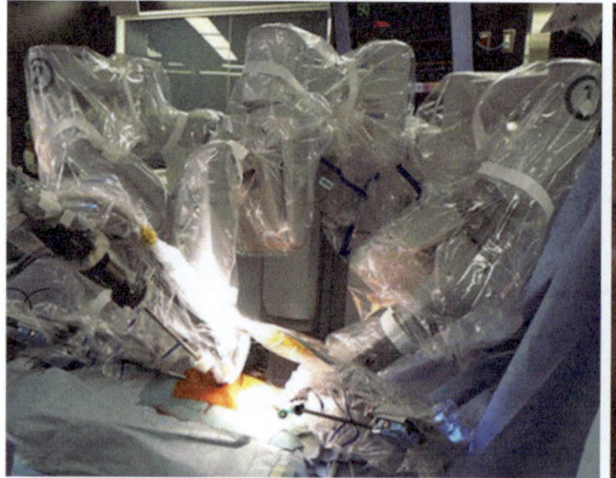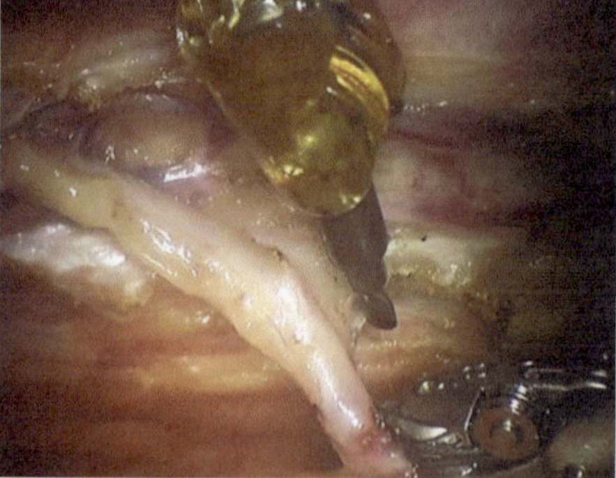

Fig. 6 Intraoperative image of the left internal mammary artery harvesting with the da Vinci Surgical System. The artery is harvested in skeletonized fashion

2.4 Other Procedures

Besides the procedures mentioned above, the da Vinci Surgical Systems are also applicable in treating ventricular septal defect and atrial tumor [10, 11]. With the invention of COR-KNOT (LSI SOLUTIONS, Victor, NY), mitral valve replacement is now performed with the assistance of the robot [12]. Robotic aortic valve surgery has also been reported [13]. Concomitant surgery, such as combining robotic mitral valve repair and coronary artery bypass grafting, is also a good option to avoid sternotomy. It is also possible to combine keyhole left atrial stapler appendectomy with robotic CABG and MVR [14, 15].

3 Tips for Achieving Safe and Successful Robotic Cardiac Surgery

Robotic cardiac surgery has unique features which differ from conventional open surgeries. We herein discuss core concepts and tips to achieve successful and safe keyhole cardiac surgeries.

3.1 Avoidance of Knot-Tying

Although the da Vinci Surgical System provides precise and artistic movements, knot-tying using robotic arms is still a time-consuming process compared to tying by hand. In order for robotic keyhole surgery to proceed smoothly and efficiently, knot-tying should be minimized. Using continuous sutures rather than interrupted sutures is one solution. Watanabe et al. reported that barbed sutures (V-Loc, Covidien, Mansfield, MA) enable continuous suture without knot-tying in mitral valve ring annuloplasty [16].

However, there are several situations in which knot-tying is unavoidable. In such cases, the knot-tying technique should be simplified. "Figure-4 knot," described by Ishikawa et al., avoids knot loosening and provides solid ligation [17]. "Shape-memory suture with spiral," described by Seguchi et al., enables solid hangman knots without ligation [18]. The suture is useful in additional suture for atriotomy line hemostasis.

3.2 Controlling the Bleedings from the Aorta

In order to accomplish cardiac operation via total endoscopy, controlling arterial bleeding, especially from the aorta, is crucial. Incision or injection to the aorta can be avoided by using an endovascular endoballoon. However, in patients with atherosclerosis in the aorta or in countries where endoballoon is unavailable, injection of antegrade cardioplegia needle to the aorta is unavoidable. The hemostasis after extubation of the needle is technically demanding, and this is a limiting factor preventing many faculties from performing the surgery using the keyhole method.

The technique described by Watanabe et al. provides a solution to this problem [5]. In their method, a double purse-string suture with elastic string is made in advance to cardioplegia needle insertion. The two ends of the elastic sutures are clipped together with da Vinci clips. An antegrade cardioplegia needle is directly passed through the chest wall and inserted into the ascending aorta through the middle of the purse-string sutures. For aorta clamping, a transthoracic flexible aortic clamp (Cygnet, Vitalitec International, Balgheim, Germany) is used. The flexible clamp is inserted through the 2 cm service port into the transverse sinus.

Removal of the cardioplegia needle should be performed before weaning from cardiopulmonary bypass. While evacuating the needle from the aorta, the elastic purse-string suture is drawn together by sliding the clips. This provides temporary hemostasis from the cannula hole. An additional 4-0 Prolene suture (Ethicon, Raritan, NJ) is placed to ensure hemostasis.

3.3 Securing Clear Surgical Field

Sufficient and continuous atrial blood suctioning is important to achieve clear visualization and stress-free operation. Since robotic arms cannot afford to be used for suctioning and assistants have difficulty in inserting coronary suctions without interference, placing a DOBON suction catheter (Senko Medical Instrument Mfg, Tokyo, Japan) in the bottom of the atrium is useful to obtain a clear surgical field (Fig. 7). In a right atrial procedure, superior vena cava clamping is vital to avoid blood filling in the atrium. In contrast, blood from the inferior vena cava can be controlled by the drainage tube in most cases. In a patient with persistent left superior vena cava, an additional drainage tube from the left jugular vein is effective in reducing venous return from the coronary sinus.

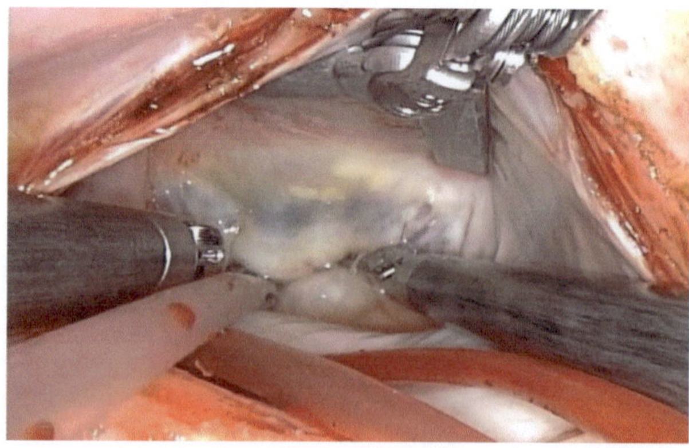

Fig. 7 Secured clear visualization of the mitral valve with posterior leaflet prolapse. Suction catheter placed in the bottom of the atrium provides a bloodless surgical field

Minimally invasive cardiac surgery via the right thoracic cavity has been reported to be technically challenging in cases with pectus excavatum (PE). Low ceiling prevents ideal intracardiac visualization. The sternal elevation with the electrical sternum lifting system, reported by Ishikawa et al., provides a fine visualization of the surgical field and relieves stress in performing robotic surgery and Minimally Invasive Cardiac surgery. In cases with severe PE, combining with the Nuss procedure is effective for correcting rib cage deformity from a small incision [19].

3.4 *Prevention of Stroke*

Prevention of operation-related stroke should be made the highest priority in all cardiac procedures. Unlike conventional open chest cardiac surgery, there are some features in robotic surgery which need specific considerations.

First is the difficulty of quick intracardiac deairing before aortic declamping. This is because ventricle compression is impossible in keyhole surgery. Therefore, sufficient and gradual filling up of the left atrium and ventricle should be accomplished during the left atrial wall closure. This could be achieved by filling up the right cardiac system and expanding the left lung. Blood will be filled antegradely to the left cardiac system from the pulmonary veins and retrogradely from the coronary veins to coronary arteries.

Second is the location of arterial line. Since uncontrollable hemorrhage from the aorta is a concern, the arterial lines for cardiopulmonary bypass are usually connected to peripheral arteries. Femoral arteries are the most common channel for feeding blood, and operations can be performed safely in most cases. However, in cases with moderate to severe atherosclerosis and plaques in the aorta, there are concerns of cholesterol embolism by the retrograde perfusion. In such cases, an additional arterial line to axillary arteries must be established.

Third is the difficulty of changing bed positioning during the procedure. When the da Vinci is docked to a patient, there is always an announcement, "Do not move the operating table for da Vinci is docked." Adherence to this instruction is important for avoiding chest wall and organ injuries while manipulating the robotic arms. However, it prevents surgeons and anesthesiologists from changing to the Trendelenburg position at aortic declamping and cardiopulmonary bypass weaning. Even though it is time-consuming, it is important to undock the robotic ports once and change the body position to avoid air embolism and maintain the cerebral circulation.

In other considerations, Nishijima et al. reported that the silent infarction of the watershed area in the right hemisphere was seen in patients who underwent cardiac operation with arterial line from femoral arteries [20]. The right hemisphere is the farthest region from the femoral arteries. In minimally invasive cardiac procedure, it is vital to maintain sufficient arterial pressure to avoid low cerebral perfusion. Furthermore, since the right hemisphere is not only farthest but also the highest region in left decubitus position, Trendelenburg positioning might be helpful to maintain circulation in the region, especially during weaning from cardiopulmonary bypass.

4 Perspectives

We herein described the basic method of robot-assisted keyhole cardiac surgeries with the da Vinci Surgical System. The robot has become widely used in mitral valve repair, tricuspid valve repair, atrial septal defect repair, and coronary artery bypass grafting. In the recent years, there have been some reports of its use in ventricular septal defect closure and valve replacements. With the evolution of camera flexibility, arm mobility, and invention of new devices, the utility of the da Vinci Surgical System is expected to broaden.

Moreover, in order to perform safe and advanced operations, concomitant advances of surgery personnel are also essential. In robotic surgery, the console surgeon is not the only one who requires a high level of skill. Patient-side surgeons, anesthesiologists, nurses, perfusionists, and mechanics also require specialized skills, and mutual respect is important. Lastly, as the operator's vision is limited to the surgical field, communication and teamwork are essential for success in utilizing this cutting-edge technology.

References

1. Ishikawa N, Watanabe G. Robot-assisted cardiac surgery. Ann Thorac Cardiovasc Surg. 2015;21:322–8.
2. Watanabe G. Successful intracardiac robotic surgery initial results from Japan. Innovations. 2010;5:48–50.
3. Ishikawa N, Watanabe G, Tomita S, Nagamine H, Yamaguchi S. Japan's first robot-assisted totally endoscopic mitral valve repair with a novel atrial retractor. Artif Organs. 2009;33:864–6.
4. Tarui T, Ishikawa N, Horikawa T, Seguchi R, Shigematsu S, Kiuchi R, et al. First major clinical outcomes of totally endoscopic robotic mitral valve repair in Japan - a single-center experience. Circ J. 2019;83(8):1668–73. https://doi.org/10.1253/circj.CJ-19-0284. Epub 2019 Jun 21.
5. Watanbe G, Ishikawa N. Alternative method for cardioplegia delivery during totally endoscopic robotic intracardiac surgery. Ann Thorac Surg. 2014;98:1129–31.
6. Ishikawa N, Watanabe G, Tarui T. No-touch aorta robot-assisted atrial septal defect repair via two ports. Interact Cardiovasc Thorac Surg. 2018;26:721–4.
7. Tarui T, Ishikawa N, Watanabe G. A novel robotic bilateral internal mammary artery harvest using double docking technique for coronary artery bypass grafting. Innovations. 2017;12:74–6.
8. Nakamura Y, Kuroda M, Ito Y, Masuda T, Nishijima S, Hirano T, et al. Left internal thoracic artery graft assessment by firefly fluorescence imaging for robot-assisted minimally invasive direct coronary artery bypass. Innovations. 2019;14:144–50.
9. Nishida S, Watanabe G, Ishikawa N, Kikuchi Y, Takata M. Beating-heart totally endoscopic coronary artery bypass grafting: report of a case. Surg Today. 2010;40:57–9.

10. Gao C, Yang M, Wang G, Xiao C, Wang J, Zhao Y. Totally endoscopic robotic ventricular septal defect repair in the adult. J Thorac Cardiovasc Surg. 2012;144(6):1404–7.
11. Tarui T, Ishikawa N, Ohtake H, Watanabe G. Totally endoscopic robotic resection of left atrial myxoma with persistent left superior vena cava. Interact Cardiovasc Thorac Surg. 2016;23:174–5.
12. Senay S, Gullu A, Kocyigit M, Degirmencioglu A, Karabulut H, Alhan C. Robotic mitral valve replacement. Multimed Man Cardiothorac Surg. 2014;16:201.
13. Badhwar V, Wei L, Cook C, Hayanga C, Daggubati R, Sengupta P, et al. Robotic aortic valve replacement. J Thorac Cardiovasc Surg. 2021;161(5):1753–9.
14. Tarui T, Ishikawa N, Kiuchi R, Watanabe G. Hybrid treatment combining robotic coronary artery bypass grafting and percutaneous catheter radiofrequency ablation. Interact Cardiovasc Thorac Surg. 2018;26:163–4.
15. Seguchi R, Ohtsuka T, Ishikawa N, Watanabe G. Bilateral endoscopic technique for left atrial appendectomy and robot-assisted mitral valve repair. Interac Cardio Vasc Thorac Surg. 2021;34:326.
16. Watanabe G, Ishikawa N. Use of barbed suture in robot-assisted mitral valvuloplasty. Ann Thorac Surg. 2015;99:342–5.
17. Ishikawa N, Watanabe G. Simple tying technique for robotic and endoscopic sutures. Innovations. 2017;12:152–3.
18. Seguchi R, Ishikawa N, Tarui T, Horikawa T, Ushijima T, Watanabe G. A novel shape-memory suture for minimally invasive thoracoscopic cardiac surgery. Innovations. 2019;14:55–9.
19. Ishikawa N, Watanabe G, Takafumi H, Tarui T, Seguchi R, Kiuchi R, et al. Combined robot-assisted mitral valve plasty and nuss procedure via small ports. Artif Organs. 2021;45:633–6.
20. Nishijima S, Nakamura Y, Yoshiyama D, Yasumoto Y, Kuroda M, Nakayama T, et al. Silent brain infarction after minimally invasive cardiac surgery with retrograde perfusion. J Card Surg. 2020;38:1927–32.

Robotic Surgery Devices in Lobectomy for Lung Malignancies with the da Vinci Xi Surgical System

Makoto Oda and Rurika Hamanaka

Abbreviations

HD	High-definition
ICG	Indocyanine green
RATS	Robot-assisted thoracic surgery
VATS	Video-assisted thoracic surgery

1 Introduction

Robotic surgery, like video-assisted thoracic surgery (VATS), has become a well-established minimally invasive technique in surgery of the lung [1–4]. The approach is safe and effective and widely used to treat malignant and benign tumors of the lung, mediastinal tumors, myasthenia gravis, diaphragmatic plication, and other diseases. Procedures that can be performed robotically include segmentectomy of the lung [5], bronchial/vascular resection and reconstruction [6], and chest wall resection and reconstruction. Robotic surgery provides several advantages, including high-definition (HD) stereoscopic visualization (Fig. 1a), improved surgical dexterity (Fig. 1b), removal of physiologic tremor, reduction of fulcrum effect, and greater surgeon comfort [7].

The da Vinci Xi surgical system (Intuitive Surgical Inc., Sunnyvale, CA, USA) utilizes four surgical arms (a camera arm and three working arms), which enables solo surgery. This chapter provides an overview of robotic devices currently available for use with the da Vinci Xi surgical system.

M. Oda (✉) · R. Hamanaka
Department of Thoracic Surgery, Shin-yurigaoka General Hospital,
Kawasaki, Kanagawa, Japan

© The Author(s), under exclusive license to Springer Nature Switzerland AG 2023
J. P. Manzano, L. M. Ferreira (eds.), *Robotic Surgery Devices in Surgical Specialties*, https://doi.org/10.1007/978-3-031-35102-0_4

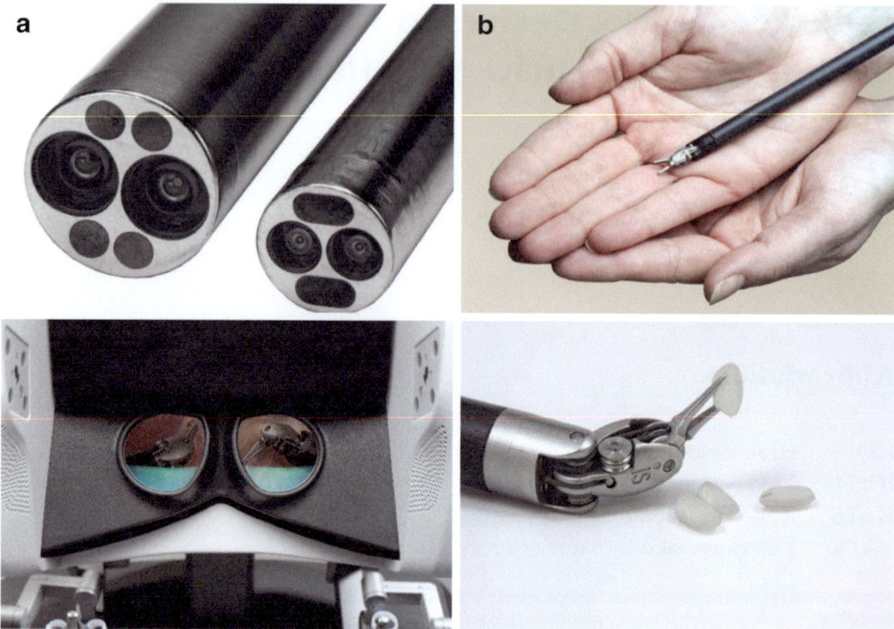

Fig. 1 Robotic endoscope (**a**) and instrument (**b**)

2 da Vinci Xi System and Approaches for Lung Cancer

The fourth-generation da Vinci Xi system was released in 2014 followed by the da Vinci X system in 2017 (Fig. 2). The da Vinci Xi system provides surgeon-controlled three-dimensional HD visualization, multi-quadrant access, Firefly™ fluorescence indocyanine green imaging (Fig. 3), integrated energy, skill simulation, vessel sealer instruments, and staplers. Three units comprise the da Vinci Xi system: patient cart, vision cart, and surgeon console (Fig. 4). The vision cart has a large HD display and serves as the integrated hub for power generation, CO_2 source, image processing, and data systems. The robotic arms are controlled by the surgeon at the surgeon console [8].

Robotic surgery for lung cancer can be performed using a utility incision without CO_2 insufflation or complete portal approach with CO_2 insufflation [7, 9] (Fig. 5). Advantages of complete portal approach over robot-assisted approach include better visualization, decreased bleeding owing to CO_2 insufflation, and smaller incisions [10]. However, it does not allow intraoperative manual finger insertion into the chest cavity for palpation.

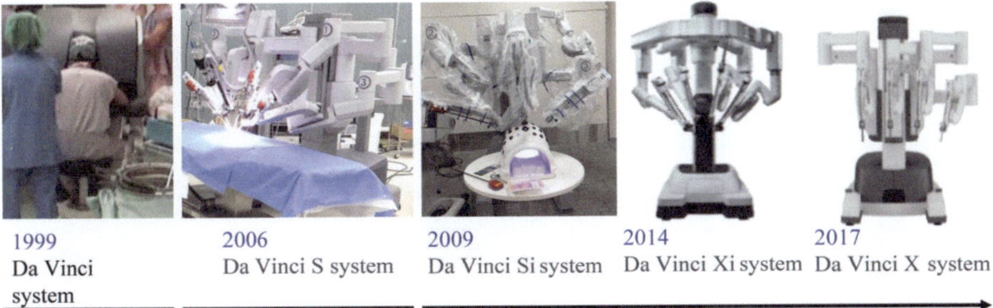

Fig. 2 Evolution of the da Vinci system

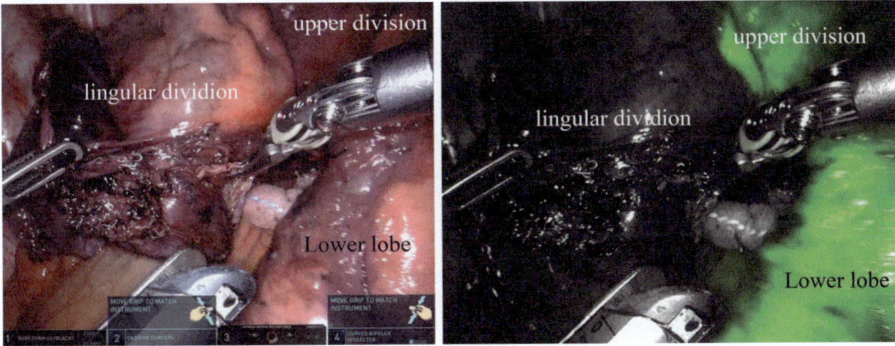

Fig. 3 Identification of the intersegmental plane between the left upper division and lingular division during left lingular segmentectomy using Firefly™ fluorescence indocyanine green imaging

Port placement for robotic lobectomy varies according to surgeon preference. A 2019 survey of high-volume robotic thoracic surgeons reported that 90% utilized a 4-arm approach and 79% used a completely 4-arm portal approach with CO_2 insufflation. In addition, most surgeons used the seventh to ninth intercostal spaces for the camera and instruments [11]. We preferentially use the port placement method used by Dylewski (Fig. 5), in which the camera port is placed at the sixth intercostal space for upper lobectomy and seventh intercostal space for middle or lower lobectomy (Figs. 6 and 7). A more cranial camera port position enables a better operative view for superior mediastinal lymph node dissection. In addition, it provides a better view of the truncus superior artery.

Adding the above two approaches of the robot-assisted procedure and complete portal procedure, pure uniportal RATS using the da Vinci Xi and its instruments has been recently reported performing all types of lung resections, including segmentectomies and (double-)sleeve and carinal resections [12].

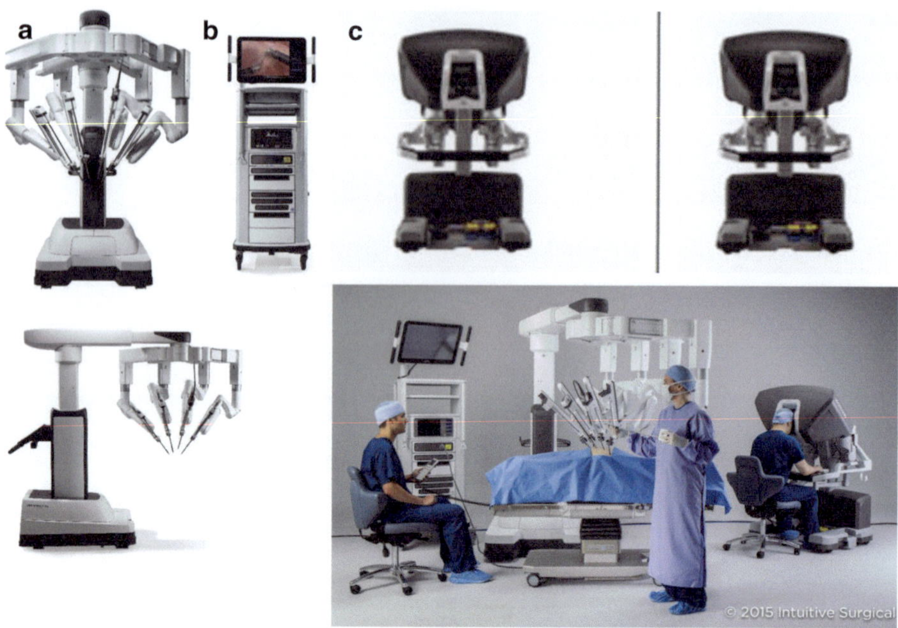

Fig. 4 The three units of the da Vinci Xi system: (**a**) patient cart, (**b**) vision cart, and (**c**) surgeon console

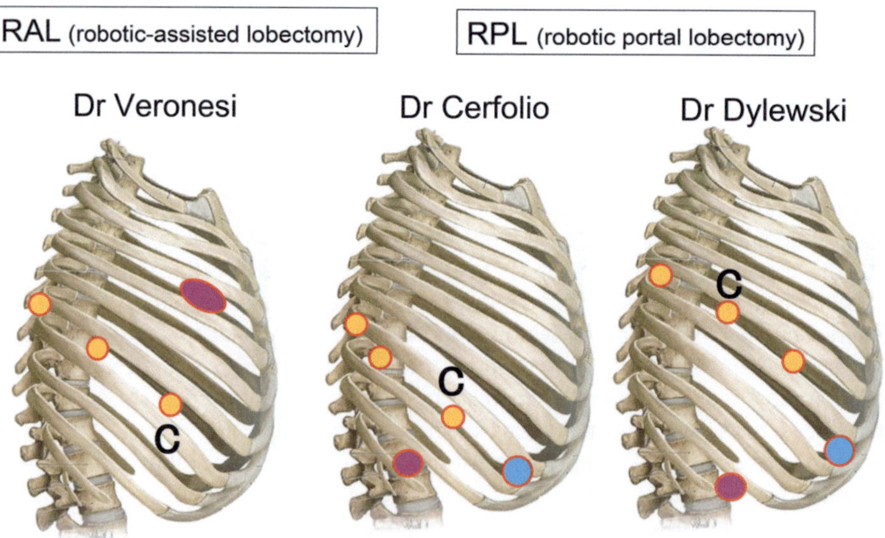

Fig. 5 Port placement for robot-assisted and completely robotic right upper lobectomy. Yellow circles indicate an 8-mm port. Blue circles indicate a 12-mm port. Purple circles indicate an 8-mm assistant port. The camera port is indicated by "C"

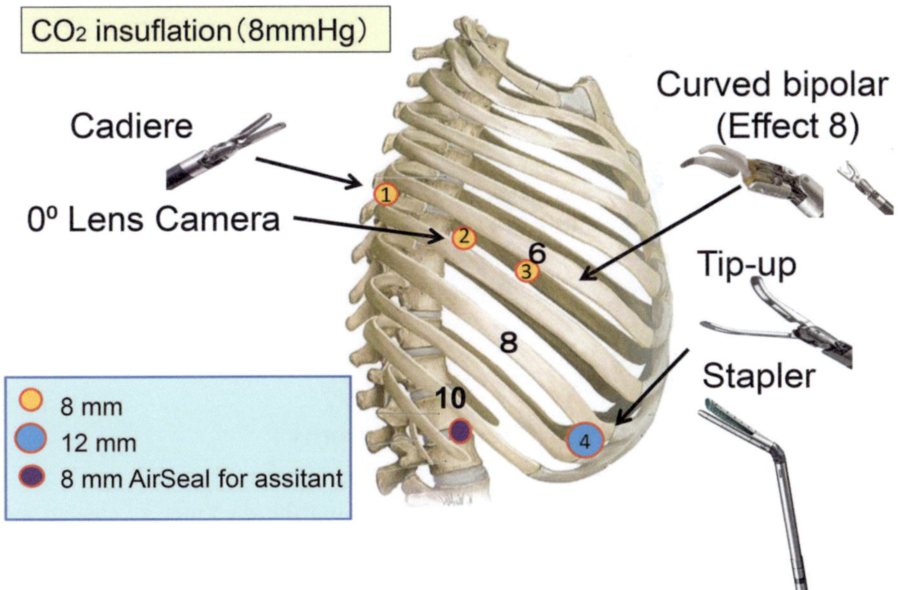

Fig. 6 A schema of port positions and their associated instruments for robotic portal lobectomy

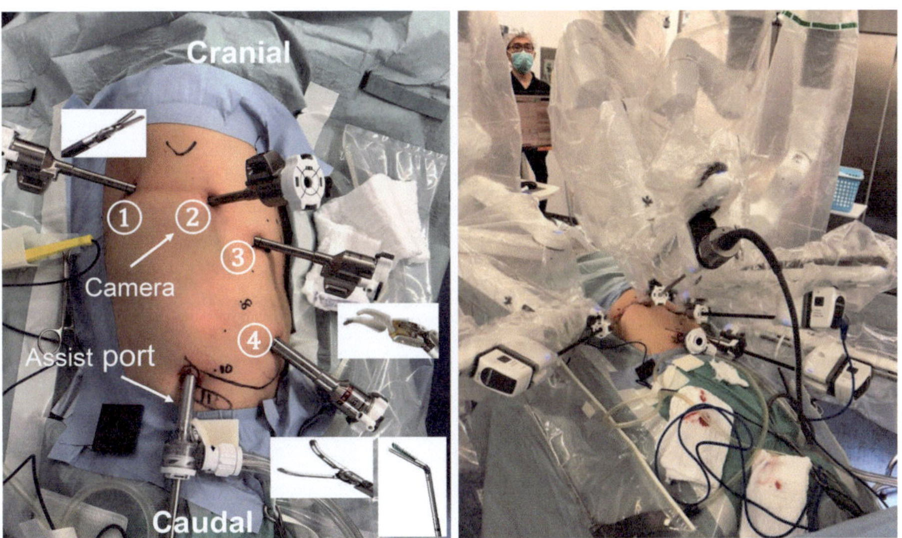

Fig. 7 Photographs in the operating room showing port positions and da Vinci Xi system

3 Robotic Endoscopes

Surgeons may select a 0° or 30° tridimensional robotic endoscope to use during robotic surgery. Both provide clear three-dimensional HD visualization (Fig. 1a) and are controlled by the surgeon console. However, the use of the 0° endoscope is more intuitive, and it has less of a fulcrum effect, which decreases intercostal nerve damage and related postoperative pain. Nonetheless, some surgeons prefer the 30° endoscope. Either endoscope can be placed in any arm of the Xi and X systems, unlike the previous da Vinci systems (original, S, Si), in which the endoscope can be placed in only one arm.

4 Instruments Used in Robotic Lobectomy

The various instruments for robotic lobectomy using the da Vinci Xi system are listed in Table 1. With one robotic arm holding the camera, a second is used to control tissue-grasping instruments such as the Cadiere forceps and fenestrated bipolar grasper. Instruments for surgical dissection, such as monopolar and bipolar cautery devices, are controlled using the third arm (Fig. 8). The fourth arm is typically used for lung retraction [13]; we also use it for stapling (Fig. 6).

Table 1 Instruments of the da Vinci Xi system

Monopolar cautery
Curved scissors
Spatula
Hook
Bipolar cautery
Maryland forceps
Long bipolar grasper
Curved bipolar dissector
Fenestrated bipolar grasper
Force bipolar
Clip applier
Medium-large clip
Small clip
Grasper
Tip-up fenestrated grasper
Cadiere forceps
Advanced instruments
Vessel sealer extender
SynchroSeal

- ## Monopolar

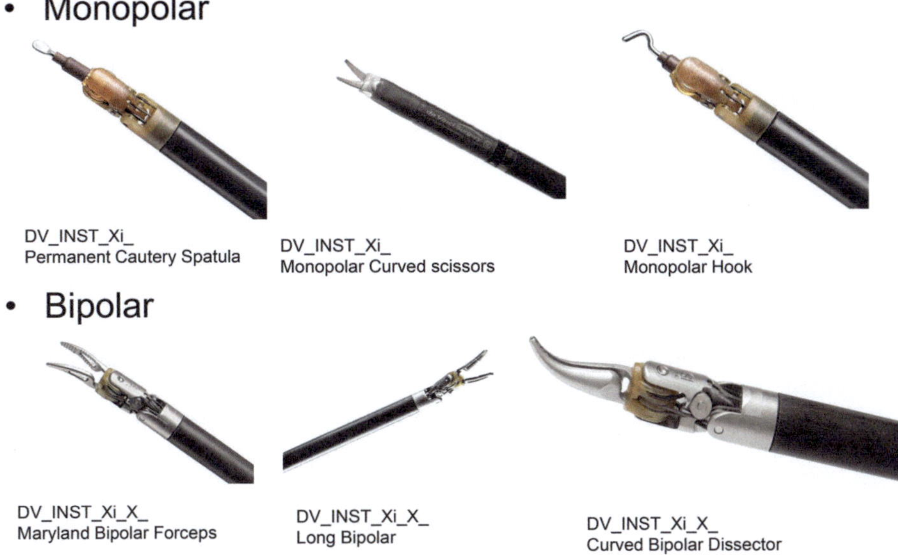

- ## Bipolar

Fig. 8 Monopolar and bipolar instruments

4.1 Robotic Ports

Eight- and twelve-millimeter ports are used with the da Vinci Xi system. Most instruments can be passed through 8-mm ports except for staplers, which require a 12-mm port because of their larger diameter. Instruments and endoscopes can be manipulated through the ports without causing much trauma to the chest wall to minimize postoperative wound pain. This enables earlier ambulation, decreases length of hospital stay, and allows faster recovery in general.

4.2 Energy Devices

Energy devices are used to dissect tissues, including the pulmonary ligament, lymph nodes, and perivascular and peribronchial tissue, and to coagulate and divide small vessels. Monopolar devices include the cautery spatula, curved scissors, and hook (Fig. 8). Bipolar devices include the Maryland bipolar forceps, long bipolar grasper, and curved bipolar dissector (Fig. 8).

Monopolar devices have a risk of stray energy transfer [14, 15] and should be used with caution around the phrenic, vagal, and recurrent laryngeal nerves. Stray energy transfer by a monopolar L-hook can be reduced by lowering the power setting, utilizing the low-voltage cut mode (instead of coagulation mode), and avoiding open air activation [14].

Bipolar devices are used to dissect, grasp, and transect tissue and achieve hemostasis [16]. Bleeding tissue can be grasped and cauterized. These devices have little risk of stray energy transfer and can be safely used near nerves. We preferentially use the curved bipolar dissector because it can dissect tissue more smoothly than other bipolar devices; however, its bipolar tip is shorter than those of the Maryland bipolar forceps and long bipolar grasper.

4.3 Fourth Arm

In the fourth arm, the tip-up fenestrated grasper (Fig. 9) is used to retract the lung and provide an appropriate surgical field like an assistant surgeon would in open surgery and VATS. This enables solo surgery. Since we also perform stapling with the fourth arm, staplers are exchanged with the tip-up fenestrated grasper when needed. Therefore, we place a 12-mm port with a plastic reducer as the fourth arm port at the beginning of surgery. The plastic reducer for the tip-up fenestrated grasper is initially placed inside the 12-mm port and used until the stapler is needed.

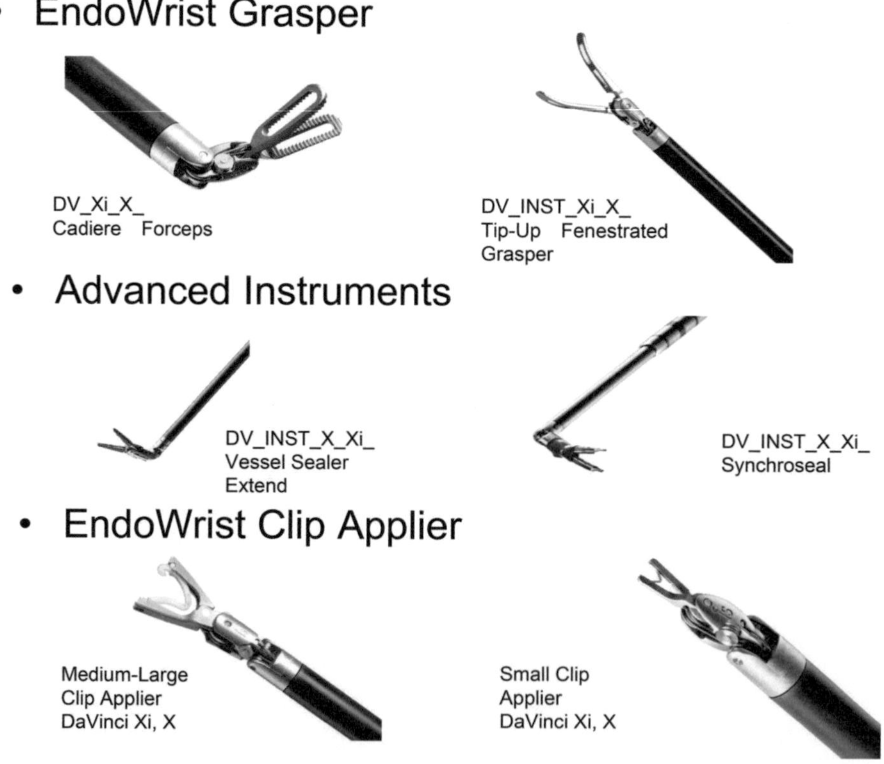

Fig. 9 Graspers, advanced instruments, and clip appliers

Then, the grasper and reducer are removed, leaving the 12-mm port for stapler insertion. The other three ports do not usually require instrument exchange, which decreases operation time.

4.4   Advanced Instruments and Clip Appliers

Advanced instruments and clip appliers are listed in Table 1 and shown in Fig. 9. The Vessel Sealer Extend can be used as an alternative to bipolar devices to seal lymphatic vessels up to 7 mm in diameter [16]. Furthermore, some surgeons prefer using it to divide incomplete fissures between lobes because of its ability to seal air leakage.

Double medium-large plastic and small metal clips are useful to achieve hemostasis of vascular bundles (Figs. 9 and 10). However, migration of a hemostatic clip into the bladder has been reported as a complication of robotic prostatectomy [17]. Medium-large plastic clips are used to ligate the proximal side of a vessel before cutting. To prevent clip migration, a small metal clip is placed adjacent (Fig. 10). For smaller diameter vessels, two small metal clips are used.

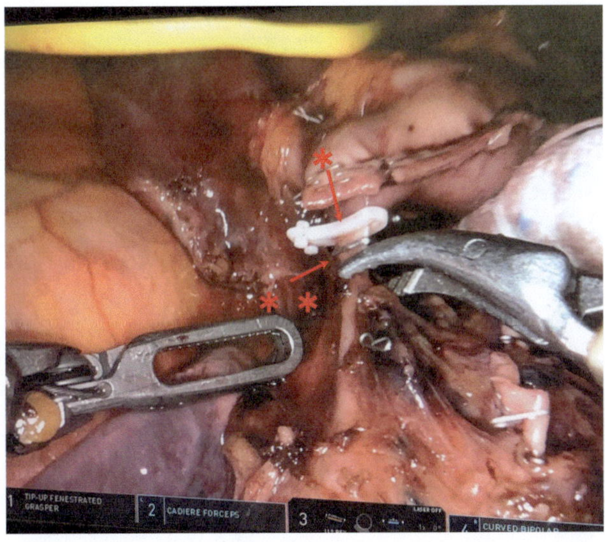

Fig. 10 Intraoperative photograph of da Vinci clips. The single asterisk denotes a medium-large plastic clip ligating the proximal side of a vessel before cutting. The double asterisk indicates a small metal clip placed adjacent to the plastic clip to prevent migration

5 Stapling Devices

With the da Vinci Xi system, robotic staplers are controlled directly by the console surgeon. The surgeon may select an EndoWrist™ or SureForm™ stapler (Table 2, Fig. 11) [18]. Straight- and curved-tip types are available for both. Staplers with a curved tip are useful for passing through pulmonary vessels and bronchi, whereas the straight-tip type is useful for transecting pulmonary parenchyma and incomplete fissures. As noted above, robotic staplers require a 12-mm robotic port for insertion and use, while the other robotic instruments can be used through an 8-mm port.

The EndoWrist™ stapler has several different length and tip combinations: 45 mm and straight, 30 mm and straight, and 30 mm and curved. Combinations for the SureForm™ stapler include 60 mm and straight, 45 mm and straight, and 45 mm and curved. For both staplers, staple cartridges are selected according to stapler length, stapler tip, and length of staple desired (Table 3). SureForm™ staples are shown in Fig. 12.

Differences between the EndoWrist™ and SureForm™ staplers are shown in Table 2 and Fig. 11. The tip of the EndoWrist™ staplers rotates as an ellipse, 54° vertically and 108° horizontally. The tip of the SureForm™ stapler rotates as a cone (120°). Because the SureForm™ stapler tip is thinner, it passes through vessels and bronchi more easily and safely with less tension to vessels and bronchi. With the EndoWrist™ stapler, the anvil side of the stapler is opened and closed. In contrast, the staple side of the stapler is opened and closed with the SureForm™ stapler. that

Table 2 Characteristics of the EndoWrist™ and SureForm™ staplers

	EndoWrist™	SureForm™
Articulation	Vertical 54°, Horizontal 108°	120° Cone
Thickness of anvil	Thicker	Thinner
Stapler reload exchange	More difficult	Easier
Stapler jaw alinement	Smart clamp	I-beam
Stapler shaft	Reusable (50 applications)	Disposable

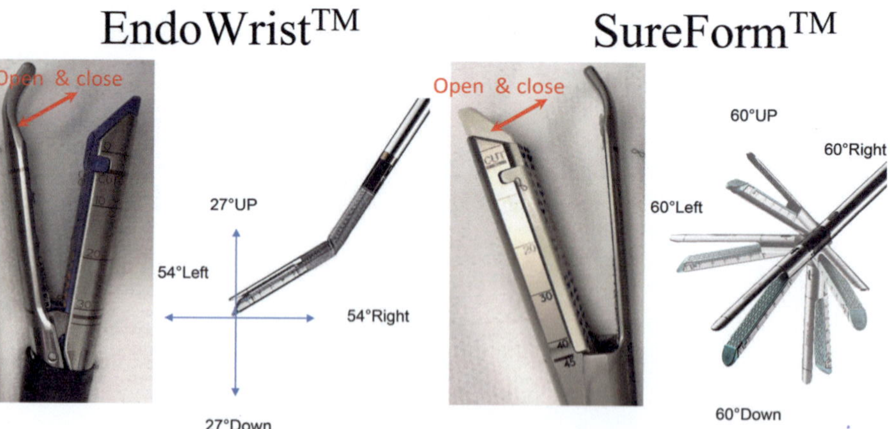

Fig. 11 EndoWrist™ and SureForm™ staplers

Table 3 da Vinci Xi system stapler cartridges used in our hospital

			1st stage	2nd stage	3rd stage	4th stage
EndoWrist	30 curved	Gray	O			
		White	O	O		
		Blue	O			
		Green	O	O		
	45 straight	Blue	O			
		Green	O			
SureForm	45 curved	White			O	O
		Blue			O	O
		Green			O	O
	60 straight	Blue		O		
		Green		O	O	(O)
		Black		O	O	(O)

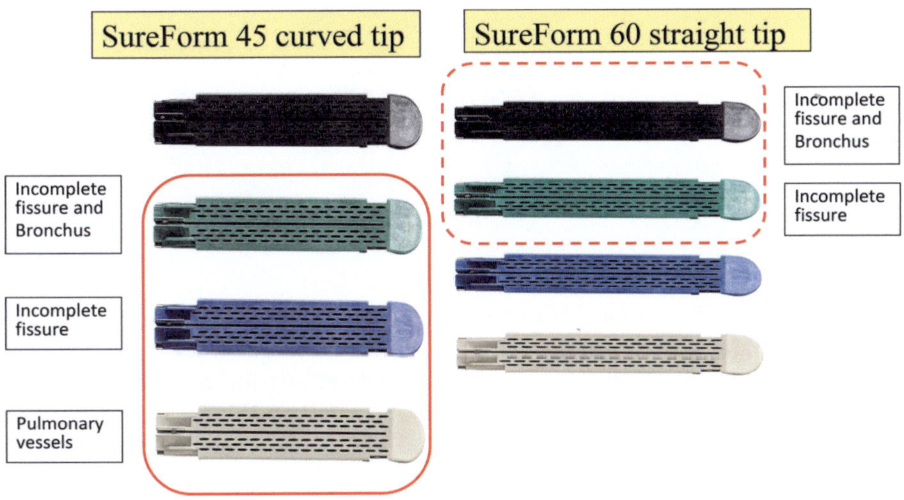

Fig. 12 SureForm™ staplers

makes SureForm™ staplers more safely used for vessels. Therefore, we prefer to use the SureForm™ stapler. In our experience, most stapling can be performed using only the 45 mm SureForm™ curved-tip stapler (Table 3).

Because the stapler's working end is long, a 12-mm port should be placed as caudal as possible [18, 19] (Fig. 13). Two ports (one anterior and one posterior) can be useful to provide a variety of stapler angles [18]. On the other hand we use only

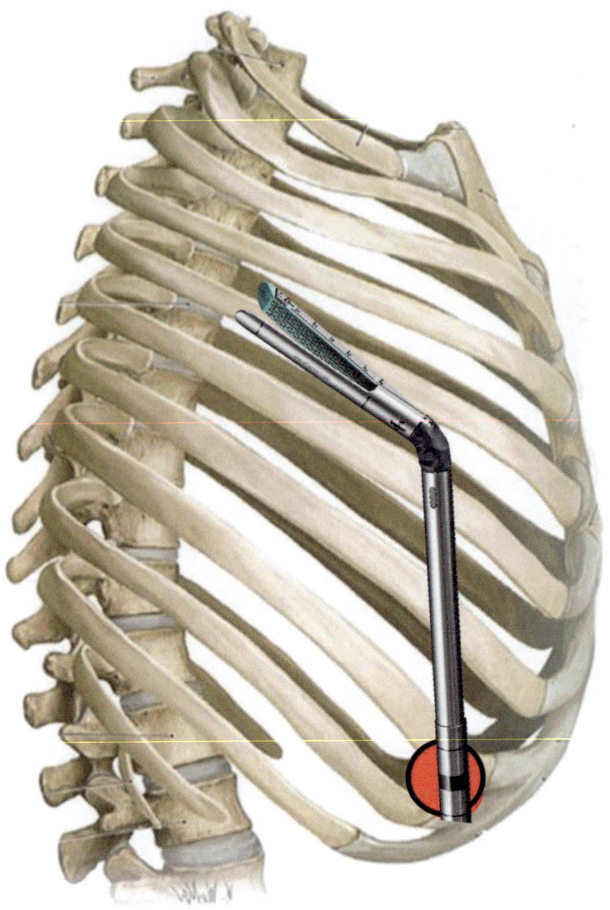

Fig. 13 A 12-mm port is required for the use of the robotic stapler. The port should be placed as caudal as possible because the working end is long

one 12-mm port (Figs. 6 and 13) and the other ports can be 8-mm by using the vessel loop technique [20] or using moving the ground technique when necessary.

The use of robotic staplers has been associated with significantly lower risks of perioperative bleeding, conversion to open surgery, and possibly air leak and overall complications compared with the use of handheld staplers; moreover, it does not appear to increase total costs [21].

6 Conclusion

This chapter provided an overview of robotic devices currently available for use with the da Vinci Xi surgical system, which can be used to perform numerous types of robot-assisted and completely robotic lung surgeries, including lobectomy, segmentectomy, and other types of resection. Further advances in robotic technology will increase utilization of minimally invasive thoracic surgery and increase quality of care.

References

1. Kent M, Wang T, Whyte R, Curran T, Flores R, Gangadharan S. Open, video-assisted thoracic surgery, and robotic lobectomy: review of a national database. Ann Thorac Surg. 2014;97:236–42; discussion 242–4.
2. Li JT, Liu PY, Huang J, Lu PJ, Lin H, Zhou QJ, et al. Perioperative outcomes of radical lobectomies using robotic-assisted thoracoscopic technique *vs.* video-assisted thoracoscopic technique: retrospective study of 1,075 consecutive p-stage I non-small cell lung cancer cases. J Thorac Dis. 2019;11:882–91. https://doi.org/10.21037/jtd.2019.01.78.
3. Liang H, Liang W, Zhao L, Chen D, Zhang J, Zhang Y, et al. Robotic versus video-assisted lobectomy/segmentectomy for lung cancer: a meta-analysis. Ann Surg. 2018;268:254–9. https://doi.org/10.1097/SLA.0000000000002346.
4. Cerfolio RJ, Ghanim AF, Dylewski M, Veronesi G, Spaggiari L, Park BJ. The long-term survival of robotic lobectomy for non-small cell lung cancer: a multi-institutional study. J Thorac Cardiovasc Surg. 2018;155:778–86. https://doi.org/10.1016/j.jtcvs.2017.09.016.
5. Zhang Y, Chen C, Hu J, Han Y, Huang M, et al. Early outcomes of robotic versus thoracoscopic segmentectomy for early-stage lung cancer: a multi-institutional propensity score-matched analysis. J Thorac Cardiovasc Surg. 2020;160:1363–72. https://doi.org/10.1016/j.jtcvs.2019.12.112.
6. Qiu T, Zhao Y, Xuan Y, Qin Y, Niu Z, Shen Y, et al. Robotic sleeve lobectomy for centrally located non-small cell lung cancer: a propensity score-weighted comparison with thoracoscopic and open surgery. J Thorac Cardiovasc Surg. 2020;160:838–846.e2. https://doi.org/10.1016/j.jtcvs.2019.10.158.
7. Veronesi G, Novellis P, Bottoni E, Alloisio M. Robotic lobectomy: right upper lobectomy. Oper Tech Thorac Cardiovasc Surg. 2017;21:249–68.
8. Terra RM, Leite PHC, Dela Vega AJM. Global status of the robotic thoracic surgery. J Thorac Dis. 2021;13:6123–8. https://doi.org/10.21037/jtd-19-3271.
9. Cerfolio R, Louie BE, Farivar AS, Onaitis M, Park BJ. Consensus statement on definitions and nomenclature for robotic thoracic surgery. J Thorac Cardiovasc Surg. 2017;154:1065–9. https://doi.org/10.1016/j.jtcvs.2017.02.081.
10. Ramadan OI, Wei B, Cerfolio RJ. Robotic surgery for lung resections-total port approach: advantages and disadvantages. J Vis Surg. 2017;3:22. https://doi.org/10.21037/jovs.2017.01.06.
11. Oh DS, Tisol WB, Cesnik L, Crosby A, Cerfolio RJ. Port strategies for robot-assisted lobectomy by high-volume thoracic surgeons: a nationwide survey. Innovations. 2019;14:545–52. https://doi.org/10.1177/1556984519883643.
12. Gonzalez-Rivas D, Bosinceanub M, Motas N, Manolache V. Uniportal robotic-assisted thoracic surgery for lung resections. Eur J Cardiothorac Surg. 2022;62:ezac410. https://doi.org/10.1093/ejcts/ezac410.
13. Cerfolio RJ, Cichos KH, Wei B, Minnich DJ. Robotic lobectomy can be taught while maintaining quality patient outcomes. J Thorac Cardiovasc Surg. 2016;152:991–7. https://doi.org/10.1016/j.jtcvs.2016.04.085.
14. Overbey DM, Carmichael H, Wikiel KJ, Hirth DA, Chapman BC, Moore JT, et al. Monopolar stray energy in robotic surgery. Surg Endosc. 2021;35:2084–90. https://doi.org/10.1007/s00464-020-07605-5.

15. Wikiel KJ, Overbey DM, Carmichael H, Chapman BC, Moore JT, Barnett CC, et al. Stray energy transfer in single-incision robotic surgery. Surg Endosc. 2021;35:2981–5. https://doi.org/10.1007/s00464-020-07742-x.
16. Wikiel KJ, Robinson TN, Jones EL. Energy in robotic surgery. Ann Laparosc Endosc Surg. 2020;6:9. https://doi.org/10.21037/ales.2020.03.06.
17. Turini GA, Brito JM, Leone AR, Golijanin D, Miller EB, Pareek G, et al. Intravesical hemostatic clip migration after robotic prostatectomy: case series and review of the literature. J Laparoendosc Adv Surg Tech A. 2016;26:710–2. https://doi.org/10.1089/lap.2015.0506.
18. Pearlstein DP. Robotic lobectomy utilizing the robotic stapler. Ann Thorac Surg. 2016;102:e591–3. https://doi.org/10.1016/j.athoracsur.
19. Galetta D, Casiraghi M, Pardolesi A, Borri A, Spaggiari L. New stapling devices in robotic surgery. J Vis Surg. 2017;3:45. https://doi.org/10.21037/jovs.2017.02.03.
20. Cerfolio RJ, Bryant AS, Skylizard L, Minnich DJ. Initial consecutive experience of completely portal robotic pulmonary resection with 4 arms. J Thorac Cardiovasc Surg. 2011;142:740–6. https://doi.org/10.1016/j.jtcvs.2011.07.022.
21. Zervos M, Song A, Li Y, Lee SH, Oh DS. Clinical and economic outcomes of using robotic versus hand held staplers during robotic lobectomy. Innovations. 2021;16:470–6. https://doi.org/10.1177/15569845211040814.

Robotic Devices in Urology

Marcio Covas Moschovas, João Pádua Manzano, and Vipul Patel

1 Introduction

The concept of using a robotic platform to assist surgical procedures was initially created in military medicine to improve the surgical care of wounded soldiers on the battlefield. The objective of using this technology was to improve the standard of care from the "Golden Hour" to the "Golden Minute" by bringing the operative room condition to the battlefield instead of losing valuable time transferring bleeding soldiers to local hospitals [1, 2]. In this scenario, faster treatment could be provided inside the conflict zone while minimizing the risks of losing surgeons and medical staff in the war. Surgeons could operate on several soldiers wounded in different geographic locations without being exposed to danger and losing time in transportation.

Although the robotic-assisted surgery concept began in the 1960s, it wasn't until the 1990s that the first project was effectively carried out by the US Defense Department in association with various startup companies [3]. After several years of technological advancement, especially in the three-dimensional field, the first robotic-assisted surgery was performed in 1997 in Belgium, with a robotic platform called "Mona" (da Vinci® precursor) [4, 5]. In the same year, the da Vinci® (Intuitive Surgical, Sunnyvale, USA) robot was cleared in the USA by the FDA, but only for visualizing and retracting tissues. Three years later, in 2000, this robot was cleared for a general surgery approach to Nissen fundoplication and cholecystectomy.

M. C. Moschovas (✉) · V. Patel
AdventHealth Global Robotics Institute, Celebration, FL, USA

University of Central Florida (UCF), Orlando, FL, USA
e-mail: vipul.patel.md@flhops.org

J. P. Manzano
Department of Surgery, Universidade Federal de São Paulo, São Paulo, Brazil
e-mail: jmanzano@unifesp.br

J. P. Manzano, L. M. Ferreira (eds.), *Robotic Surgery Devices in Surgical Specialties*, https://doi.org/10.1007/978-3-031-35102-0_5

Two decades after the first robotic surgical procedure, the technology has evolved through successive consoles and proved advantageous over conventional open and laparoscopic procedures [6–9]. Robotic surgery played an important role in urology, especially for approaching the surgical treatment of prostate cancer. Therefore, in this chapter we described different robotic devices currently being used in the urologic field.

2   da Vinci® Platform Evolution

Initially designed to approach coronary artery surgery, the da Vinci® robot gained popularity in urologic surgeries after Binder and colleagues performed the first robotic-assisted radical prostatectomy (RARP) in Frankfurt (in 2000) [10, 11]. Since then, several da Vinci® robotic models have been released, each with continued technological improvements including ergonomics, instruments, high-definition scopes, Endo-wrist™ technology, and single-port surgery [12, 13]. Currently, the da Vinci® is the most common technology used in robotic surgery worldwide.

2.1   da Vinci® Standard

This is the first unit used after the FDA approved robotic surgery in the USA. The da Vinci® Standard had some limitations due to its archaic technology. It lacked bipolar instruments and three-arm configuration, which limited hemostasis and range of motion to work in different quadrants [12].

2.2   da Vinci® S

Introduced to the market in 2006, this robot presented some improvements compared to the da Vinci® standard. This model had longer robotic arms which improved its range of motion, and four arms which provided the option of using an extra instrument during surgery. In addition, the implementation of bipolar energy enhanced hemostasis performance during the surgical procedure. Finally, the creation and adoption of high-definition (HD) scopes led robotic surgery imaging to a superior level [12].

2.3   *da Vinci® Si*

Three years later in 2009, Intuitive Surgical (Sunnyvale, USA) launched another generation of the da Vinci® robot. Named the da Vinci® Si, this model presented some modifications and upgrades, including finger-base clutching, Firefly™ technology with indocyanine green fluorescence, and scope improvements. In addition, this generation provided dual-console benefits, which enhanced training and teaching methods.

2.4   *da Vinci® Xi*

The Xi system (Fig. 1) was released in 2014 and presented improvements in the arm design and trocar placement. This platform has thinner arms with modified articulations, which reduces the external clashing and allows different types of docking for the same procedure (side docking or between the legs). In addition, all ports are 8 mm in diameter and the camera can be placed at all four arms, which offers a dynamic visualization in procedures accessing different quadrants, such as nephroureterectomies or partial nephrectomies. The docking is performed with laser guidance, which indicates the correct positioning to optimize the internal and external space during the surgery. Finally, this platform allows docking with an integrated OR table that can be moved during the procedure without undocking and repositioning the patient (Trumpf Medical, Germany) [12].

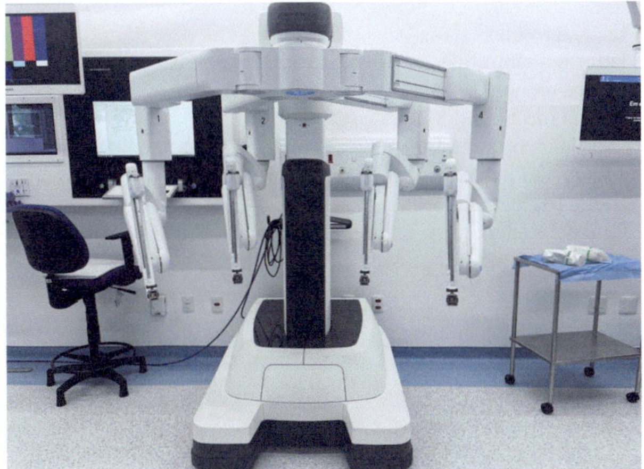

Fig. 1 da Vinci® Xi model system—Intuitive Surgical

2.5 *da Vinci® X*

Cleared by the FDA in 2017, this platform is a hybrid between the Si and Xi technologies, mixing the Si arm configuration and cart model with the Xi 8 mm dynamic scope. Therefore, this unit does not have the same versatility provided by the Xi in terms of reduced external clashing and multiquadrant procedure. However, the Xi platform offers the advantages of the Xi instruments and scope with reduced costs, which opens robotic surgery access to centers with financial limitations to invest in this technology.

2.6 *da Vinci® SP*

The da Vinci® SP robot (Figs. 2, 3, and 4) was initially designed based on laparoendoscopic single site surgery (LESS), which associates the concept of minimally invasive surgery with a single incision to place the trocar. However, the laparoscopic and initial robotic approach to LESS did not gain traction due to its steep learning curve, lack of standardized technique, and reduced number of well-designed studies describing encouraging outcomes [14–20]. In this scenario, improvements in the robotic approach to LESS started with the SP 1098 platform: a pure single-port system consisting of a flexible scope and two flexible instruments controlled by the Xi system. Some groups reported feasible and safe procedures performed with the SP 1098 platform, including partial nephrectomy, radical prostatectomy, and perineal radical prostatectomy [21, 22]. However, only after

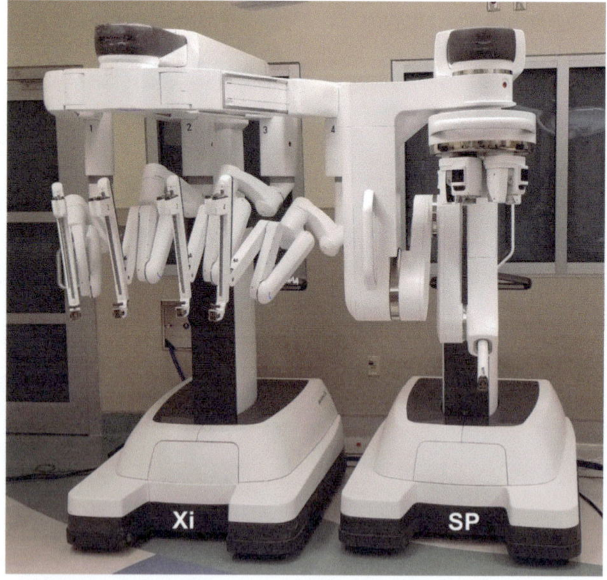

Fig. 2 da Vinci® Platforms—Intuitive Surgical—comparison between the Xi and SP robots, side by side. Left: da Vinci® Xi model system. Right: da Vinci® SP model system

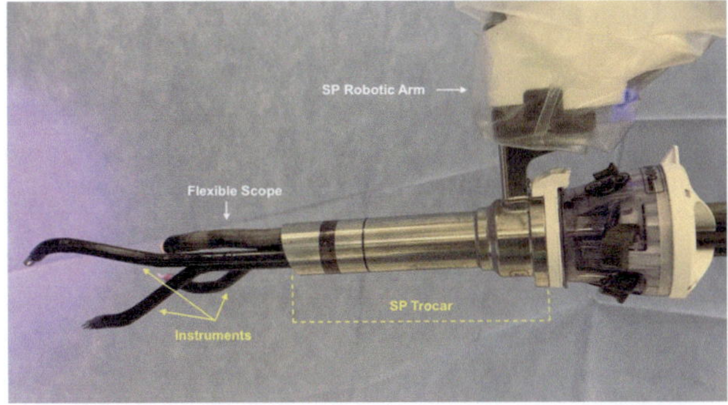

Fig. 3 da Vinci® SP model system—Intuitive Surgical—single-arm attached to trocar

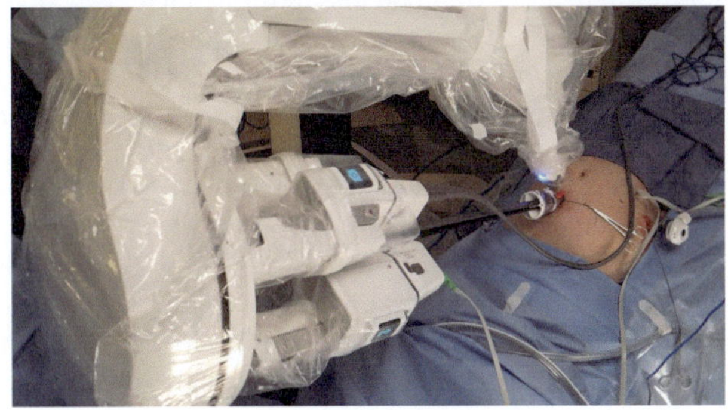

Fig. 4 da Vinci® SP model system—Intuitive Surgical—single-arm robot after docking

releasing the final version of the da Vinci® SP robot that the robotic single-port surgery begins its expansion throughout multiple referral centers.

The da Vinci® SP was cleared by the FDA in 2018 and consists of a single trocar that houses three biarticulated instruments and one flexible scope. Since the first clinical report of this robot, several authors have described the outcomes in different types of urologic procedures. Recently, the SP has had updates in the number of pedals and scope definition [14, 16–20, 23–25].

3 Building a Robotic Program

Despite the robotic platform model, it is crucial to develop a robotic program to integrate all surgical teams and nursing staff to improve outcomes and optimize the robot use [26]. In addition, it is imperative to study the limitations of each robot according to the demand and type of surgeries performed at each center. In this scenario, the da Vinci® SP still has some limitations because it is only available in the USA and Korea, and only a few specialties are cleared by the FDA to use it in humans, while the previous generations are available worldwide and can be used in all surgical specialties.

4   Current Systems Available for Urological Procedures

Robotic surgery has been widely used in urology to approach malignant and benign diseases of adults and pediatric patients [27]. The multiport da Vinci® system still comprises most robots used to approach urologic surgeries. The platform model varies among centers according to the financial condition and surgical volume of each institution. Despite the modifications previously described between multiport generations, the operative performance and outcomes are similar between the most recent platforms (da Vinci® Xi) and the previous models (da Vinci® Si) [13, 28].

Different groups compared the outcomes of SP and Xi robots in patients who underwent radical prostatectomy [22, 25, 29]. Some authors described advantages for the SP in terms of blood loss, postoperative pain, opioid use, and early discharge. In our experience, comparing two groups of patients with similar preoperative characteristics, we did not find these advantages and we had a higher operative time for the SP group [25]. However, it is crucial to highlight that all current articles are based on retrospective analysis with potential risks of bias. In addition, due to the SP's recent use in most centers, none of the articles have reported the long-term functional and oncological outcomes of this robot. Therefore, we still need prospective and randomized control trials to evaluate the actual benefits of the SP platform over its multiport antecessors.

Other platforms such as Revo-I®, Versius®, Senhance®, Hugo®, and Toumai® have recently appeared on the market, with articles describing outcomes published in peer-reviewed journals [30, 31]. However, before comparing these new platforms with the da Vinci® technology, Revo-I®, Versius®, Senhance®, Hugo®, and Toumai® must be technically and scientifically validated. Other non-laparoscopic systems are also available for urologic diseases, such as The Focal One® HIFU device, for prostate cancer focal treatment, and Avicenna Roboflex® for nephrolithiasis endoscopic treatment.

4.1   Versius Robot

Developed by Cambridge Medical Robotics Ltd. (Cambridge, UK), the Versius surgical system (Fig. 5) had its first project in 2014 and received the European CE mark in March 2019 [32]. It consists of human-like arms with shoulder, elbow, and wrist placed individually on portable carts. The surgeon can receive haptic feedback from the handles. It utilizes fully articulated 5 mm diameter instruments that feature seven degrees of freedom. The surgeon's console has an open design, facilitating communication with staff, and requires polarized glasses for HD 3D vision.

The system was used in a preclinical trial, in which surgeons successfully performed kidney, prostate, and lymphadenectomy surgeries on porcine models and cadavers. Several clinical studies with gastrointestinal, gynecological, and urological surgeries have been recently published [32, 33].

Fig. 5 Versius surgical system—Cambridge Medical Robotics Ltd. (Cambridge, UK)

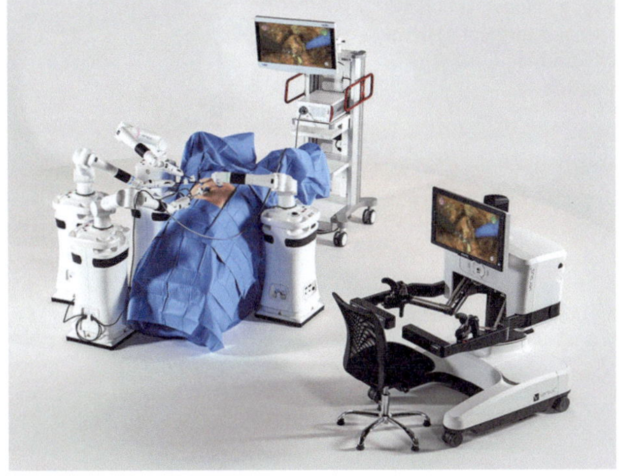

The Versius system is already established as a surgical tool in Europe, India, Australia, and the Middle East centers. At the end of 2021, it received regulatory approval from the Brazilian National Health Surveillance Agency, opening the way for sales in the rapidly growing Brazilian market. Brazil will be the 11th country to use the Versius system for surgeries in adults.

4.2 Hugo Robot

Medtronic has obtained European approval (CE mark) to use its Hugo® surgical robot (Figs. 6 and 7) for urological and gynecological procedures, paving the way for the system to make its continental debut in several countries [34].

Hugo® performed its first human procedure in June 2021, a minimally invasive prostatectomy in Santiago, Chile [35]. It has since expanded into Latin America, with gynecological surgeries in Panama City, Panama. Medtronic also announced its first operation with Hugo® RAS System in the Asia-Pacific region, through a prostatectomy in Chennai, India.

The robotic platform consists of modular surgical arms on wheeled carts. All company's systems are linked to a global patient registry, which tracks results and feeds back data into the platform.

Fig. 6 Hugo® robotic-assisted surgical system—Medtronic plc—surgeon console

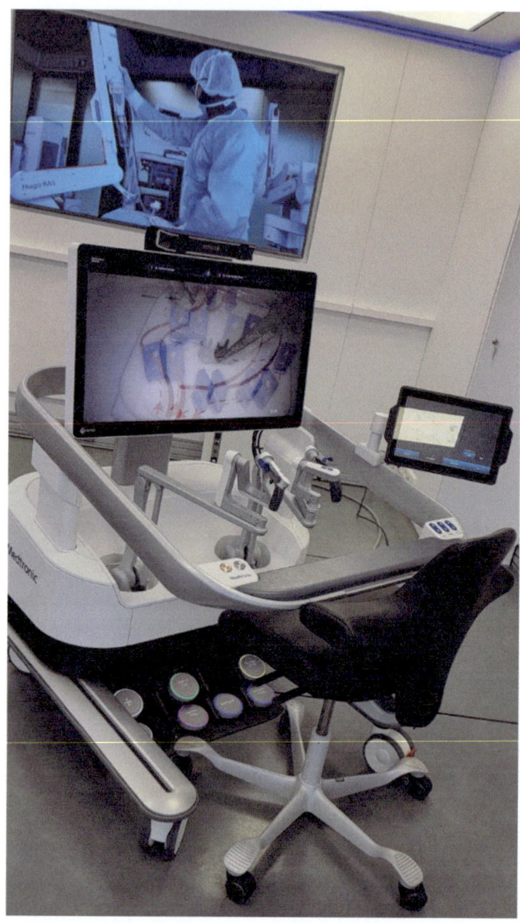

Fig. 7 Hugo® robotic-assisted surgical system—Medtronic plc—modular surgical arms on wheeled carts

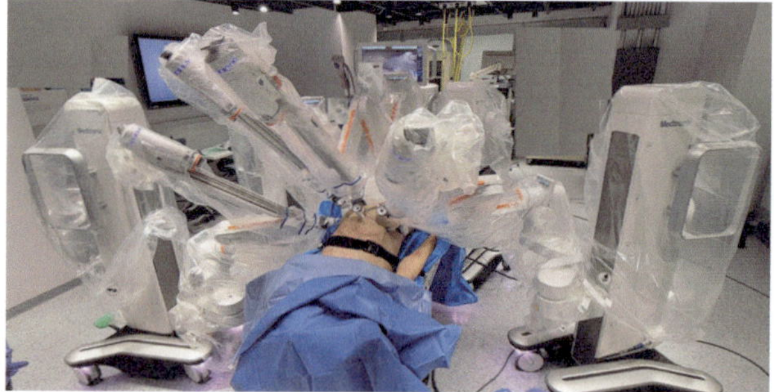

4.3   Revo-I Robot

The Revo-I is a surgical platform developed by Meere Company Inc. (Yongin, Korea), a company founded in 1984, a manufacturer of high-tech equipment, which in 2007 started developing robotic surgical platforms. In 2015, version 5 of Revo-I was approved in preclinical tests and trials. In August 2017 it received approval for use in humans by the Korean Ministry of Food and Medicine Safety.

This is a master-slave system, which is very similar to the da Vinci Si system. It features a patient cart with four articulated arms, a surgeon's console with a binocular 3D HD closed vision system, and a control cart. The 3D HD endoscope is 10 mm in diameter. The 7.4 mm diameter instruments are entirely handful, providing seven degrees of freedom, and are reusable up to 20 times.

Finally, in 2018, the first human study using the Revo-I was published reporting a robot-assisted Retzius-sparing radical prostatectomy [36].

4.4   Senhance Robot

The Senhance® Surgical System was initially developed by the Italian company Sofar (Milan, Italy), called TELELAP ALF-X advanced robotic system, and received CE mark certification in 2016 for abdominal surgeries. Subsequently, acquired by TransEnterix Surgical Inc. (Morrisville, NC, USA), in October 2017, Senhance® became the first robotic system to receive FDA clearance since the da Vinci authorization in 2000.

The Senhance® Surgical System is a multiport robotic system that takes advantage of innovative new technologies, such as camera manipulation controlled by the surgeon's eye movements through an infrared eye-tracking system and haptic feedback from instruments, which helps with a smooth transition for laparoscopy surgeons.

The multiport system comprises up to four independent robotic arms on separate carts. The surgeon is ergonomically seated on an open console, operating on a 3D high-definition monitor using polarized glasses.

The use of Senhance® for radical prostatectomy and other urological procedures has recently been described in Europe [37].

4.5   Toumai Robot

MicroPort® Medical Group Co. (Shanghai, China), a company that traditionally produced drug-eluting stents in 36 countries, started in 2014 the development of medical robots. Since then, it has been engaged in the research and development of endoscopic surgical robots.

In November 2019, the Toumai™ endoscopic surgery robot successfully completed its first surgery, a robot-assisted laparoscopic radical prostatectomy (RALRP), at Dongfang Hospital in Shanghai [38].

In February 2021 the start of a clinical trial using the Toumai® Robotic Endoscopic Surgery System was announced. In January 2021, Microport reported the successful completion of a complex partial nephrectomy to treat a complete Endophytic renal tumor at Renji Hospital, affiliated with Shanghai Jiao Tong University. The team led by Dr. Wei Xue, Head of the Urology Department, performed the operation. Since then, the Toumai® Endoscopic Robot has been used in several urological surgeries, such as radical prostatectomies and partial nephrectomies, demonstrating its clinical feasibility. There is still no scientific publication to validate these results.

4.6   Prostate Cancer Focal Treatment

The Focal One® HIFU device is the first medical device designed specifically for the focal treatment of prostate cancer [39]. It was the latest developments in high-intensity focused ultrasound technology coupled with a robotic arm and image fusion software to respond to all the specificities of focal PCa treatment (Fig. 8).

Fig. 8 Focal One®—
EDAP TMS

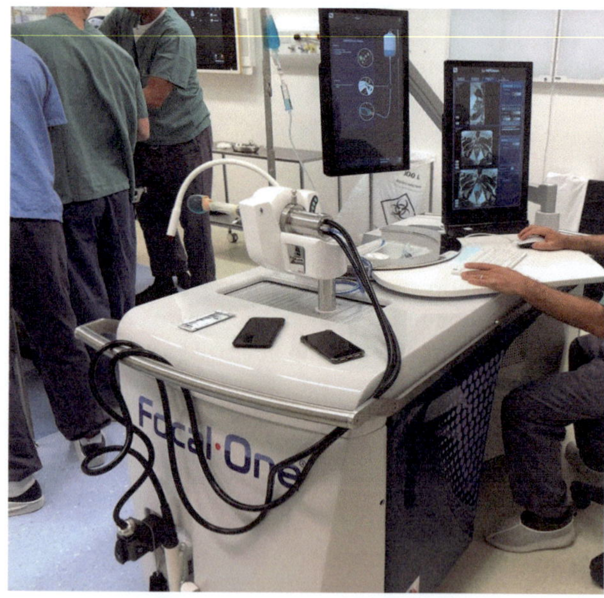

4.7   Robotic Devices for Retrograde Intrarenal Surgery

Robotic systems are not limited to laparoscopic surgery. In 2008, robotic FURS was first reported using the Sensei-Magellan system designed for interventional cardiology [40]. However, with this device, the ureteroscope was only passively manipulated, which was the main reason this project was discontinued after 18 clinical cases. Avicenna Roboflex™ (Elmed, Ankara, Turkey) was specially developed for FURS.

The surgeon sits at an open console manipulating a standard flexible ureteroscope with HD video technology. The handpiece of the scope is attached to a robotic manipulator enabling rotation, insertion, and scope deflection. Touchscreen functions and foot pedals provide irrigation, activation, and control of the laser fiber and fluoroscopy. The Avicenna Roboflex has had a CE mark since 2014, and FDA approval is in preparation. The multi-centric experience reports of the Avicenna Roboflex are promising [41, 42].

5   Technological Improvements Triggered by Robotic Surgery

In addition to the enhancements of consecutive platforms, robotic surgery has also spurred the development of new technologies to facilitate preoperative surgical planning while optimizing intraoperative performance.

5.1   Three-Dimensional (3D) Imaging Reconstruction

The 3D imaging reconstruction allows more accurate visualization and understanding of the anatomic planes between the tumor, surrounding vessels, and other organs [43]. During the preoperative routine, CT (computerized tomography) or MRI (magnetic resonance imaging) images are used to create a 3D anatomical reconstruction which is accessed on smartphones, on tablets, or by the robotic console (Tilepro-Isis mode).

5.2   Robotic Scope Imaging and Design

The robotic scope has been improved with high-definition 3D (three-dimensional) imaging and near-infrared technology (Firefly) [44]. After injecting intravenous indocyanine green dye, the scope detects the tissue perfusion (colored in green), and the surgeon identifies the correct surgical plane to access. This technology has an optimal application in partial nephrectomies, facilitating tumoral perfusion identification after the renal artery clamping. It has also been used in radical cystectomies to identify perfusion of the bowel segment used in the urinary diversion step.

Another modification regards the flexible scope presented by the new da Vinci® SP, which enables different angulations and visualization of different quadrants when the "cobra" mode is activated.

5.3 Intraoperative Ultrasound

Intraoperative ultrasound (US) technology has also been incorporated into robotic surgery to improve robotic-assisted partial nephrectomies. With this technology, the surgeon identifies and delineates the planes between the tumor and the renal parenchyma before the tumor removal [45]. US is also used to delineate intravenous thrombus in radical nephrectomies in patients with advanced renal tumors with vena cava thrombi [46].

5.4 Augmented Reality

Augmented reality using 3D images is another technology described in the robotic approach to urologic procedures [47]. Some renal tumors are difficult to identify even with intraoperative ultrasound assistance, especially intraparenchymal and small tumors, which usually are not evidently bulging in the cortical surface. In these cases, according to the authors, this technology enables easier identification of complex and intraparenchymal renal tumors with potential improvements in the quality of the tumor resection.

5.5 Artificial Intelligence (AI)

Artificial intelligence has been incorporated into robotic surgery in the last few years. This technology has been used to help surgeons identify the correct planes of dissection and improve surgical precision in different steps, such as suturing. Shademan and colleagues described studies with supervised autonomous soft tissue robotic suturing using AI in the open surgical setting [48]. The suturing algorithm was created based on surgical videos done by experts in intestinal anastomosis.

When comparing the expert (surgeon) anastomosis with supervised autonomous in ex vivo and porcine models, the author reported superior outcomes for the AI suturing in terms of metrics (suture spacing), pressure applied to avoid anastomosis leakage, needle repositioning, lumen reduction in some sutures such as bowel anastomosis, and completion time.

6 Current and Future Perspectives

In the last two decades, robotic surgery has been rapidly becoming more common and has been evolving with the creation of several generations of robotic platforms. After millions of patients were operated on with this technological assistance in the USA, robotic surgery has become the standard treatment of some urological diseases such as localized prostate cancer (radical prostatectomy) and kidney tumors (partial nephrectomy).

The robotic training methods have also improved, especially after the advent of the dual console (teaching console), which integrates the expert and the trainee, providing the same operative view while sharing robotic commands. In addition, the simulator quality has been enhanced with new software and programs that allow a step-by-step surgical training.

In Brazil, robotic training was restricted to a few centers in the early days of robotic surgery, following bureaucratic guidelines to authorize the certification of new generations of robotic surgeons. At that time, the certification demand was used to be larger than the services provided by the certifying company, causing delays in the qualifications of several surgeons. However, this trend has changed in the past years with increasing accessibility of this technology in different centers. Currently, for urology certification, each hospital is providing its own training and certification based on established protocols and guidelines described by the Brazilian Urologic Society (SBU) [49]. In our opinion, facilitating the certification access with obvious quality maintenance leads to robotic training inclusion and improvements.

Finally, new platforms and technologies have been created and integrated into robotic surgery [50]. We believe that the expansion of new companies on the market will reduce the costs of platforms and instruments, allowing further improvements in surgical outcomes. In addition, decreasing the final costs enables robotic surgery in centers with financial restrictions, such as public hospitals with residency programs.

7 Conclusion

In the past years, several robotic technologies have been developed and incorporated into surgical procedures with increased benefits for the patients. The methods of training and certification have also been modernized and the da Vinci® technology is still leading the market worldwide. Currently, the multiport is still the standard of care in all surgical specialties using robotic technology. We believe that competition with new platforms will further decrease surgical prices, expanding the accessibility to new generations of surgeons interested in minimally invasive surgery.

References

1. Rotondo MF, Schwab CW, McGonigal MD, et al. "Damage control": an approach for improved survival in exsanguinating penetrating abdominal injury. J Trauma. 1993;35(3):375.
2. Price BA. Anesthesia and perioperative care of the combat casualty. Textbook of military medicine. Part IV – surgical combat casualty care, R. Zajtchuk, R. F. Rellamy and C. M. Grande (eds). 287 × 220 mm. Pp. 1931. Illustrated 1995. Tacoma, Washington: TMM Publications. Br J Surg. 2005;84(6):892. https://doi.org/10.1002/bjs.1800840651.
3. Satava RM. Robotic surgery: from past to future—a personal journey. Surg Clin N Am. 2003;83(6):1491. https://doi.org/10.1016/S0039-6109(03)00168-3.
4. George EI, Brand TC, LaPorta A, Marescaux J, Satava RM. Origins of robotic surgery: from skepticism to standard of care. J Soc Laparoendosc Surg. 2018;22(4):e2018.00039. https://doi.org/10.4293/JSLS.2018.00039.
5. Himpens J, Leman G, Cadiere GB. Telesurgical laparoscopic cholecystectomy. Surg Endosc. 1998;12(8):1091. https://doi.org/10.1007/s004649900788.
6. Covas Moschovas M, Bhat S, Onol FF, et al. Modified apical dissection and lateral prostatic fascia preservation improves early postoperative functional recovery in robotic-assisted laparoscopic radical prostatectomy: results from a propensity score–matched analysis. Eur Urol. 2020;78(6):875. https://doi.org/10.1016/j.eururo.2020.05.041.
7. Moschovas MC, Bhat S, Fikret O, Travis R, Vipul P. Modified simple prostatectomy: an approach to address large volume BPH and associated prostate cancers. J Robot Surg. 2020;14(4):543. https://doi.org/10.1007/s11701-019-01038-6.
8. Moschovas MC, Chade DC, Arap MA, et al. Robotic-assisted radical cystectomy: the first multicentric Brazilian experience. J Robot Surg. 2020;14(5):703. https://doi.org/10.1007/s11701-020-01043-0.
9. Mazzone E, D'Hondt F, Beato S, et al. Robot-assisted radical cystectomy with intracorporeal urinary diversion decreases postoperative complications only in highly comorbid patients: findings that rely on a standardized methodology recommended by the European Association of Urology Guidelines. World J Urol. 2021;39(3):803. https://doi.org/10.1007/s00345-020-03237-5.
10. Binder J, Kramer W. Robotically-assisted laparoscopic radical prostatectomy. BJU Int. 2001;87(4):408. https://doi.org/10.1046/j.1464-410x.2001.00115.x.
11. Mohr FW, Falk V, Diegeler A, Autschback R. Computer-enhanced coronary artery bypass surgery. J Thorac Cardiovasc Surg. 1999;117(6):1212. https://doi.org/10.1016/S0022-5223(99)70261-8.
12. Rassweiler JJ, Autorino R, Klein J, et al. Future of robotic surgery in urology. BJU Int. 2017;120(6):822. https://doi.org/10.1111/bju.13851.
13. Bhat KRS, Moschovas MC, Onol FF, et al. Evidence-based evolution of our robot-assisted laparoscopic prostatectomy (RALP) technique through 13,000 cases. J Robot Surg. 2021;15(4):651. https://doi.org/10.1007/s11701-020-01157-5.
14. Covas Moschovas M, Bhat S, Rogers T, et al. Applications of the da Vinci single port (SP) robotic platform in urology: a systematic literature review. Minerva Urol Nephrol. 2021;73(1):6. https://doi.org/10.23736/S0393-2249.20.03899-0.
15. Moschovas MC, Seetharam Bhat KR, Onol FF, et al. Single-port technique evolution and current practice in urologic procedures. Asian J Urol. 2021;8(1):100. https://doi.org/10.1016/j.ajur.2020.05.003.
16. Covas Moschovas M, Bhat S, Onol F, Rogers T, Patel V. Early outcomes of single-port robot-assisted radical prostatectomy: lessons learned from the learning-curve experience. BJU Int. 2021;127(1):114. https://doi.org/10.1111/bju.15158.
17. Covas Moschovas M, Bhat S, Rogers T, et al. Technical modifications necessary to implement the da Vinci single-port robotic system. Eur Urol. 2020;78(3):415. https://doi.org/10.1016/j.eururo.2020.01.005.

18. Covas Moschovas M, Helman T, Reddy S, et al. Minimally invasive lymphocele drainage using the da Vinci single-port platform: step-by-step technique of a prostate cancer referral center. J Endourol. 2021;35(9):1357. https://doi.org/10.1089/end.2020.1175.

19. Noël J, Moschovas MC, Sandri M, et al. Patient surgical satisfaction after da Vinci® single-port and multi-port robotic-assisted radical prostatectomy: propensity score-matched analysis. J Robot Surg. 2021;16:473. https://doi.org/10.1007/s11701-021-01269-6.

20. Covas Moschovas M, Bhat S, Rogers T, Noel J, Reddy S, Patel V. Da Vinci single-port robotic radical prostatectomy. J Endourol. 2021;35(S2):S93. https://doi.org/10.1089/end.2020.1090.

21. Maurice MJ, Ramirez D, Kaouk JH. Robotic laparoendoscopic single-site retroperitioneal renal surgery: initial investigation of a purpose-built single-port surgical system. Eur Urol. 2017;71(4):643. https://doi.org/10.1016/j.eururo.2016.06.005.

22. Kaouk J, Aminsharifi A, Sawczyn G, et al. Single-port robotic urological surgery using purpose-built single-port surgical system: single-institutional experience with the first 100 cases. Urology. 2020;140:77. https://doi.org/10.1016/j.urology.2019.11.086.

23. Kaouk JH, Haber GP, Autorino R, et al. A novel robotic system for single-port urologic surgery: first clinical investigation. Eur Urol. 2014;66(6):1033. https://doi.org/10.1016/j.eururo.2014.06.039.

24. Covas Moschovas M, Bhat S, Rogers T, et al. Da Vinci SP platform updates and modifications: the first impression of new settings. J Robot Surg. 2021;15:977. https://doi.org/10.1007/s11701-021-01248-x.

25. Moschovas MC, Bhat S, Sandri M, et al. Comparing the approach to radical prostatectomy using the multiport da Vinci Xi and da Vinci SP robots: a propensity score analysis of perioperative outcomes. Eur Urol. 2021;79(3):393. https://doi.org/10.1016/j.eururo.2020.11.042.

26. Giedelman C, Covas Moschovas M, Bhat S, et al. Establishing a successful robotic surgery program and improving operating room efficiency: literature review and our experience report. J Robot Surg. 2021;15(3):435. https://doi.org/10.1007/s11701-020-01121-3.

27. Sheth KR, Koh CJ. The future of robotic surgery in pediatric urology: upcoming technology and evolution within the field. Front Pediatr. 2019;7:259. https://doi.org/10.3389/fped.2019.00259.

28. Abdel Raheem A, Sheikh A, Kim DK, et al. Da Vinci Xi and Si platforms have equivalent perioperative outcomes during robot-assisted partial nephrectomy: preliminary experience. J Robot Surg. 2017;11(1):53. https://doi.org/10.1007/s11701-016-0612-x.

29. Talamini S, Halgrimson WR, Dobbs RW, Morana C, Crivellaro S. Single port robotic radical prostatectomy versus multi-port robotic radical prostatectomy: a human factor analysis during the initial learning curve. Int J Med Robot Comput Assist Surg. 2021;17(2):e2209. https://doi.org/10.1002/rcs.2209.

30. Farinha R, Puliatti S, Mazzone E, et al. Potential contenders for the leadership in robotic surgery. J Endourol. 2021;36:317. https://doi.org/10.1089/end.2021.0321.

31. Koukourikis P, Rha KH. Robotic surgical systems in urology: what is currently available? Investig Clin Urol. 2021;62(1):14. https://doi.org/10.4111/icu.20200387.

32. Dixon F, Khanna A, Vitish-Sharma P, et al. Initiation and feasibility of a multi-specialty minimally invasive surgical programme using a novel robotic system: a case series. Int J Surg. 2021;96:106182. https://doi.org/10.1016/j.ijsu.2021.106182.

33. Thomas BC, Slack M, Hussain M, et al. Preclinical evaluation of the versius surgical system, a new robot-assisted surgical device for use in minimal access renal and prostate surgery. Eur Urol Focus. 2021;7(2):444–52. https://doi.org/10.1016/j.euf.2020.01.011.

34. Medtronic. n.d. https://www.medtronic.com/covidien/en-gb/robotic-assisted-surgery/hugo-ras-system.html.

35. Fierce Biotech. n.d. https://www.fiercebiotech.com/medtech/meet-hugo-medtronic-s-robotic-assisted-surgery-system-makes-global-debut-chilean-clinic.

36. Chang KD, Abdel Raheem A, Choi YD, Chung BH, Rha KH. Retzius-sparing robot-assisted radical prostatectomy using the Revo-i robotic surgical system: surgical technique and results of the first human trial. BJU Int. 2018;122(3):441–8. https://doi.org/10.1111/bju.14245.

37. Kaštelan Ž, Knežević N, Hudolin T, et al. Extraperitoneal radical prostatectomy with the Senhance Surgical System robotic platform. Croatian Med J. 2019;60(6):556–9. https://doi.org/10.3325/cmj.2019.60.556.

38. Shine. n.d. https://www.shine.cn/news/metro/1911025111.

39. Napoli A, Alfieri G, Scipione R, et al. High-intensity focused ultrasound for prostate cancer. Exp Rev Med Devices. 2020;17(5):427–33. https://doi.org/10.1080/17434440.2020.1755258.

40. Desai MM, Aron M, Gill IS, et al. Flexible robotic retrograde renoscopy: description of novel robotic device and preliminary laboratory experience. Urology. 2008;72(1):42–6. https://doi.org/10.1016/j.urology.2008.01.076.

41. Rassweiler J, Fiedler M, Charalampogiannis N, Kabakci AS, Saglam R, Klein JT. Robot-assisted flexible ureteroscopy: an update. Urolithiasis. 2018;46(1):69–77. https://doi.org/10.1007/s00240-017-1024-8.

42. Saglam R, Muslumanoglu AY, Tokatlı Z, et al. A new robot for flexible ureteroscopy: development and early clinical results (IDEAL Stage 1–2b). Eur Urol. 2014;66(6):1092–100. https://doi.org/10.1016/j.eururo.2014.06.047.

43. Bertolo R, Autorino R, Fiori C, et al. Expanding the indications of robotic partial nephrectomy for highly complex renal tumors: urologists' perception of the impact of hyperaccuracy three-dimensional reconstruction. J Laparoendosc Adv Surg Techn A. 2019;29(2):233. https://doi.org/10.1089/lap.2018.0486.

44. Bates AS, Patel VR. Applications of indocyanine green in robotic urology. J Robot Surg. 2016;10(4):357. https://doi.org/10.1007/s11701-016-0641-5.

45. di Cosmo G, Verzotti E, Silvestri T, et al. Intraoperative ultrasound in robot-assisted partial nephrectomy: state of the art. Arch Ital Urol Androl. 2018;90(3):195. https://doi.org/10.4081/aiua.2018.3.195.

46. Seetharam Bhat KR, Moschovas MC, Onol FF, et al. Robotic renal and adrenal oncologic surgery: a contemporary review. Asian J Urol. 2021;8(1):89. https://doi.org/10.1016/j.ajur.2020.05.010.

47. Porpiglia F, Checcucci E, Amparore D, et al. Three-dimensional augmented reality robot-assisted partial nephrectomy in case of complex tumours (PADUA ≥10): a new intraoperative tool overcoming the ultrasound guidance. Eur Urol. 2020;78(2):229. https://doi.org/10.1016/j.eururo.2019.11.024.

48. Cha J, Shademan A, Le HND, et al. Multispectral tissue characterization for intestinal anastomosis optimization. J Biomed Opt. 2015;20(10):106001. https://doi.org/10.1117/1.JBO.20.10.106001.

49. Portal da Urologia. n.d. https://portaldaurologia.org.br/medicos/wp-content/uploads/2021/04/O.

50. Covas Moschovas M, Kind S, Bhat SK, Noel J, Sandri M, Rogers TP, Moser D, Brady I, Patel V. Implementing the da Vinci SP® without increasing positive surgical margins: experience and pathological outcomes of a prostate cancer referral center. J Endourol. 2021;36:493. https://doi.org/10.1089/end.2021.0656. PMID: 34963334.

Robotic Devices in Surgery of the Digestive System

Bruno Zilberstein, Danilo Dallago De Marchi, Andrea Vieira Martins, Rodrigo Moises de Almeida Leite, and Gustavo Guimarães

The Robot is a working tool to be applied in Minimally Invasive Surgery [1]. Although an important series of Robots is being created, in this chapter, we will be exclusively commenting on the instruments in Robotic Surgery of the Digestive System, of the "Da Vinci" Robot, whether of the Si, X, or Xi model. These models are made up of three components: Patient Cart, Console, and Vision cart (Figs. 1, 2, and 3).

These robotic systems are currently the most used worldwide with more than 5000 units sold [4].

The instruments are similar for the three models, with changes in the relationship between the clamps in their fitting on the robot's arms and the optics. In the Si model the optic is 12 mm, while in the Xi and X models the optic is 8 mm.

The Da Vinci Robot (Si, Xi, and X) has four arms, one of which is always dedicated to optics, which can be 0° or 30° [5].

B. Zilberstein (✉) · D. D. De Marchi · A. V. Martins · R. M. de Almeida Leite · G. Guimarães
Oncological Surgical Division of Beneficencia Portuguesa de Sao Paulo Hospital, Sao Paulo, Brazil

© The Author(s), under exclusive license to Springer Nature Switzerland AG 2023

J. P. Manzano, L. M. Ferreira (eds.), *Robotic Surgery Devices in Surgical Specialties*, https://doi.org/10.1007/978-3-031-35102-0_6

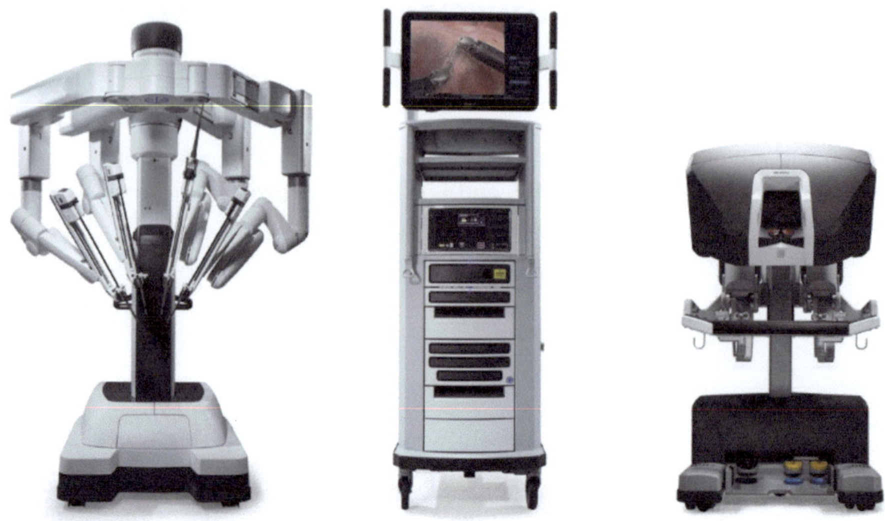

Fig. 1 Xi Robot: Patient Cart, Vision cart, and Console. (From Intuitive Surgical, 2023 [2, 3])

Fig. 2 X Robot: Console. (From Intuitive Surgical, 2023 [2, 3])

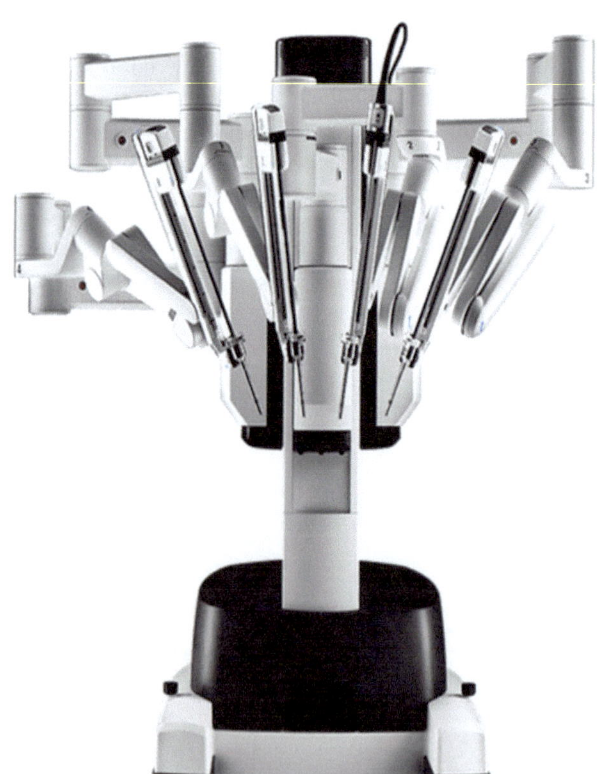

Fig. 3 Si Robot: Console.
(From Intuitive Surgical,
2023 [2, 3])

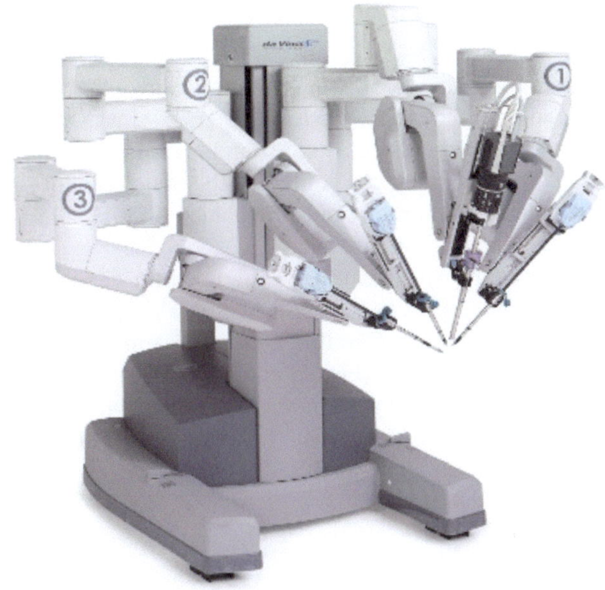

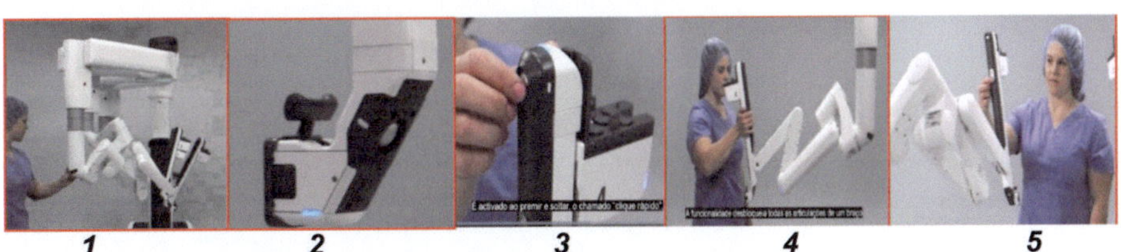

Fig. 4 Robot Xi. (From Intuitive Surgical, 2023 [2, 3])

1   Terms Used in Robotic Surgery

Draping: draping the robot.
   Docking: taking the patient's cart to the patient.
   Undocking: move the patient's cart away.
   On site: to check if the vision cart is connected to the internet network.

1. Boom rotation: The button is located on arms 1 and 4; it turns the robot arms to the right or left.
2. Port clutch: A button on the robot's arm that performs various movements (up and down and left and right).
3. Clutch: A button on the robot arm that performs movement in the remote center.
4. Grab movie: Grabs and holds and performs rough arm movements.
5. Clearance patient: A button on the robot arm where the surgeon gains more space to operate (Fig. 4).

2   Optics or Endoscopes

Regardless of the Si or X or Xi system, the optics can be 0° or 30°. The optics vary depending on the robot model.

For the Si system, this optic can be 12 mm or 8.5 mm. That's why, unlike other Robot models, in the case of the Si, the optics cannot be changed during the surgical procedure and normally must be placed on a 12 mm long trocar, since the Robot's arm is attached to the trocar.

Also in the Si system, there is a need for decoupling and inverting the optics in case it is necessary to change the camera's field of view. For real-time fluorescence image visualization (Firefly), in this system it is necessary to use another green-colored handle optics (Figs. 5 and 6).

For the X and Xi system, the optics are 8 mm and can be placed on any of the Robot's trocars as they are all 8 mm (Figs. 7, 8 and 9).

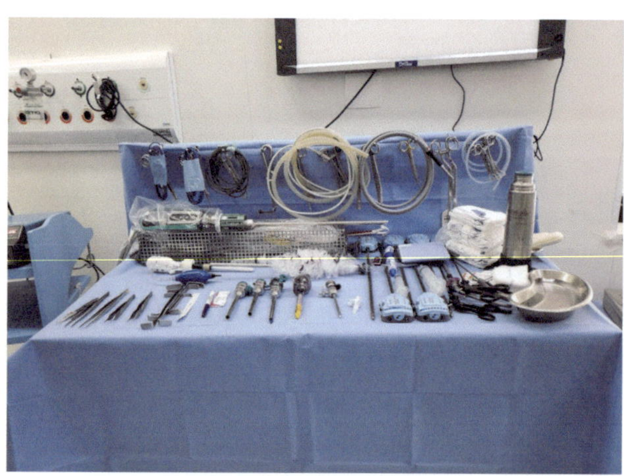

Fig. 5 Robotic surgery table, Robot Si. (From the author's archive [6])

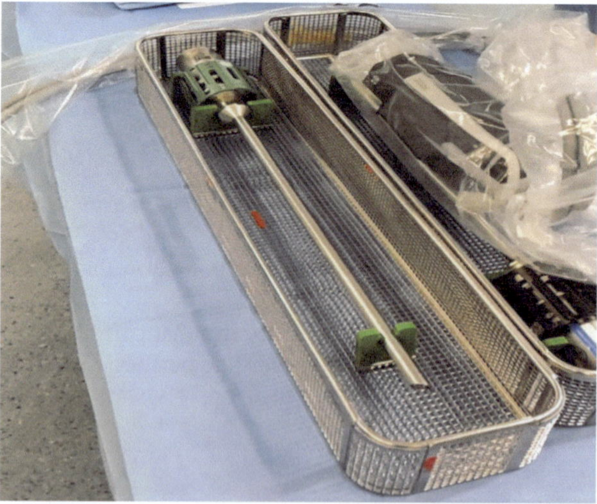

Fig. 6 12 mm. Scope. (From the author's archive [6])

In this case, the Firefly system is automatic and the inversion of the image is activated on the Robot console without the need to decouple the optics (Fig. 10).

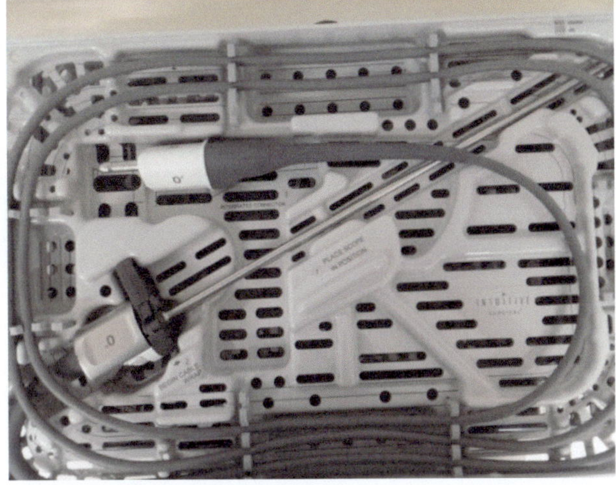

Fig. 7 30° Scope. (From the author's archive [6])

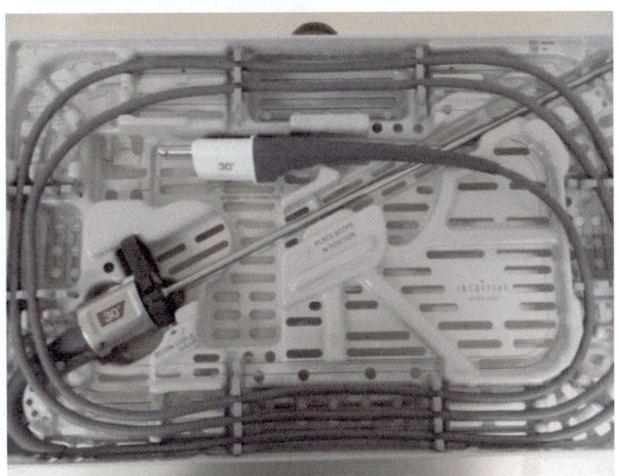

Fig. 8 0° Scope. (From the author's archive [6])

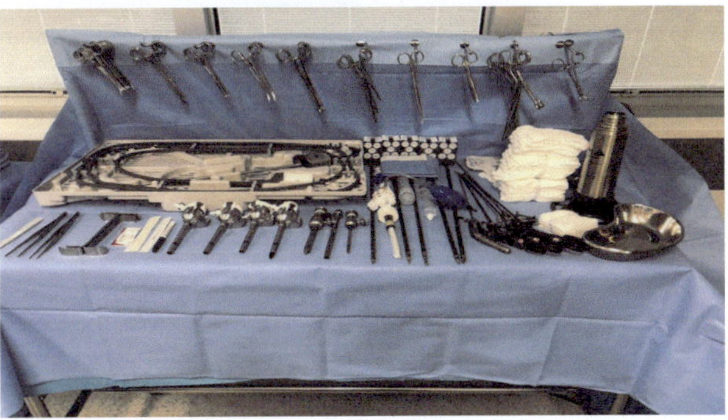

Fig. 9 Table mounted for robotic surgeries Robot Xi and X. (From the author's archive [6])

Fig. 10 Robot Xi. (From authors' archive [7])

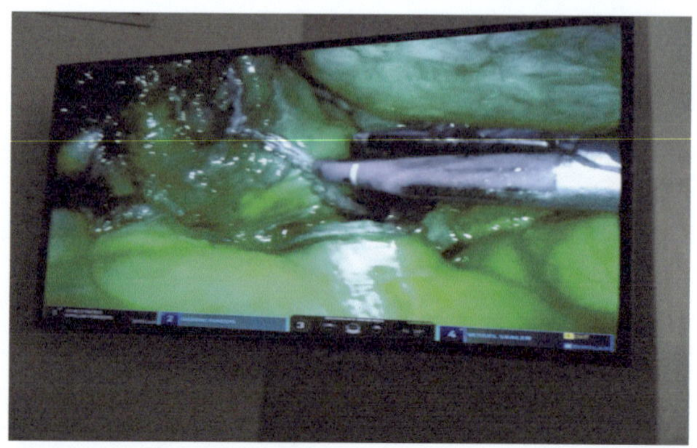

Fig. 11 8 mm Trocar Robot Si. (From the author's archive [6])

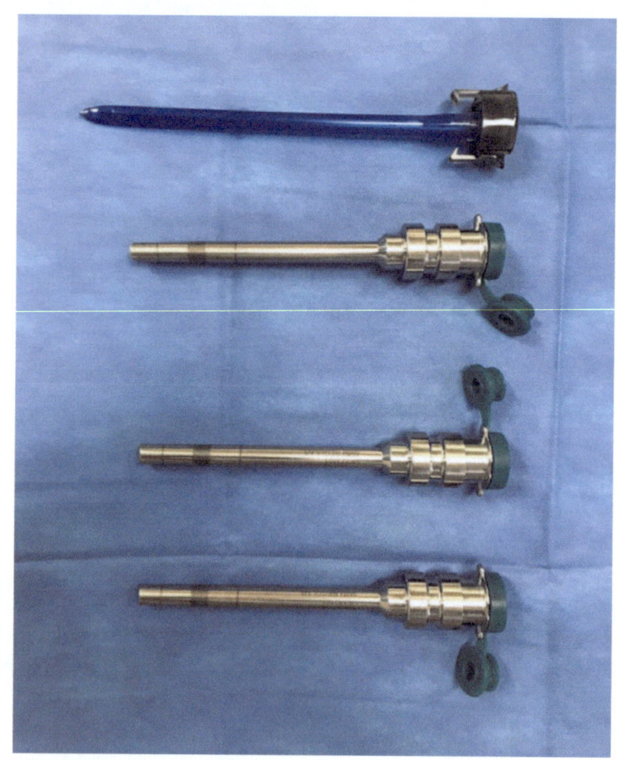

3 Cables and Trocars

See Figs. 11, 12, 13, 14, and 15.

Fig. 12 12 mm Disposable Trocar. (From the author's archive [6])

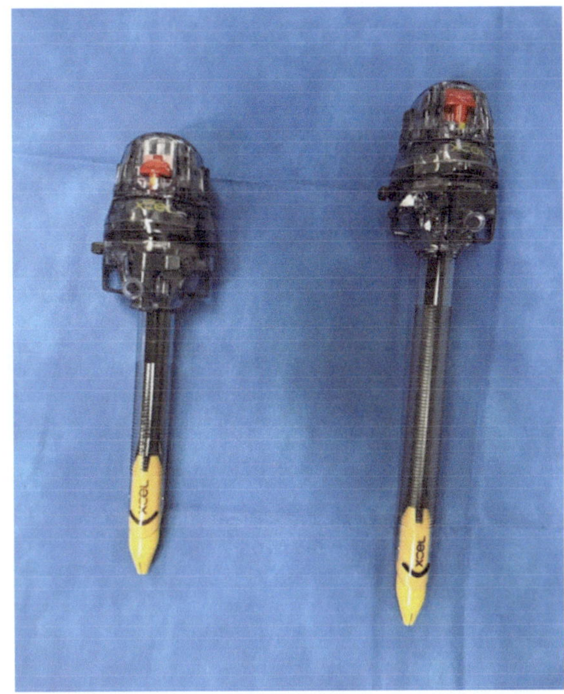

Fig. 13 Monopolar and bipolar cables. (From the author's archive [6])

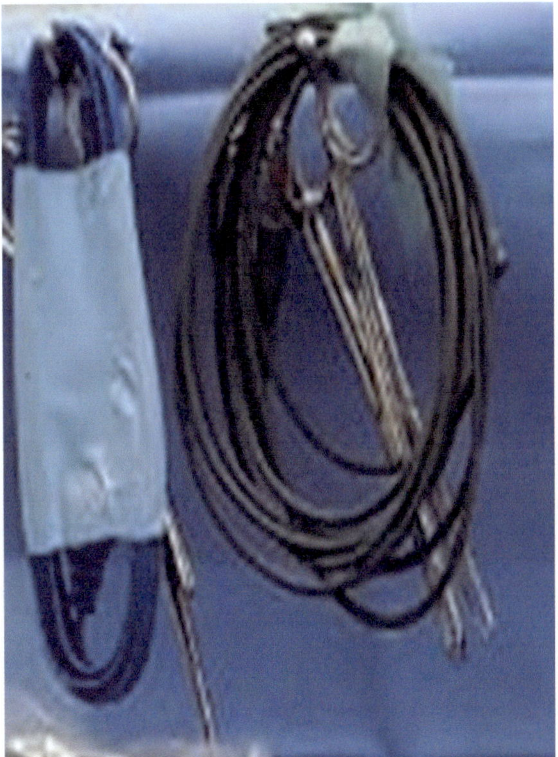

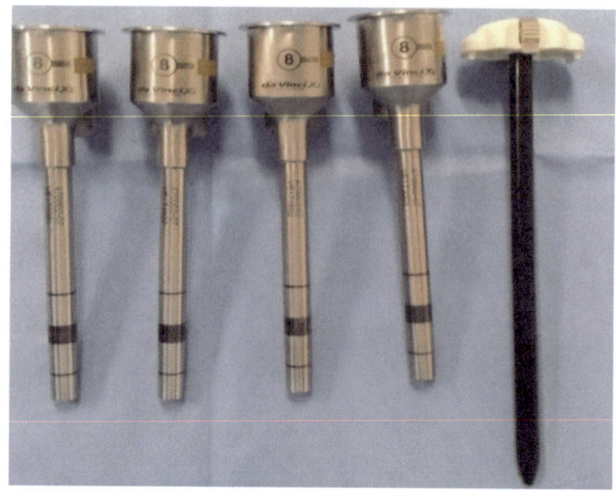

Fig. 14 Robot Xi e X Trocars. (From the author's archive [6])

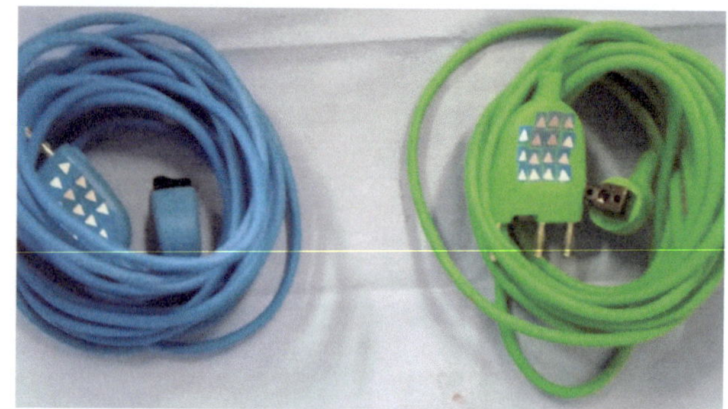

Fig. 15 Bipolar (blue) and monopolar (green) cables. (From the author's archive [6])

4 Robotic Tweezers

The tweezers are sterilized and have limited usage time given by the manufacturer. After that they are discarded.

4.1 *Grasping Forceps*

All of them have the "endowrist" manipulation capability (articulated movement in seven directions), that is, they can be freely manipulated in various angles and directions.

Cardiere: Forceps; serrated and fenestrated forceps, weak jaw closure, atraumatic. It is the most used grasping forceps in digestive surgery.

Prograsp: Forceps; serrated and fenestrated forceps of strong grasp, rarely used in digestive surgery.

Tip-up fenestrated: Serrated and fenestrated tweezers, delicate, which can be used as a counter-needle holder or pair of tissue apprehensions (Figs. 16, 17, and 18).

There are also **Tenaculum** and **Cobra-Grasper**; grasping forceps which, due to their design, are not recommended in digestive surgery (Figs. 19 and 20).

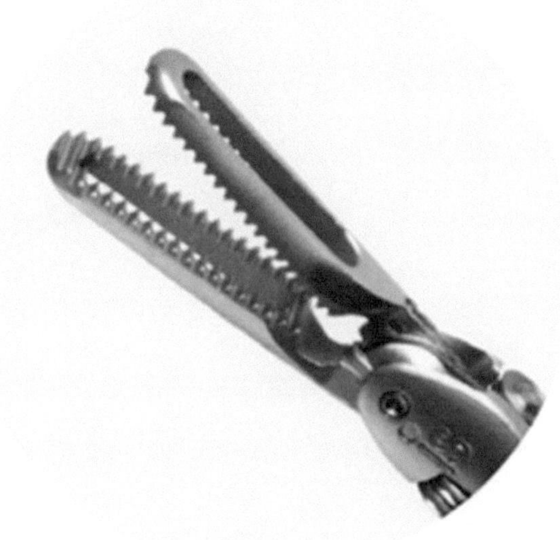

Fig. 16 Cardiere. (From Intuitive Surgical, 2023 [2, 3])

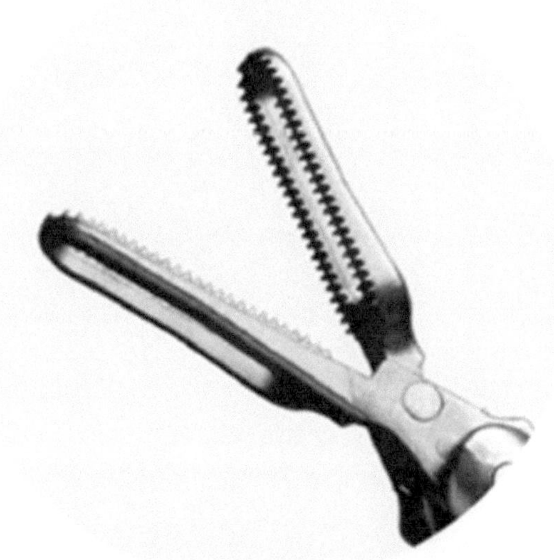

Fig. 17 Pograsp. (From Intuitive Surgical, 2023 [2, 3])

Fig. 18 Tip-up fenestrated. (From Intuitive Surgical, 2023 [2, 3])

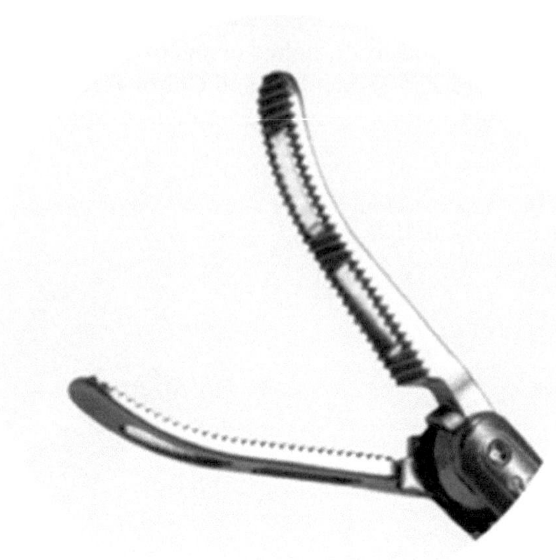

Fig. 19 Tenaculum. (From Intuitive Surgical, 2023 [2, 3])

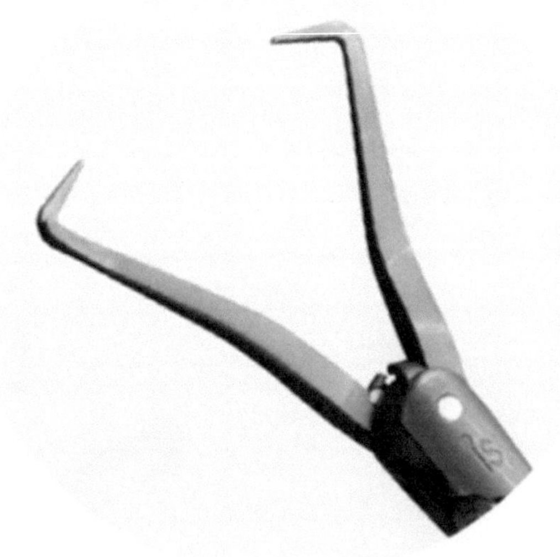

Fig. 20 Cobra-Grasper.
(From Intuitive Surgical,
2023 [2, 3])

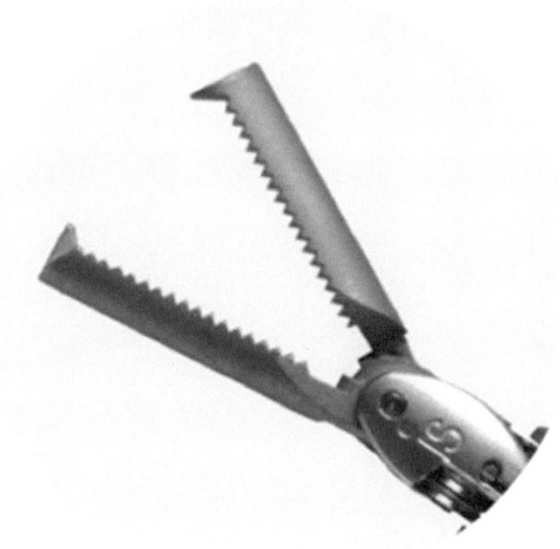

4.2 Power Clamps: Monopolar and Bipolar

Fenestrated bipolar: It is similar to Cardiere, however, more delicate and has a lower apprehension power (endowrist mobility) and has bipolar energy.

Maryland bipolar: They are used as a grasping forceps and allows for bipolar coagulation (endowrist mobility). Due to its fine tip, it has a greater risk of tissue damage if used as a grasping forceps and, therefore, must be used for dissection and delicate coagulation (Figs. 21 and 22).

Monopolar cautery Hook: There is "hook" forceps that has the mobility of the endowrist and therefore lends itself to delicate dissections of viscera and vessels, obeying their curvatures and recesses. Widely used in esophagectomy, gastrectomy, and pancreatectomy.

Monopolar curved scissors: It is an endowrist mobility scissors, used for cutting and cautery and fine dissection. In abdominal hernia operations, whatever the region, it becomes a very useful instrument.

Monopolar spatula cautery: It is a delicate spatula, with endowrist movement, and which lends itself to blunt dissections. The cautery power is used in pancreatectomies and hepatectomies and whenever a blunt dissection is desired (Figs. 23, 24, and 25).

Harmonic energy clamp: Corresponds to ultrasonic scissors. The allow cutting and coagulation and is widely used for dissection. It has the disadvantage of not having an endowrist which can limit its application in more restricted spaces.

Fig. 21 Fenestrated bipolar. (From Intuitive Surgical, 2023 [2, 3])

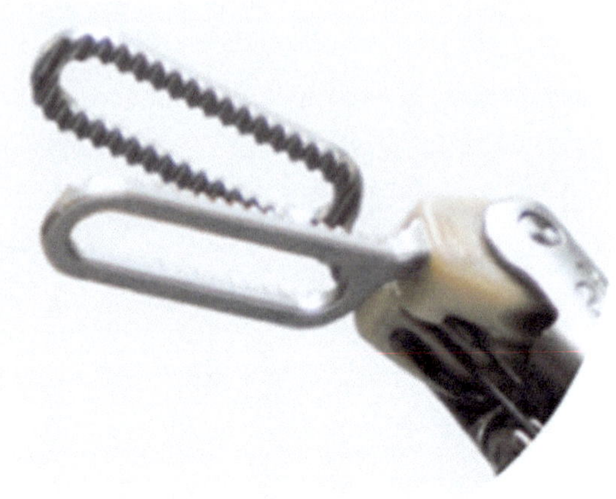

Fig. 22 Maryland bipolar. (From Intuitive Surgical, 2023 [2, 3])

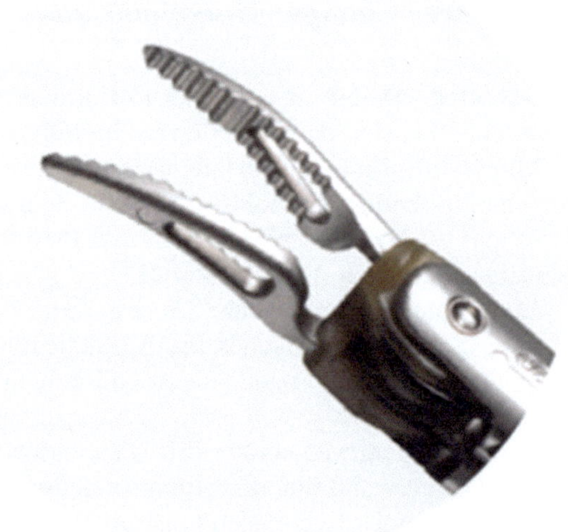

Fig. 23 Monopolar
cautery hook. (From
Intuitive Surgical, 2023
[2, 3])

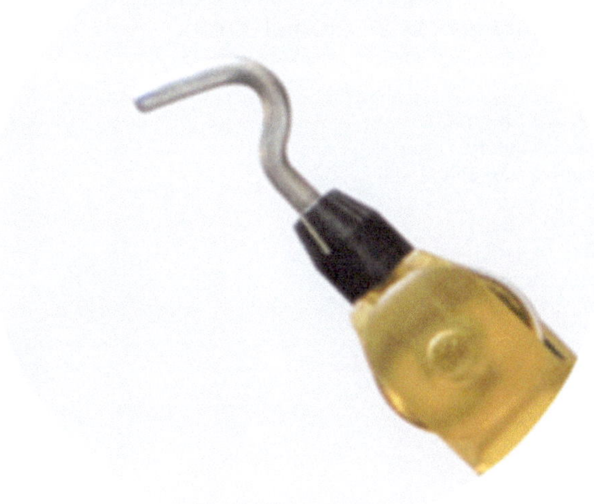

Fig. 24 Monopolar curved
scissors. (From Intuitive
Surgical, 2023 [2, 3])

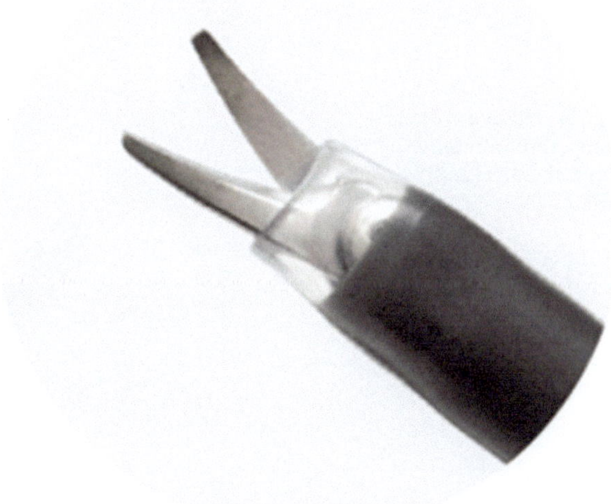

Vessel Sealer: The bipolar energy clamp that can seal vessels up to 7 mm. It has an endowrist and used for dissection, but is too coarse for fine dissection. Very useful for performing colectomies or bariatric surgery of the "sleeve gastrectomy" type (Sleeve) (Figs. 26, 27, 28, and 29).

Fig. 25 Monopolar spatula cautery. (From Intuitive Surgical, 2023 [2, 3])

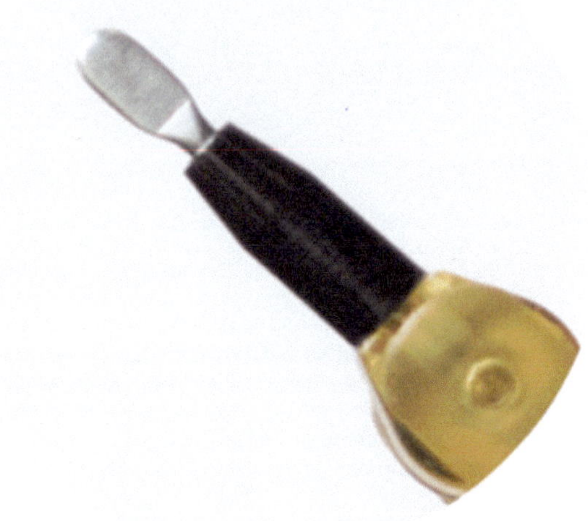

Fig. 26 Harmonic energy clamp. (From Intuitive Surgical, 2023 [2, 3])

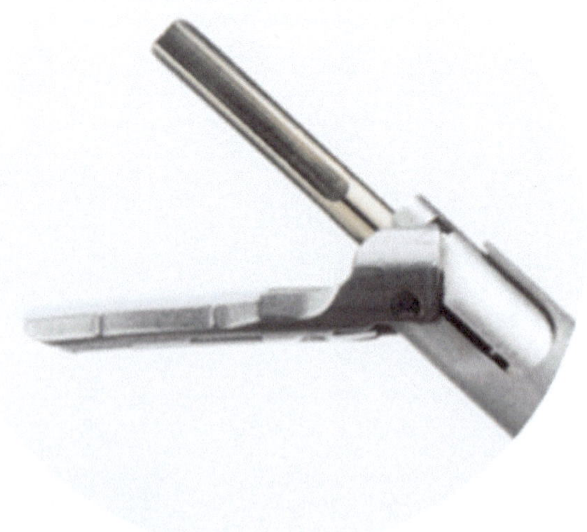

Fig. 27 Vessel Sealer. (From Intuitive Surgical, 2023 [2, 3])

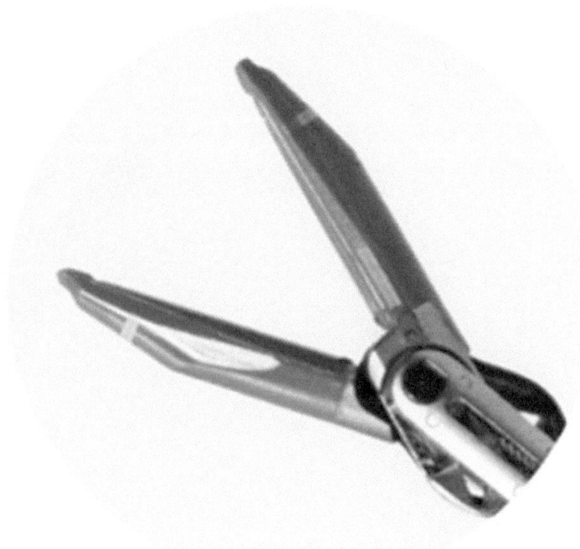

Fig. 28 Vessel Sealer Extend. (From Intuitive Surgical, 2023 [2, 3])

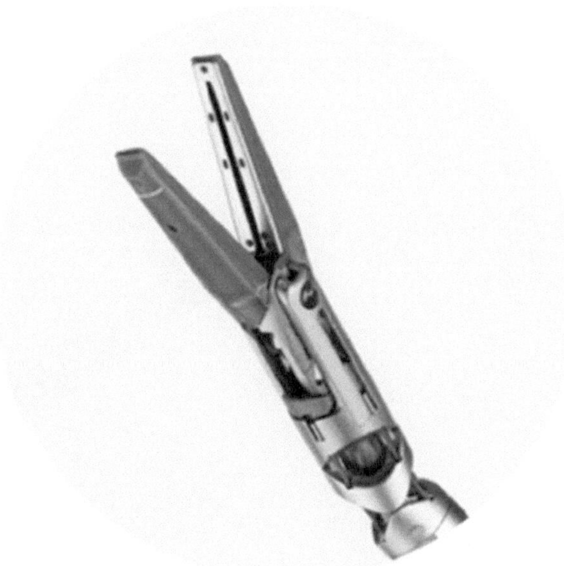

Fig. 29 SynchroSeal. (From Intuitive Surgical, 2023 [2, 3])

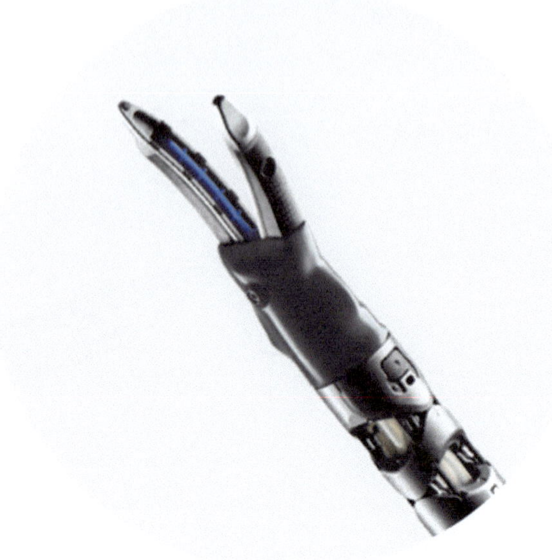

Fig. 30 Big clipper. (From Intuitive Surgical, 2023 [2, 3])

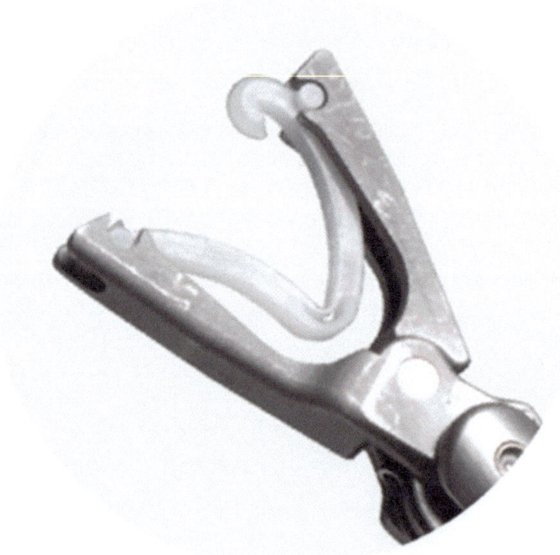

4.3   Robotic Clippers

Robotic clippers: Instruments for applying clips for ligation of vessels, with three sizes, small, medium, and large (Figs. 30, 31, and 32).

Fig. 31 Medium clipper.
(From Intuitive Surgical,
2023 [2, 3])

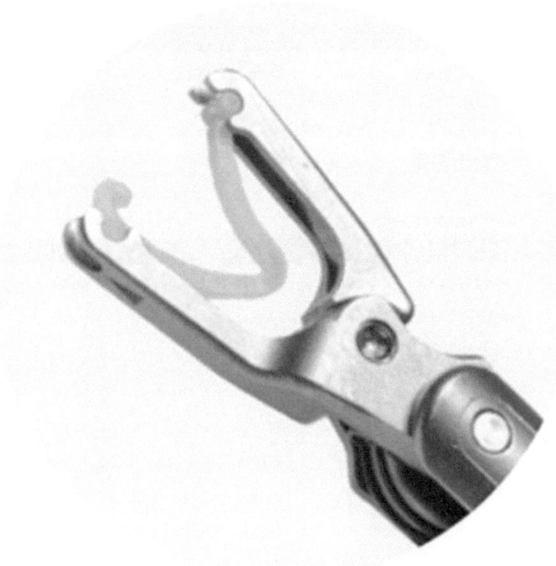

Fig. 32 Small clipper.
(From Intuitive Surgical,
2023 [2, 3])

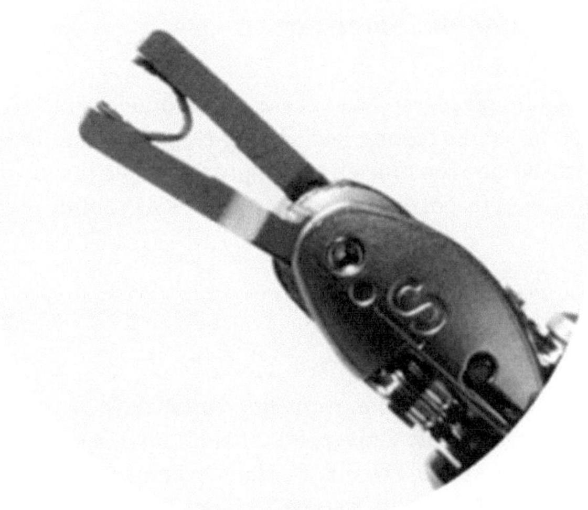

SureForm stapler instruments

	Item code	Product description		Qty/box	Uses
	480460	SureForm 60 instrument		6	Single use
	480445	SureForm 45 instrument		6	Single use
	480545	SureForm 45 curved-tip instrument		6	Single use

SureForm stapler reloads

	Item code	Product description		Qty/box	Uses
	48360W	Reload, SureForm 60, 2.5 white	6-row	12	1 firing
	48360B	Reload, SureForm 60, 3.5 blue	6-row	12	1 firing
	48360G	Reload, SureForm 60, 4.3 green	6-row	12	1 firing
	48360T	Reload, SureForm 60, 4.6 black	6-row	12	1 firing
	48345M	Reload, SureForm 45, 2.0 gray	6-row	12	1 firing
	48345W	Reload, SureForm 45, 2.5 white	6-row	12	1 firing
	48345B	Reload, SureForm 45, 3.5 blue	6-row	12	1 firing
	48345G	Reload, SureForm 45, 4.3 green	6-row	12	1 firing
	48345T	Reload, SureForm 45, 4.6 black	6-row	12	1 firing

Fig. 33 Models and characteristics of robotic staplers. (From Intuitive Surgical, 2023 [2, 3])

4.4   Robotic Staplers

Robotic staplers: They correspond to automatic staplers with lateral movements that allow the cutting and sealing of tissues and large vessels. It has the advantage that the surgeon himself can apply the staple line using the benefit of the endowrist; however, its cost in our country makes its routine use difficult (Fig. 33).

4.5   Needle Holder

All have articulated movements (endowrist).

Large Needle Driver: For smaller diameter wires up to 3-0.

Mega Needle Driver: For larger diameter wires.

Mega Suturecut Needle Driver: There is a needle holder that can also cut the suture thread. Its use requires a lot of attention so that there is no accidental cutting of the suture thread during the performance of the same (Figs. 34, 35, 36, 37, 38, and 39).

Fig. 34 Large Needle Driver. (From Intuitive Surgical, 2023 [2, 3])

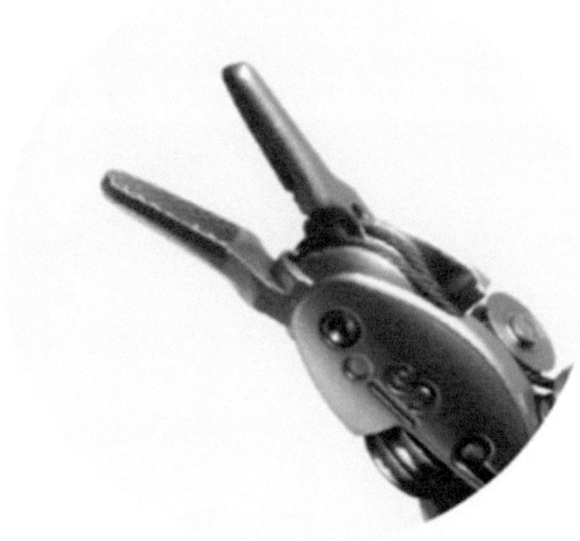

Fig. 35 Mega Needle Driver. (From Intuitive Surgical, 2023 [2, 3])

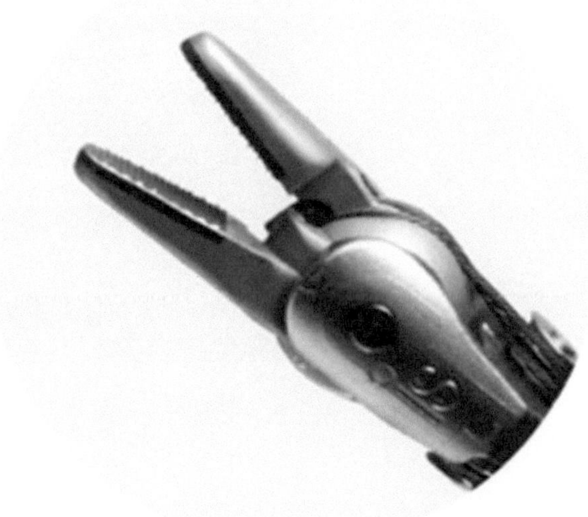

Fig. 36 Mega SutureCut Needle Driver. (From Intuitive Surgical, 2023 [2, 3])

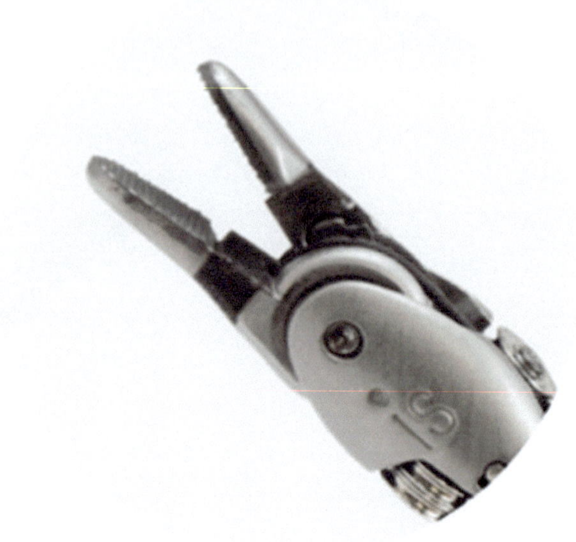

Fig. 37 Si Robotic clamps. (From the author's archive [7])

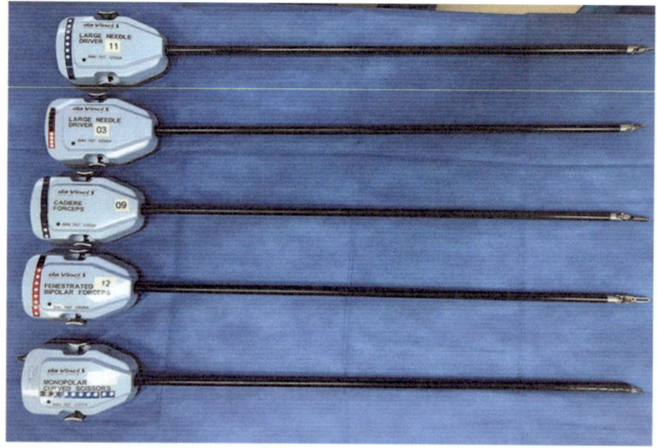

Fig. 38 Xi and X Robotic clamps. (From the author's archive [7])

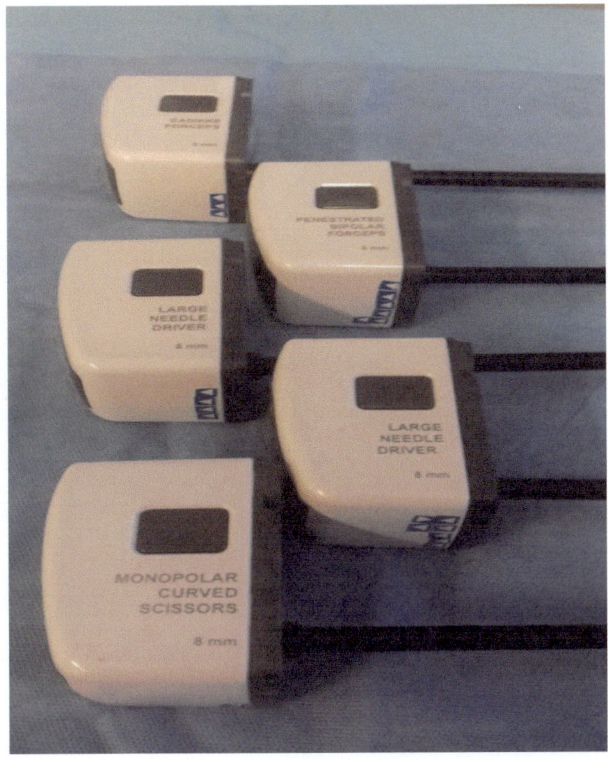

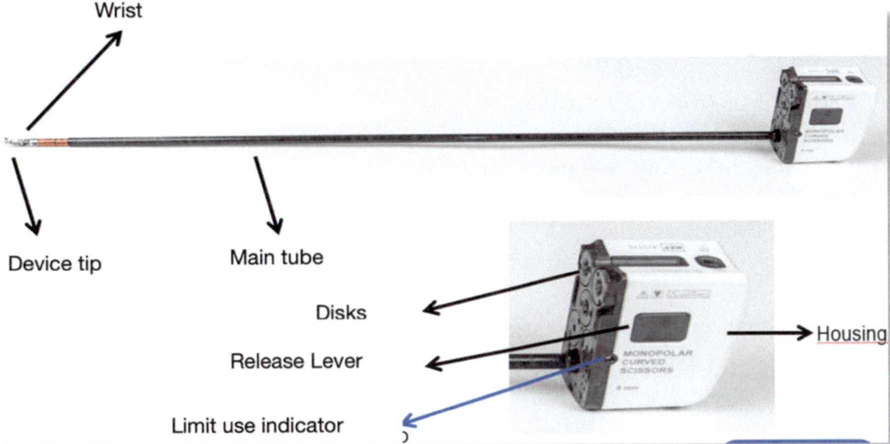

Fig. 39 Xi and X Robotic clamp. (From the author's archive [7])

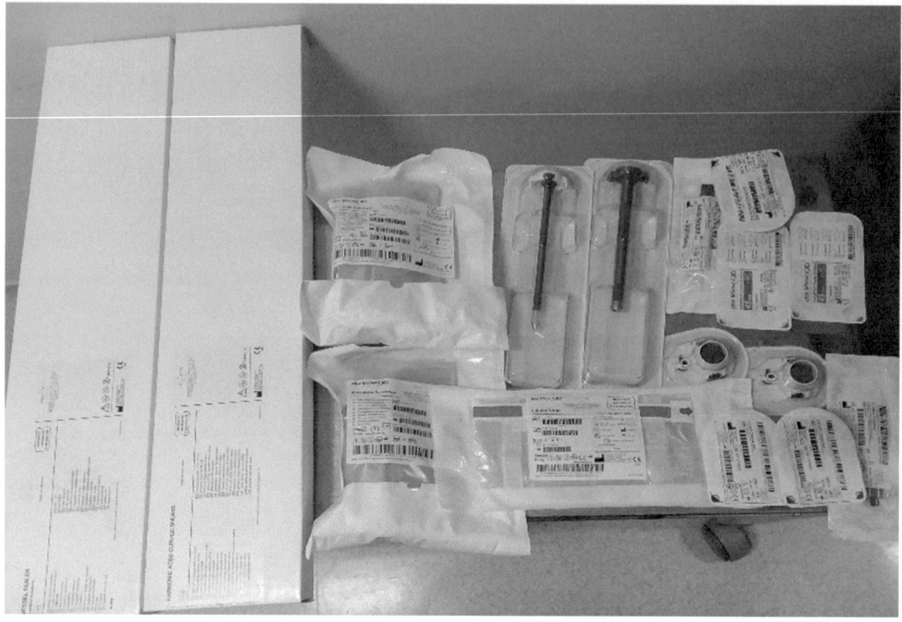

Fig. 40 Disposable robotic surgery kit. (From the author's archive [6, 7])

5 Robotic Surgery Kit

Robotic surgeries, in addition to the use of tweezers and optics, require disposable supplies:

- 4 arm drapes (robot arm cover);
- 1 column cover;
- 4 cannulas for trocars 5–8 mm;
- 1 scissor tip protector (tip cover);
- 1 shutter (bladeless).

  Single use tweezers:

- 1 harmonic ace clamp (single use);
- 1 vessel sealer clamp (single use) (Fig. 40).

6 Non-robot Instruments Needed for a Robotic Procedure

In addition to the Robot's own instruments, it is necessary to add instruments specific to video laparoscopy surgery:

- Verres needle to perform pneumoperitoneum;
- Laparoscopic forceps for use during the operative act by the assistant surgeon;
- Small surgery box to perform the punctures;
- A complete video laparoscopy box is mandatory in case of conversion.

7 Sterile Materials

For digestive tract surgeries, it is recommended:

- Normal video laparoscopy box;
- Obese video laparoscopy box;
- Small surgery box;
- Conventional digestive system surgery box;
- Single laparoscopic needle holder;
- 5 mm permanent loose trocar;
- Ultracision Cable;
- Nathanson retractor;
- Purple laparoscopic hemolock (normal and obese);
- Green laparoscopic hemolock;
- Laparoscopic Clipper 300 and 400;
- Thermos bottle + clothesline;
- Cuba kidney and cupula;
- 1 pair of long Langenbecks + 1 pair of short Langenbecks;
- Adson forceps with tooth and 1 Adson forceps without tooth;
- 1 Laparoscopic aponeurosis kit (Figs. 41, 42, 43, and 44).

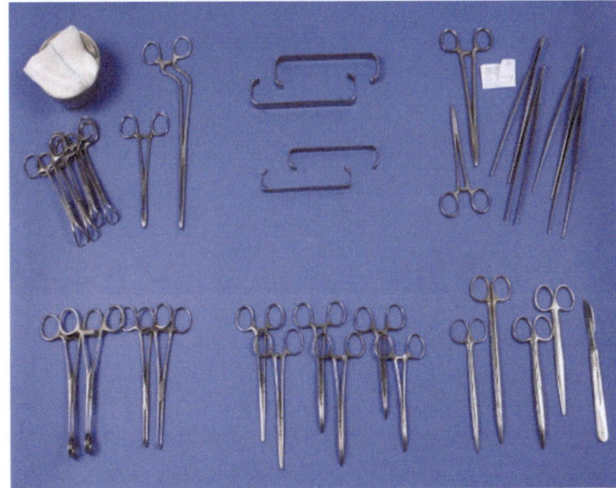

Fig. 41 Conventional tweezers. (From the author's archive [7])

Fig. 42 Laparoscopic forceps. (From the author's archive [7])

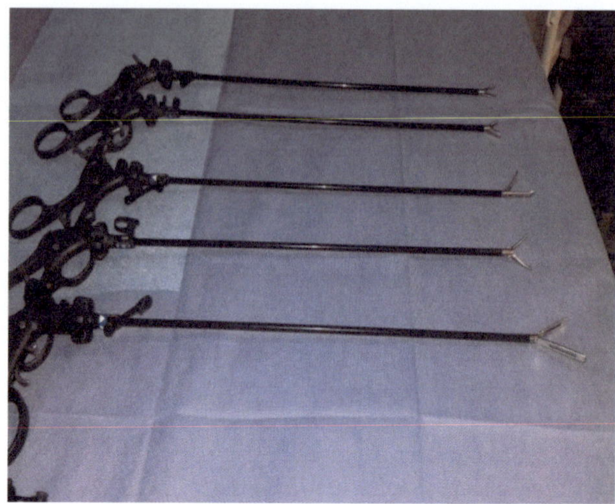

Fig. 43 Laparoscopic needle holder. (From the author's archive [7])

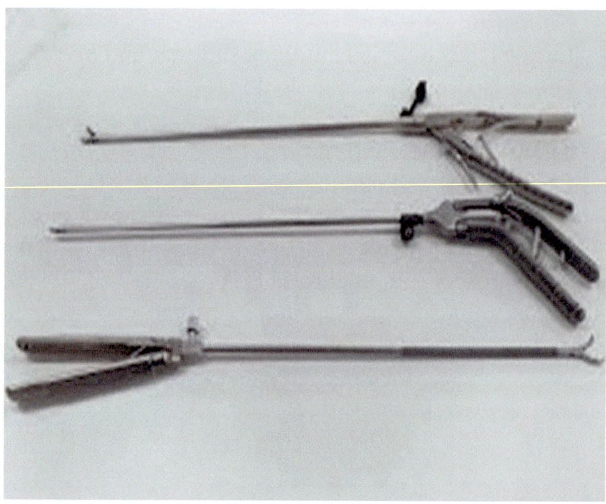

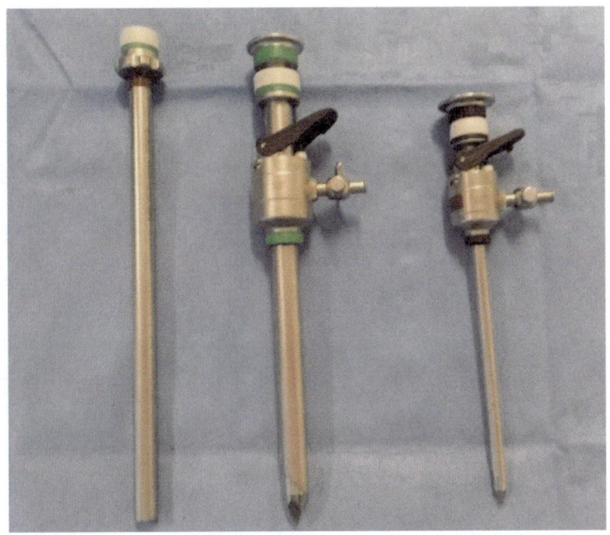

Fig. 44 Laparoscopic Trocars 10 mm and 5 mm. (From the author's archive [7])

8 Disposable Materials and Orthoses, Prostheses, and Special Materials

For digestive tract surgeries, it is recommended:
Disposable materials may vary by procedure and surgical technique.

– Wires;
– Antiallergic gloves;
– Probes;
– Drains;
– Dressings;
– 300 and 400 clipping loads;
– Disposable Trocars;
– Loads of purple and green;
– Parts collector;
– Staplers;
– Veress needle;
– Incision retractor (Figs. 45, 46, 47, 48, 49, 50, and 51).

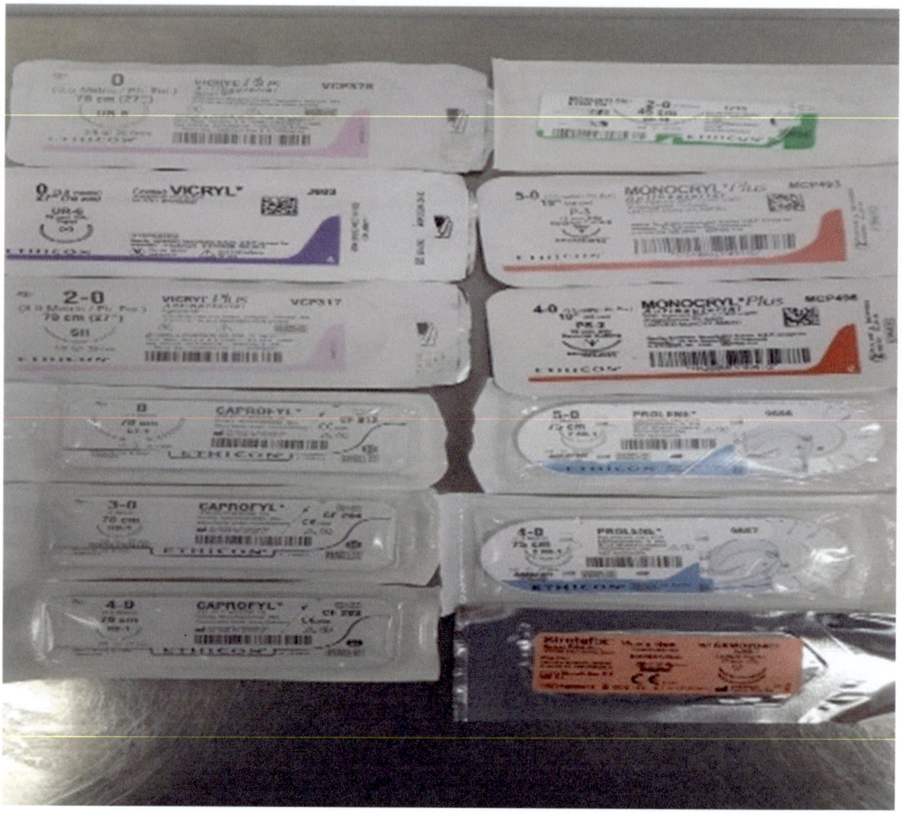

B. Zilberstein et al.

Fig. 45 Wires. (From the author's archive [7])

Fig. 46 Clipping loads.
(From the author's
archive [7])

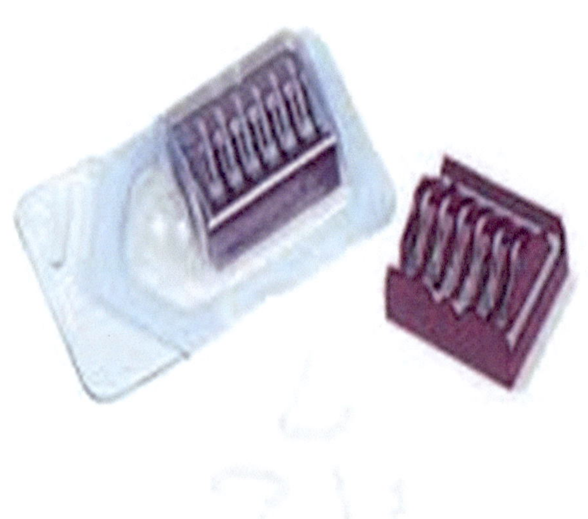

Fig. 47 Verres needle. (From the author's archive [7])

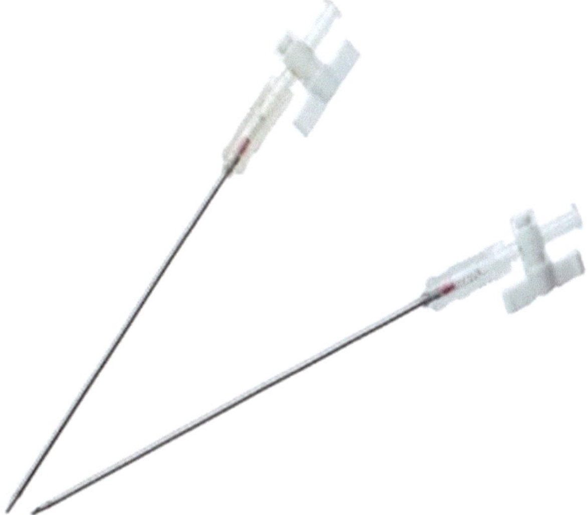

Fig. 48 Disposable trocars. (From the author's archive [7])

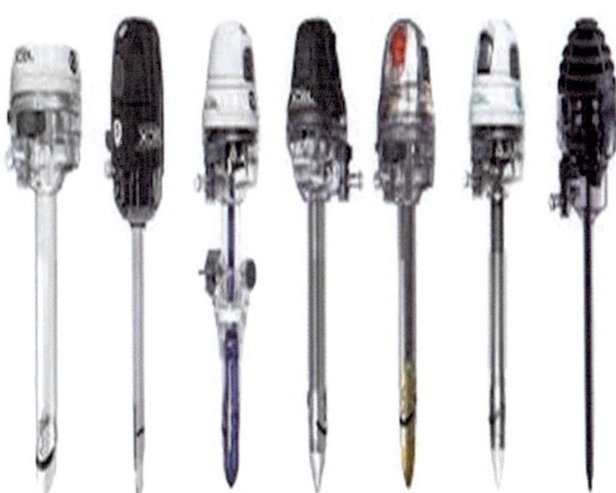

Fig. 49 Parts collector. (From the author's archive [7])

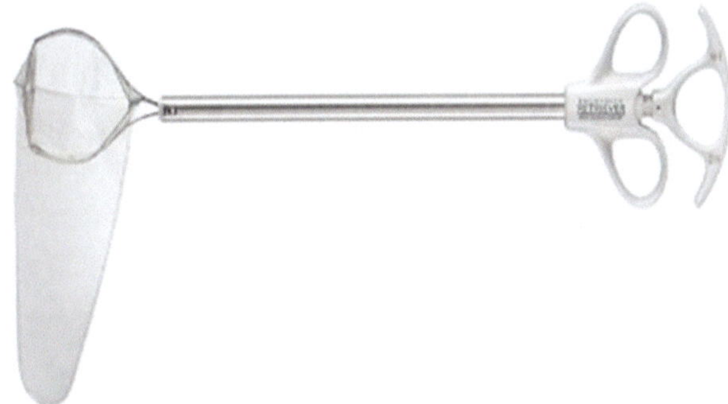

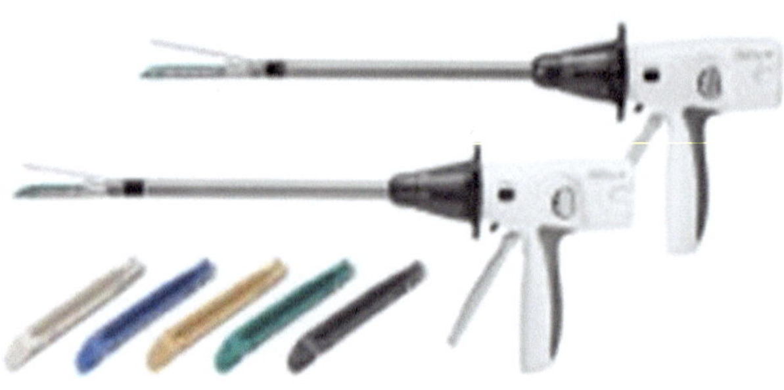

Fig. 50 Staplers. (From the author's archive [7])

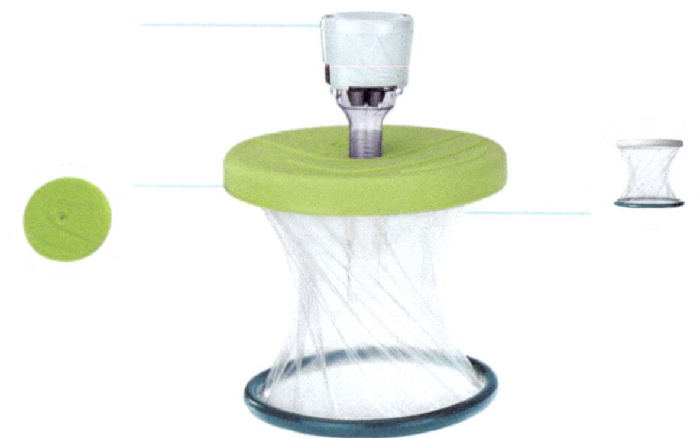

Fig. 51 Incision retractor. (From the author's archive [7])

References

1. Morrell ALG, Charles Morrell-Junior A, Morrell AG, et al. Technical essential aspects in robotic colorectal surgery: mastering the Da Vinci Si and Xi platforms. Rev Col Bras Cir. 2021;48:e20213007. https://doi.org/10.1590/0100-6991e-20213007. Published 2021 Sep 24.
2. Xi. Sistema Manual do Usuário. https://www.strattner.com.br/wp-content/uploads/2020/11/05_IU_Xi_IS4000.pdf.
3. Da Vinci X/Xi instrument & accessory catalog. 2020. https://www.intuitive.com/en-us/-/media/ISI/Intuitive/Pdf/xi-x-ina-catalog-no-pricing-us-1052082.pdf.
4. Ngu JC, Tsang CB, Koh DC. The da Vinci Xi: a review of its capabilities, versatility, and potential role in robotic colorectal surgery. Robot Surg. 2017;4:77–85. https://doi.org/10.2147/RSRR.S119317. Published 2017 Jul 28.
5. Azizian M, Liu M, Khalaji I, DiMaio S. The da Vinci surgical system. In: The encyclopedia of medical robotics; 2018. p. 3–28.
6. Lucia A, Martins AV. Guia prático de enfermagem em cirurgia robótica. 2020.
7. Guimaraes G. Cirurgia Robótica: princípios e fundamentos. Editora Universitária Ciências Médicas de Minas Gerais; 2022.

Robotic Devices in Head and Neck Surgery

Andressa Teruya Ramos and Renan Bezerra Lira Lira

1 Platforms Available

1.1 da Vinci: Intuitive (Models Si, X, Xi, and SP)

The first platform to gain space in the market and remain a successful model in the specialty was the da Vinci robot, created with the objective of presenting good reproducibility, with an accreditation and security system for the use of the tool and thus standardize the procedures performed. It is a multiportal linear system that uses four articulated robotic arms and endoscopic cameras with 3D visualization, allowing the magnification of the image and high definition of the operative field. The surgeon remains on the console and has control of optics, movement and angulation of the tweezers, precision of movements, and ergonomics [1].

The latest model produced by the company, Single Port (SP), has the main advantage of keeping all devices coming out of the same portal and improving the mobility and angle of optics [2]. The SP has already been tested for use in robotic head and neck surgeries mainly in the USA and Asian countries but is not yet available in Brazil [3, 4].

At first, every head and neck surgeon who would like to obtain their certification as robotic surgeons had to perform their training and qualification in the USA. Since 2021, Brazil has the only center outside the USA where certification is provided in the specialty, through the postgraduate degree in robotic head and neck surgery of the private hospital [5].

A. T. Ramos (✉) · R. B. L. Lira
Department of Head and Neck Surgery, Hospital Beneficiência Portuguesa de São Paulo,
São Paulo, Brazil

J. P. Manzano, L. M. Ferreira (eds.), *Robotic Surgery Devices in Surgical
Specialties*, https://doi.org/10.1007/978-3-031-35102-0_7

1.2   Versius: Cambridge Medical Robotics

The system has as advantage the modular design with independent arms, facilitating the positioning of the robot for the onset of surgery (docking). The commands are also performed by the surgeon on the console [6]. There are no published reports related in the literature about use in head and neck surgeries.

1.3   Hugo: Medtronic

As well as Versius, Hugo is mobile and modular; it has four separate arms that can be relocated in the operating room as needed [7]. It is still underexplored in head and neck surgeries.

1.4   Flex Robotic System: Medrobotics

The Flex Robotic System is the first flexible system specifically designed for use in head and neck surgery, authorized by the FDA (Food and Drug Administration) for transoral surgeries. Consisting of a single arm for control the flexible endoscopic optic. The other tweezers attach to the mouth opener and the surgeon is close to the patient, handling the tweezers. This system is a device that is intended for robot-assisted visualization and surgical site access to the oropharynx, hypopharynx, and larynx in adults ($\geq$ 22 years of age). Also provides accessory channels for compatible flexible instruments used in surgery [8].

2   Clinical Applications

2.1   Transoral Robotic Access TORS

Transoral robotic access is used for resection of lesions of the oropharynx (lingual tonsils, tonsillar tonsils, tongue base, soft palate), supraglottic larynx, hypopharynx, and parapharyngeal space [9]. The oropharynx is the main site affected with the greatest number of cases, that's why it will be highlighted in this chapter (Fig. 1).

Transoral robotic resection for early oropharynx tumors has established itself as a feasible and oncologically safe technique, being initially disseminated by Gregory Weinstein in 2010 at the University of Pennsylvania where he has also dedicated himself to certifying head and neck surgeons around the world to use the da Vinci robot [10] (Fig. 2).

The incidence of HPV-related oropharynx tumors has increased significantly in the last decade, mainly driven by white men, young adults with no history of

Fig. 1 Possible areas of transoral resection

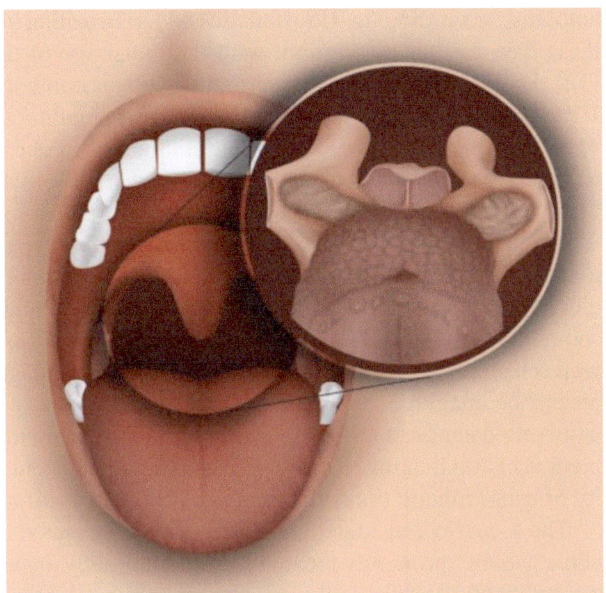

Fig. 2 Early-stage tonsil cancer tonsil tumor exposure after mouth opener placement

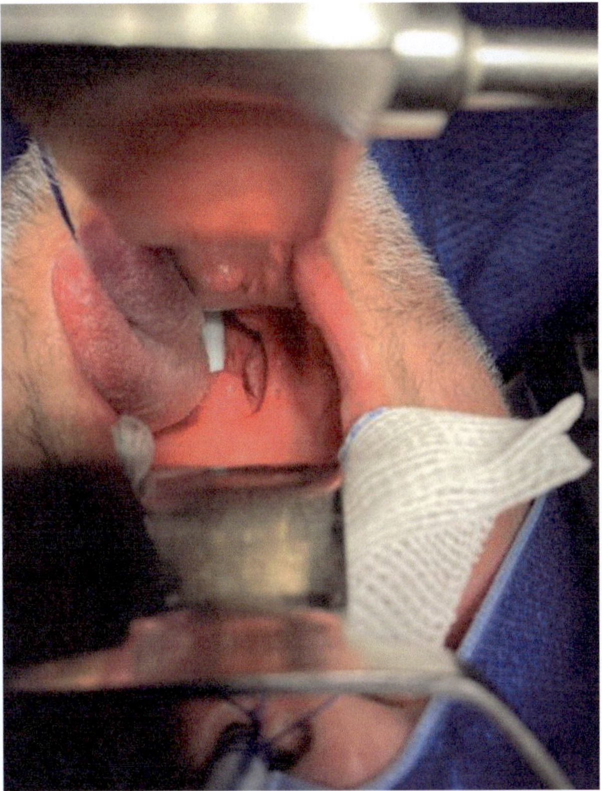

smoking, according to US statistics [11]. Brazilian data from 2021 corroborate these data for our population, with the mean age of diagnosis being 59 years old [12]. Despite having a better prognosis when compared to tumors not related to HPV [11], at this time the same pattern of treatment can be performed exclusively with radiotherapy or surgery for initial tumors and chemotherapy concomitant with radiotherapy or surgical treatment, and for selected cases of locally advanced tumors there is the possibility of the use of neoadjuvant chemotherapy [13].

Surgical therapy for early tumors is safe and comparable with IMRT (intensity-modulated radiation therapy), while advanced tumors that have involved large surgical resections and association with adjuvant chemotherapy and radiotherapy should be avoided due to higher morbidity [13]. In this context, patients should be well selected for surgical treatment with adequate imaging and if possible magnetic resonance imaging to estimate the actual dimensions of the tumor, signs of vascular and bone damage, and lymph node extracapsular extravasation, and thus for treatment decision making. Recent studies question current treatments and the possibility of using robotic transoral surgery (TORS) also for advanced cases [14] (Fig. 3).

The scenario considered pandemic for HPV-related oropharynx tumors in young adult patients promotes the search for minimally invasive techniques, with lower morbidity and consequently less impact on the quality of life of patients who should remain with the sequelae resulting from treatment for a long period [14]. Patients with HPV-negative tumors, in the early stages, were also shown to be good

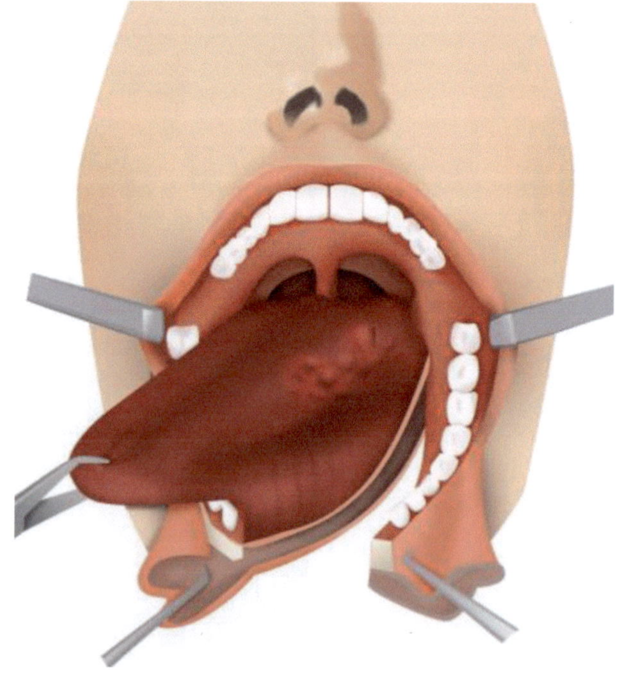

Fig. 3 Mandibulotomy for oropharyngeal tumor resection when there is no access to the robot

candidates for surgical treatment with adjuvant radiotherapy when compared to the treatment with upfront chemotherapy and radiotherapy [15].

Patients with cervical lymph node metastasis without primary site identified on physical examination or complementary tests such as PET-CT (occult primary) may be submitted to physical examination under narcosis with the use of a robot, having multiple biopsies performed. It is possible to proceed with resection with tonsillar tonsillectomy and ipsilateral lingual if necessary [16]. When locating the primary tumor, the therapy of choice is directed, which decreases the irradiated field and consequently the sequelae resulting from the treatment that, in this region, has implications in the rehabilitation of breathing, speech, and swallowing [17].

Hypopharynx and supraglottic larynx lesions are less frequent but also considered challenging because their structures are closely related to speech and swallowing. The consequences of the treatment, surgical or with radiotherapy/chemotherapy, can lead to severe dysfunctions requiring an alternative food route and tracheostomy [17]. Robotic transoral resection aims to provide a good oncological treatment with adequate margins with a better functional result, consequently improving the quality of life [17].

Using this same approach, it is also possible to treat benign pathologies such as resection of lingual tonsils for the treatment of sleep apnea and treatment of Eagle syndrome with removal of the styloid process [18]. Patients with tumors in the parapharyngeal space also benefit from transoral access [19]. Compared to conventional surgery that includes parotidectomy combined or not with access mandibulotomy, the use of TORS decreases the manipulation of complex regional neurovascular structures with potential for high complications such as facial paralysis and trismus [20]. It is noteworthy that the resection of parapharyngeal tumors requires high knowledge of local anatomy and familiarity with the use of the robotic platform, with its realization at the beginning of the learning curve not being indicated.

2.2   *Vestibular Approach*

Access to the anterior cervical region was standardized by Kocher, keeping in his honor the name of the cross-sectional incision, first described in 1912, being indicated for the surgical treatment of thyroid pathologies, parathyroid scans, and congenital malformations such as resection of thyroglossal cyst (Sistrunk surgery) [21]. This approach almost hasn't changed over the decades, but driven by the aesthetic and social appeal due the scar [21], remote access began to be studied.

The vestibular access, the space between the mucous part of the lower lip and the mandible, proved to be an alternative, being a discrete incision in the mucosa, not apparent in the anterior cervical region (Figs. 4, 5, and 6).

With this method, the surgeon makes a workspace (pocket) from the chin to the thyroid store with the use of laparoscopic material, insufflating carbon dioxide to form the workspace, and it can be performed with or without the robot's assistance.

Fig. 4 View of the vestibular access with the trocars

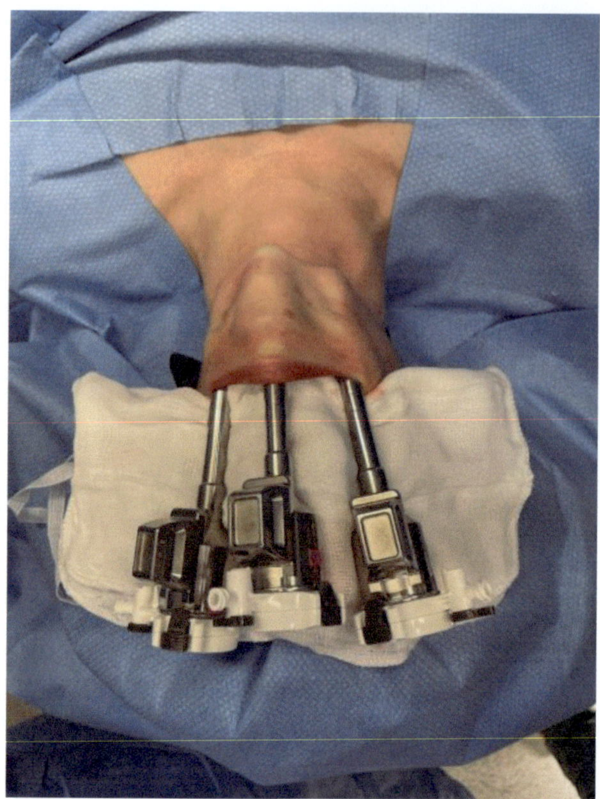

Fig. 5 Vestibular incision after 30 days of surgery

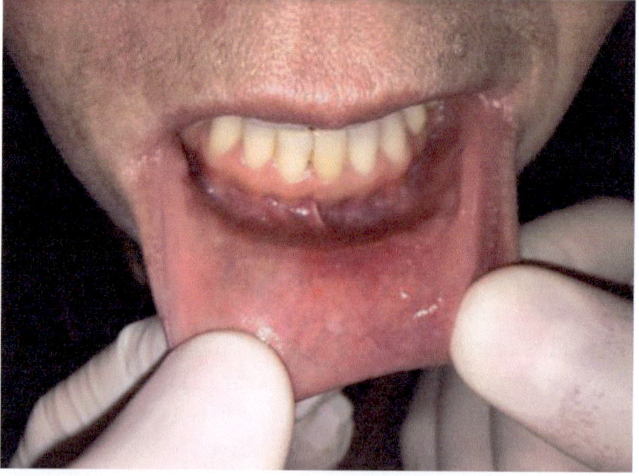

The use of this approach makes it possible to perform partial or total thyroidectomies, parathyroidectomies, and neck dissection of level VI lymph nodes [22]. The main contraindications are related to the restricted space and operative field,

Fig. 6 Cervical aspect after 30 days of surgery

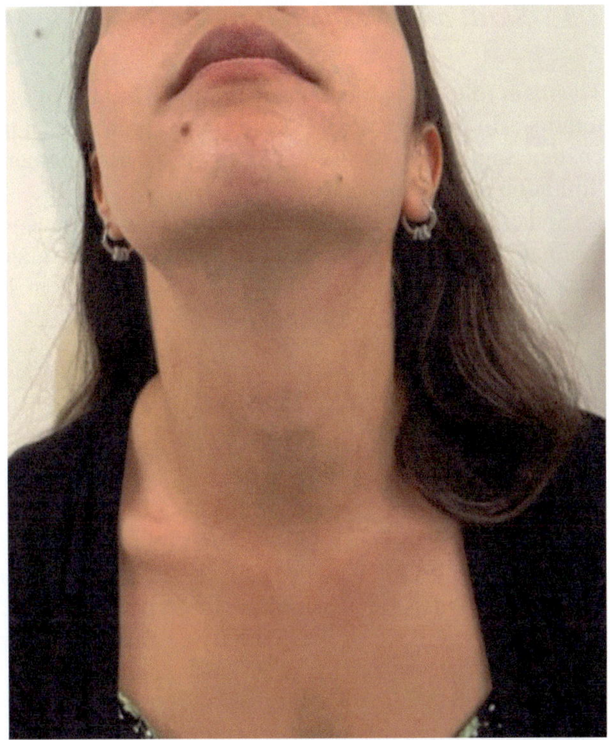

Fig. 7 Cavity after pocket done with thyroid isthmus visualization. *I* Isthmus

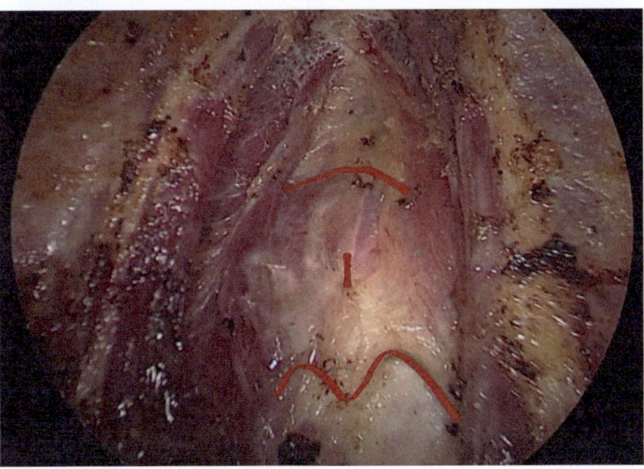

voluminous nodules, extensive tumors, and the presence of metastases to the lateral cervical lymph nodes, which limits the benefits of the technique and should be avoided [23].

Through the same access it is possible to perform thyroplasty to reduce thyroid cartilage for aesthetic purposes, in order to feminize the neck [24] (Fig. 7).

2.3 Skull and Nasopharynx Base

The main role of the robotic surgery in the treatment of skull base and nasopharynx tumors is in the resection of recurrent nasopharyngeal tumors, a surgery considered challenging due to the sequelae of previous treatment, difficulty in access, and limitation of the workspace [25].

Some combined endoscopic transnasal and transoral robotic approaches may facilitate tumor exposure and resection with adequate margins, as evidenced in various cases with good local disease control, 86% in 2 years [19].

2.4 Lateral Cervical Tumors

The most used remote access for cervical surgeries is the retroauricular access (Fig. 8), in which the jugulo-carotid space is accessed through the subplatysmal flap (Fig. 9). This approach allows the performance of thyroidectomies, mainly voluminous goiters that could not be resected by the transoral technique, as well as cervical emptying and resection of the salivary glands [26, 27] (Figs. 8 and 9).

Retroauricular access was initially used in video-assisted surgeries and later in robotic surgery, especially in Asian countries for patients with a propensity to develop hypertrophic or keloid scars [27]. Korean initial studies have observed good flap control for the treatment of benign or malignant pathologies of submandibular glands [28], which is a procedure considered rapid and important for the mastery of the technique and reduction of surgical time. Then, it was compared with the conventional technique with robotics, and no significant differences were found between the amount of resected lymph nodes and postoperative complications [29, 30], which at first would be the most feared divergences by the surgeons of the specialty. It was also carried out in Brazil almost a decade ago, demonstrating safety and reproducibility in Western countries and in our population (Fig. 10) [31, 32].

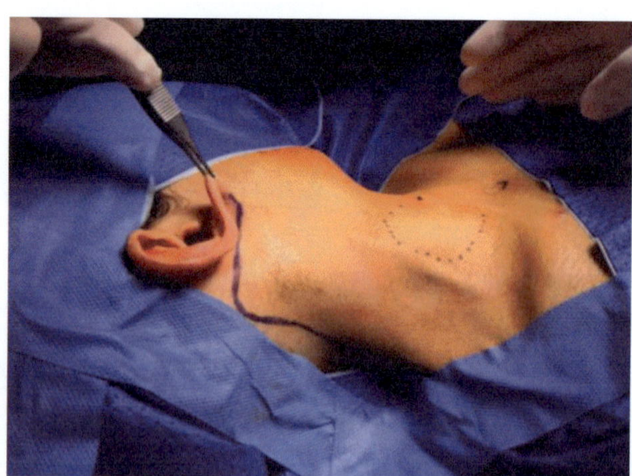

Fig. 8 Retroauricular incision

Fig. 9 Subplatysmal flap

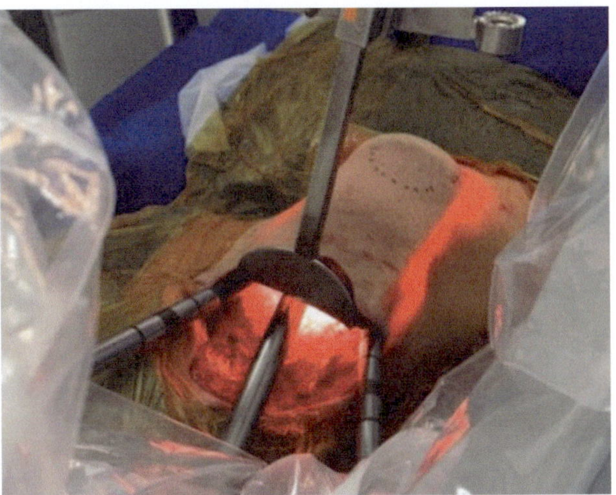

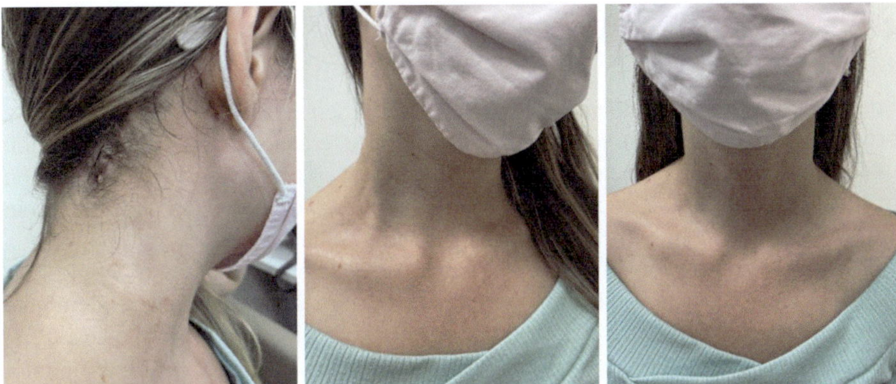

Fig. 10 Cervical aspect after 30 days of right neck dissection surgery

Based on the experience of the robot use, it was possible to also apply it in the surgical treatment of pathologies of the parotid gland and delicate surgery due to manipulation of the facial nerve and its branches that permeate the gland.

The first robotic parotidectomies were performed in Asia in 2013 and 2014, and the experience was reported as successful [33, 34]. Using the retroauricular facelifting incision, it is possible to easily access the parotid store, associated with magnified three-dimensional visualization, dexterity gain, and surgical precision help in the identification and preservation of the facial nerve, the use of intraoperative nerve monitoring being maintained as in the conventional approach [35].

Since facial nerve paralysis was the most feared complication of parotidectomy, even when compared with groups of conventional surgery with video-assisted and robotic surgery, there was no difference in the incidence of permanent nerve injury and other complications, but it presented longer operative and hospital stay [36].

3   Limitations of Use

Among the limitations of the use of the robot are as follows: it can be punctuated by the need for specific training of techniques, mastery of oncological pathologies for precision in surgical indication, and certification with Intuitive, nowadays the holder of the right to use the da Vinci platform, the most used in the world. Not only should the medical team be prepared, but also the entire team in the operating room, before and after surgery, and they should conduct specialization and updating courses in the area.

Currently, Brazilian health insurances still do not cover their use due to the non-inclusion in the ANS List and should be funded exclusively by the patient. The cost of new technologies limits the spread of robot use, but this reality has been proven accessible as large hospitals have competitive values among themselves. The average cost for using the da Vinci Xi robot using two tweezers is 5000 reais.

4   Prospects for the Future

Several technology companies have launched their own robotic platforms, a promising and competitive scenario that favors price reduction and the dissemination of the tool among the specialty. There is a prospect of expansion in the proportion of surgeries with remote access to conventional ones and improvement of the use in parotidectomy and surgical treatment of paragangliomas [37].

The great innovation of Intuitive that favors our specialty is the Single-Port model, which provides in the same portal the tweezers and the camera, reducing the area necessary for dissection, but losing part of the grip strength in the tweezers. This model is still tied to high costs, being used in some reference hospitals and not yet available in Brazil. Some experiences show the use and possible benefits in lateral transoral and cervical surgeries [2, 3].

References

1. Intuitive. n.d.. https://www.intuitive.com/en-us/products-and-services/da-vinci/systems.
2. Yang TL, Li H, Holsinger FC, Koh YW. Submandibular gland resection via the trans-hairline approach: a preclinical study of a novel flexible single-port surgical system and the surgical experiences of standard multiarm robotic surgical systems. Head Neck. 2019;41(7):2231–8. https://doi.org/10.1002/hed.25692. Epub 2019 Mar 21. PMID: 30896063.
3. Tae K. Transoral robotic thyroidectomy using the da Vinci single-port surgical system. Gland Surg. 2020;9(3):614–6. https://doi.org/10.21037/gs.2020.03.37. PMID: 32775248; PMCID: PMC7347821.
4. Park YM, Kim DH, Kang MS, Lim JY, Choi EC, Koh YW, Kim SH. The first human trial of transoral robotic surgery using a single-port robotic system in the treatment of laryngo-pharyngeal

cancer. Ann Surg Oncol. 2019;26(13):4472–80. https://doi.org/10.1245/s10434-019-07802-0. Epub 2019 Sep 9. PMID: 31502020.

5. Cirurgia Robótica. n.d.. https://cirurgiarobotica.ensinoeinstein.com/cirurgia-robotica/cirurgia_robotica_em_cabeca_e_pescoco/.

6. Orosco RK, Arora A, Jeannon JP, Holsinger FC. Next-generation robotic head and neck surgery. ORL J Otorhinolaryngol Relat Spec. 2018;80(3–4):213–9. https://doi.org/10.1159/000490599. Epub 2018 Nov 7. PMID: 30404095.

7. Medtronic. n.d.. https://www.medtronic.com/covidien/en-gb/robotic-assisted-surgery/hugo-ras-system/products-and-system.html.

8. Olaleye O, Jeong B, Switajewski M, Ooi EH, Krishnan S, Foreman A, Hodge JC. Trans-oral robotic surgery for head and neck cancers using the Medrobotics Flex® system: the Adelaide cohort. J Robot Surg. 2022;16(3):527–36. https://doi.org/10.1007/s11701-021-01270-z. Epub 2021 Jul 7. PMID: 34232448.

9. Tamaki A, Rocco JW, Ozer E. The future of robotic surgery in otolaryngology - head and neck surgery. Oral Oncol. 2020;101:104510. https://doi.org/10.1016/j.oraloncology.2019.104510. Epub 2019 Dec 13. PMID: 31841882.

10. Quon H, O'Malley BW Jr, Weinstein GS. Transoral robotic surgery and a paradigm shift in the management of oropharyngeal squamous cell carcinoma. J Robot Surg. 2010;4(2):79–86. https://doi.org/10.1007/s11701-010-0194-y. Epub 2010 Jun 29. PMID: 27628771.

11. Santos Carvalho R, Scapulatempo-Neto C, Curado MP, de Castro Capuzzo R, Marsico Teixeira F, Cardoso Pires R, Cirino MT, Cambrea Joaquim Martins J, Almeida Oliveira da Silva I, Oliveira MA, Watanabe M, Guimarães Ribeiro A, Caravina de Almeida G, Reis RM, Ribeiro Gama R, Lopes Carvalho A, de Carvalho AC. HPV-induced oropharyngeal squamous cell carcinomas in Brazil: prevalence, trend, clinical, and epidemiologic characterization. Cancer Epidemiol Biomark Prev. 2021;30(9):1697–707. https://doi.org/10.1158/1055-9965. EPI-21-0016. Epub 2021 Jun 21. PMID: 34155066.

12. National Comprehensive Cancer Network (NCCN). NCCN Clinical practice guidelines in oncology. Head and neck cancers version 2. Plymouth Meeting, PA: NCCN; 2022.

13. Nichols AC, Theurer J, Prisman E, Read N, Berthelet E, Tran E, Fung K, de Almeida JR, Bayley A, Goldstein DP, Hier M, Sultanem K, Richardson K, Mlynarek A, Krishnan S, Le H, Yoo J, MacNeil SD, Winquist E, Hammond JA, Venkatesan V, Kuruvilla S, Warner A, Mitchell S, Chen J, Corsten M, Johnson-Obaseki S, Eapen L, Odell M, Parker C, Wehrli B, Kwan K, Palma DA. Radiotherapy versus transoral robotic surgery and neck dissection for oropharyngeal squamous cell carcinoma (ORATOR): an open-label, phase 2, randomised trial. Lancet Oncol. 2019;20(10):1349–59. https://doi.org/10.1016/S1470-2045(19)30410-3. Epub 2019. Erratum in: Lancet Oncol. 2019;20(12): e663. PMID: 31416685.

14. Ferris RL, Flamand Y, Weinstein GS, Li S, Quon H, Mehra R, Garcia JJ, Chung CH, Gillison ML, Duvvuri U, O'Malley BW Jr, Ozer E, Thomas GR, Koch WM, Gross ND, Bell RB, Saba NF, Lango M, Méndez E, Burtness B. Phase II randomized trial of transoral surgery and low-dose intensity modulated radiation therapy in resectable p16+ locally advanced oropharynx cancer: an ECOG-ACRIN Cancer Research Group Trial (E3311). J Clin Oncol. 2022;40(2):138–49. https://doi.org/10.1200/JCO.21.01752. Epub 2021 Oct 26. PMID: 34699271; PMCID: PMC8718241.

15. Bollig CA, Morris B, Stubbs VC. Transoral robotic surgery with neck dissection versus nonsurgical treatment in stage I and II human papillomavirus-negative oropharyngeal cancer. Head Neck. 2022;44(7):1545–53. https://doi.org/10.1002/hed.27045. Epub 2022 Apr 1. PMID: 35365915; PMCID: PMC9324989.

16. Civantos FJ, Vermorken JB, Shah JP, Rinaldo A, Suárez C, Kowalski LP, Rodrigo JP, Olsen K, Strojan P, Mäkitie AA, Takes RP, de Bree R, Corry J, Paleri V, Shaha AR, Hartl DM, Mendenhall W, Piazza C, Hinni M, Robbins KT, Tong NW, Sanabria A, Coca-Pelaz A, Langendijk JA, Hernandez-Prera J, Ferlito A. Metastatic squamous cell carcinoma to the cervical lymph nodes from an unknown primary cancer: management in the HPV era. Front Oncol. 2020;10:593164. https://doi.org/10.3389/fonc.2020.593164. PMID: 33244460; PMCID: PMC7685177.

17. Sokoya M, Chowdhury F, Kadakia S, Ducic Y. Combination of panendoscopy and positron emission tomography/computed tomography increases detection of unknown primary head and neck carcinoma. Laryngoscope. 2018;128(11):2573–5. https://doi.org/10.1002/lary.27268.

18. Gordis TM, Cagle JL, Nguyen SA, Newman JG. Human papillomavirus-associated oropharyngeal squamous cell carcinoma: a systematic review and meta-analysis of clinical trial demographics. Cancers. 2022;14(16):4061. https://doi.org/10.3390/cancers14164061. PMID: 36011055; PMCID: PMC9406828.

19. Karatzanis AD, Psychogios G, Zenk J, et al. Comparison among different available surgical approaches in T1 glottic cancer. Laryngoscope. 2009;119:1704–8.

20. Dziegielewski PT, Kang SY, Ozer E. Transoral robotic surgery (TORS) for laryngeal and hypopharyngeal cancers. J Surg Oncol. 2015;112(7):702–6.

21. Cammaroto G, Stringa LM, Zhang H, Capaccio P, Galletti F, Galletti B, Meccariello G, Iannella G, Pelucchi S, Baghat A, Vicini C. Alternative applications of trans-oral robotic surgery (TORS): a systematic review. J Clin Med. 2020;9(1):201. https://doi.org/10.3390/jcm9010201. PMID: 31940794; PMCID: PMC7019293.

22. Mendelsohn AH. Transoral robotic assisted resection of the parapharyngeal space. Head Neck. 2015;37(2):273–80. https://doi.org/10.1002/hed.23724.

23. Vural A, Negm H, Vicini C. Robotic surgery of skull base. In: Cingi C, Bayar Muluk N, editors. All around the nose. Cham: Springer; 2020. https://doi.org/10.1007/978-3-030-21217-9_80.

24. Dubhashi SP, Subnis BM, Sindwani RD. Theodor E. Kocher. Indian J Surg. 2013;75:383–4. https://doi.org/10.1007/s12262-012-0469-9.

25. Juarez MC, Ishii L, Nellis JC, Bater K, Huynh PP, Fung N, Darrach H, Russell JO, Ishii M. Objectively measuring social attention of thyroid neck scars and transoral surgery using eye tracking. Laryngoscope. 2019;129(12):2789–94. https://doi.org/10.1002/lary.27933. Epub 2019 Mar 22. PMID: 30900247.

26. Lira RB, Ramos AT, Nogueira RMR, de Carvalho GB, Russell JO, Tufano RP, Kowalski LP. Transoral thyroidectomy (TOETVA): complications, surgical time and learning curve. Oral Oncol. 2020;110:104871. https://doi.org/10.1016/j.oraloncology.2020.104871. Epub 2020 Jun 30. PMID: 32619928.

27. Lira RB, De Cicco R, Rangel LG, Bertelli AA, Duque Silva G, de Medeiros Vanderlei JP, Kowalski LP. Transoral endoscopic thyroidectomy vestibular approach: experience from a multicenter national group with 412 patients. Head Neck. 2021;43(11):3468–75. https://doi.org/10.1002/hed.26846. Epub 2021 Aug 12. PMID: 34382715.

28. Vilaseca I, Blanch JL, Bernal-Sprekelsen M. Transoral laser surgery for hypopharyngeal carcinomas. Curr Opin Otolaryngol Head Neck Surg. 2012;20(2):97–102. https://doi.org/10.1097/MOO.0b013e32834fa8fe.

29. Lira RB, Kowalski LP. Robotic head and neck surgery: beyond TORS. Curr Oncol Rep. 2020;22(9):88. https://doi.org/10.1007/s11912-020-00950-7. PMID: 32643128.

30. Tsang RK, To VS, Ho AC, Ho WK, Chan JY, Wei WI. Early results of robotic assisted nasopharyngectomy for recurrent nasopharyngeal carcinoma. Head Neck. 2015;37(6):788–93. https://doi.org/10.1002/hed.23672.

31. Koh YW, Chung WY, Hong HJ, Lee SY, Kim WS, Lee HS, Choi EC. Robot-assisted selective neck dissection via modified face-lift approach for early oral tongue cancer: a video demonstration. Ann Surg Oncol. 2012;19(4):1334–5. https://doi.org/10.1245/s10434-011-2155-8. Epub 2011. PMID: 22187119.

32. Lee HS, Park DY, Hwang CS, Bae SH, Suh MJ, Koh YW, Choi EC. Feasibility of robot-assisted submandibular gland resection via retroauricular approach: preliminary results. Laryngoscope. 2013;123(2):369–73. https://doi.org/10.1002/lary.23321. Epub 2012 May 1. PMID: 22549880.

33. Tae K, Ji YB, Song CM, Jeong JH, Cho SH, Lee SH. Robotic selective neck dissection by a postauricular facelift approach: comparison with conventional neck dissection. Otolaryngol Head Neck Surg. 2014;150:394–400.

34. Sukato DC, Ballard DP, Abramowitz JM, Rosenfeld RM, Mlot S. Robotic versus conventional neck dissection: a systematic review and metaanalysis. Laryngoscope. 2019;129(7):1587–96.
35. Lira RB, Chulam TC, Kowalski LP. Safe implementation of retroauricular robotic and endoscopic neck surgery in South America. Gland Surg. 2017;6(3):258–66. https://doi.org/10.21037/gs.2017.03.17. PMID: 28713697; PMCID: PMC5503934.
36. Kowalski LP, Lira RB. Anatomy, technique, and results of robotic retroauricular approach to neck dissection. Anat Rec. 2021;304(6):1235–41. https://doi.org/10.1002/ar.24621. Epub 2021 Mar 26. PMID: 33773074.
37. Shin YS, Choi EC, Kim CH, Koh YW. Robot-assisted selective neck dissection combined with facelift parotidectomy in parotid cancer. Head Neck. 2014;36(4):592–5. https://doi.org/10.1002/hed.23441. Epub 2014 Jan 30. PMID: 23929700.

Robotic Devices in Pediatric Surgery

Adriano Almeida Calado and Daniel G. DaJusta

1 Introduction

In many pediatric surgical subspecialties, the field of laparoscopic continues to advance. The benefits of laparoscopic surgery, such as the decrease in postoperative pain, decrease in narcotic use, improved recovery, and decreased blood loss, have helped propel the popularity over open surgery. Thus, laparoscopic procedures for excision of organs or cancer, such as cholecystectomy, nephrectomy, splenectomy, or adrenalectomy, have become the standard of care. The two main limiting factors associated with the continued expansion of the field remain the learning curve and, of course, availability of the appropriate instruments. Becoming proficient at laparoscopic surgery is much more difficult than open surgery. The skills required to perform a surgery with a limited two-dimensional view of a camera and long instruments with limited articulation and inverted motion require a long learning curve when compared to open surgery. This has limited the application of laparoscopic to complex reconstructive surgery with only a handful of skilled experience surgeons being able to achieve success in such cases but no widespread use. Complex laparoscopic cases such as prostatectomies, pyeloplasty, or Nissen fundoplication did not seem bound to overtake their open counterpart. That has changed with the introduction of the robot in the field of laparoscopy.

While robotic surgery is still a form of laparoscopic surgery, it does offer many advantages over standard laparoscopy which mainly help decrease the learning curve associated with laparoscopic procedures. It also facilitates the application of laparoscopy to the complex reconstructive procedure that involves difficult tasks such as a significant amount of suturing for anastomosis and working on tight spaces. These advantages include the 3D vision with 10 times magnification of the

A. A. Calado (✉) · D. G. DaJusta
Department of Urology, Pernambuco University, Recife, Pernambuco, Brazil
e-mail: adriano.calado@upe.br; Daniel.DaJusta@NationwideChildrens.org

© The Author(s), under exclusive license to Springer Nature
Switzerland AG 2023
J. P. Manzano, L. M. Ferreira (eds.), *Robotic Surgery Devices in Surgical Specialties*, https://doi.org/10.1007/978-3-031-35102-0_8

robotic EndoWrist instruments that allow for seven degrees of movement freedom and tremor reduction, and finally, in stark contrast to standard laparoscopy, the movements of the arms under the view of the camera are not inverted. Among the many benefits that these advantages create is the decrease in the learning curve for both novice and experienced laparoscopic surgeons. It has also made it easy for experienced open surgeons to transition to laparoscopic procedures. Nevertheless, the robot does come with the drawback of cost as well as surgeons sometimes also complain of the lack of tactile feedback.

In the field of pediatric surgery, robotic pyeloplasty is a good example of how robotics can help popularize the laparoscopic approach (Figs. 1 and 2). In 1993 laparoscopic pyeloplasty was initially described and over time showed similar success rates as well as the common benefits associated with laparoscopic surgery when compared to open surgery. Yet 10 years after its introduction in 2004, it only represented less than 20% of the case in patients between 13 and 18 years of age. Robotic pyeloplasty was initially described in 2004, yet 10 years later in 2015 robotic pyeloplasty accounted for over 80% of the case done in this age group across the USA [1]. The use of the robotic platform has also grown in younger patients. This ultimately serves as an example of how this technology, despite its cost, can make laparoscopic surgery more widespread among pediatric surgical specialties. This has become especially true for the more complex reconstructive surgeries. Yet another important limiting factor that cannot be understated is the limited number of cases when compared to the adult world, which makes demonstrating a real benefit over open surgery or standard laparoscopic surgery much more difficult. This limitation has led to a decreased focus on creating pediatric-specific machines and instruments, leaving pediatric surgeons no choice but to adapt to using technology made for adults.

Anesthesia considerations for robotic surgery are very similar compared with other minimal invasive approaches that involve pneumoperitoneum. Efforts to minimize insufflation pressure (<10 mmHg) and reduce flow rate are necessary in children as the ratio to peritoneal surface is larger relative to body weight and the systemic absorption of carbon dioxide may be higher. In addition, increased intraperitoneal pressure can lead to increased peak inspiratory pressure and

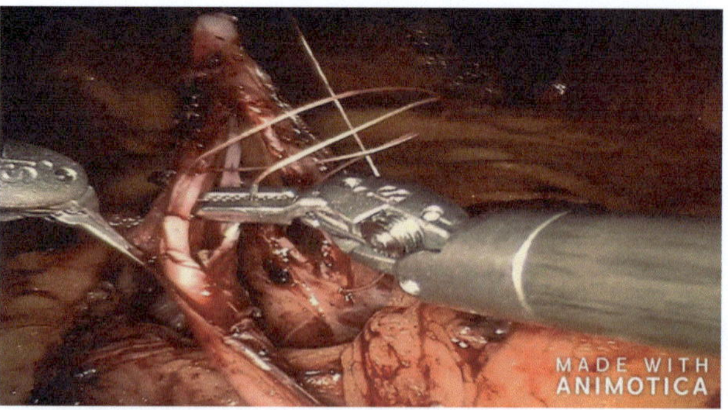

Fig. 1 Surgical field during pyeloplasty in a child with a horseshoe kidney

Fig. 2 Stent placement during pyeloplasty in a child with a horseshoe kidney

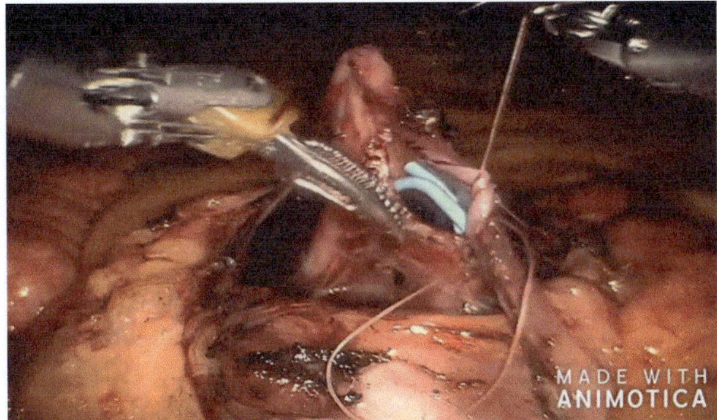

decreased pulmonary compliance as well as decreased cardiac output and renal perfusion and increased renal vascular resistance.

Between the available technology for robotic laparoscopic surgery, the da Vinci robot continues to be the leading machine in the market. Most surgical procedures performed in the current published pediatric surgery subspecialty literature have been done with this platform. Over the past few years, new devices have become available and even newer devices are currently being developed. These new devices offer the possibility for single-site surgery, flexible scopes, tactile feedback, increased maneuverability, machine learning concepts, and even the ability for machine-independent suturing. The goal of this chapter is to discuss a few of these platforms and their applications in the field of pediatric surgery subspecialties.

2 da Vinci Robotic Platform

2.1 How It Works

The da Vinci robot has now gone through four generations with the introduction of the latest version, the Xi. The machine is comprised of three parts: The first part is the surgeon console where the surgeon sits and controls the arms in the patient cart. The patient cart is the second part, which houses the four robotic arms and is placed near the patient where each arm can be connected to the robotic trocars. Finally, the vision cart serves to connect the console to the patient cart and provide the necessary support for the 3D high-definition vision system. Currently, this version only offers 8 mm trocars for both camera and instruments. The camera does provide the usual three-dimensional view with ten times magnification, while most instruments provide a wristed motion with seven degrees of freedom. Trocar position has also evolved from the previous version that relies upon triangulation like standard laparoscopic surgery to an inline configuration. More recently, the single-port version of the Xi has been introduced although not specifically approved for pediatric use. Whether a single 25 mm incision is beneficial in children is unclear.

2.2   Indications

Currently, the da Vinci platform has been used in a variety of pediatric surgical subspecialties with urology leading the way. Nevertheless, it has been used by many other pediatric subspecialties including general surgery, cardiothoracic surgery, otorhinolaryngology, as well as pediatric gynecology in a variety of minimally invasive procedures.

In urology, the most commonly performed procedure continues to be pyeloplasty. As mentioned before, the advent of robotics has helped popularize this approach in the USA. Other complex procedures have followed, such as extravesical (Lich-Gregoir) ureteral reimplantation, and more recently complex bladder procedures, such as bladder neck reconstruction (Fig. 3), Mitrofanoff (Figs. 4, 5, and 6), and enterocystoplasty (Figs. 7 and 8).

2.3   Contraindication

The main relative contraindication of using this platform relates to the workspace. Again, the da Vinci system has been designed with the adult patient in mind. As pediatric surgeons have tried to adapt this technology to use in children, they continue to push the boundaries of what can be done. But trying to safely perform robotic surgery on the smallest of patients has been one of the biggest challenges. Meehan found that in patients weighing less than 5 kg, there was an increase in arm collision and an increase in the need to convert to open surgery [2]. Nevertheless, surgery has been performed safely and with excellent results in patients weighing less than 10 kg [3]. Most of the above literature was based on the previous version of the da Vinci, and while the trocar size remains the same at 8 mm, the current

Fig. 3 Bladder neck dissection during reconstruction

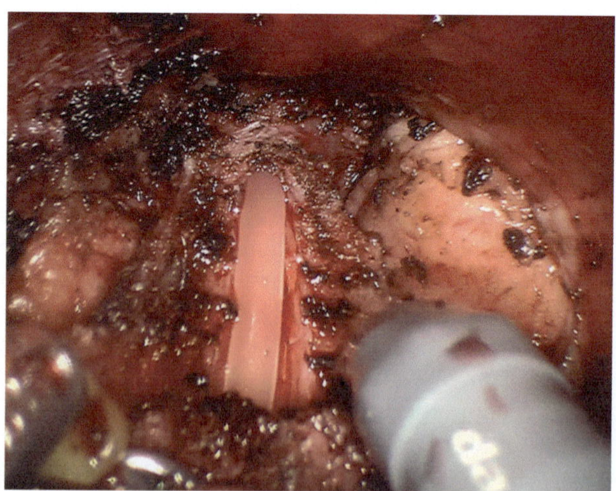

Fig. 4 Detrusor tunnel for Mitrofanoff channel

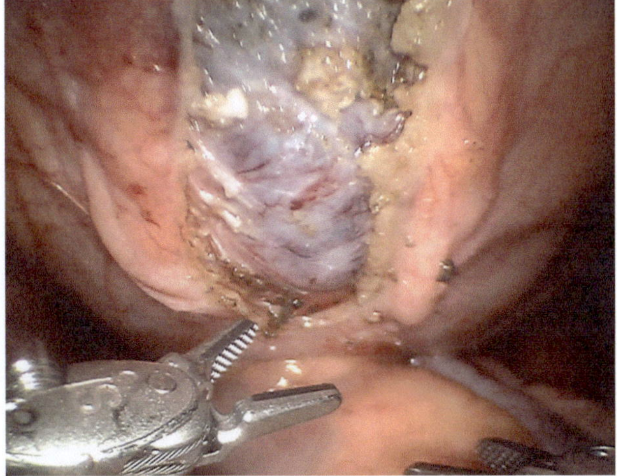

Fig. 5 Mitrofanoff mucosal anastomosis

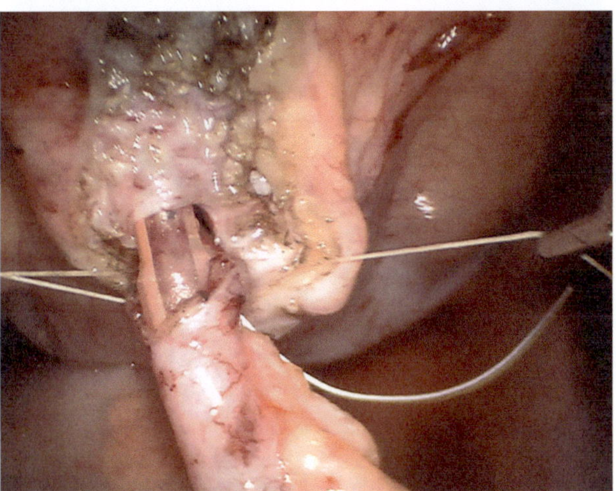

version does allow for a much closer port position with a decrease in arm collision; thus, it is likely feasible to perform surgery in patients less than 5 kg. The authors have performed surgery in infants less than 6 months with an average weight of 7 kg [4]. Additionally, a recent study did show feasibility for robotic pyeloplasty in infants with an average age of 1.6 months, but it did not provide information on patient weight [5].

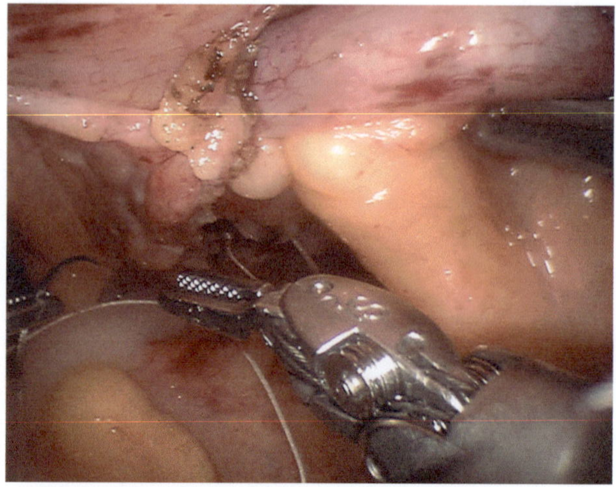

Fig. 6 Mitrofanoff implanted after detrusor closed

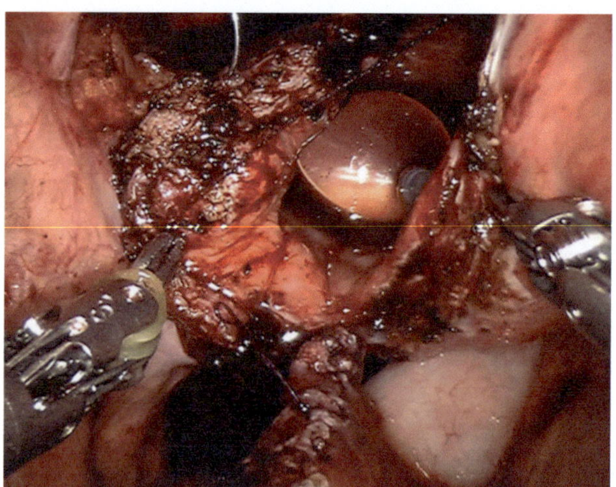

Fig. 7 Cystostomy during augmentation cystoplasty

2.4   Perspectives

As discussed previously and likely in many of the articles reported herein, in an era of rising health-care expenditures, aside from outcomes, procedural costs will continue to play a role in deciding appropriate treatment of disease.

Recently with the introduction of the single port (SP) platform which offers a special patient cart for single-site surgery. This platform allows 1 articulating camera and 3 articulating arms to be introduced through a single 25 mm trocar. The instrument offers similar maneuverability with seven degrees of freedom, but it requires more intra-abdominal space to deploy the arms than the standard Xi counterpart, which makes it less appealing to the pediatric world where there is limited intra-abdominal space. This technology has been used for single-site

Fig. 8 Completed
ileocystoplasty

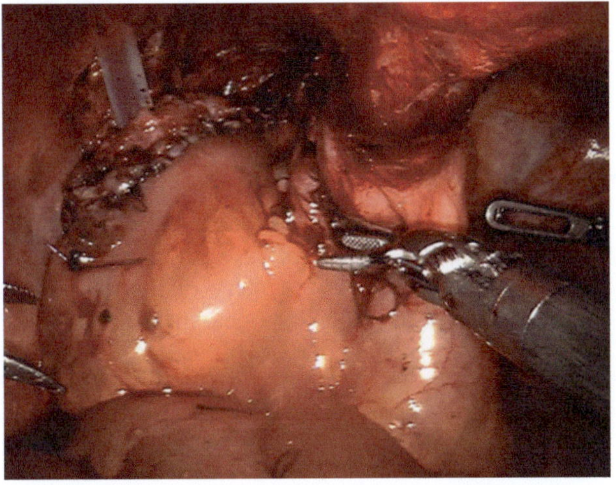

cholecystectomy in the pediatric population with success. An initial series of pyelo-plasty using this platform has been described and compared to the standard multi-port robotic technique. It did show that operative and console time is similar. It also showed initial results to be comparable. But it did not show a specific benefit of single port over multiport [6].

3   Other Devices

3.1   *Senhance Surgical Robotic System*

While this is the only other system that has gained approval for surgery in the pediatric population in Europe, little to no data has been published regarding feasibility and outcomes. So far in the field of pediatric surgery, only animal studies showing potential feasibility have been published [7]. The system consists of a surgeon console where the surgeon controls the arms. One of the touted advantages is that the camera uses eye-tracking control; thus, the camera will continuously move to place what the surgeon is looking at in the center of the field. Additionally, each arm comes in a separate cart which provides a more flexible and smaller footprint for this machine when compared to the larger patient cart in the da Vinci that has all four arms integrated. While this platform offers 5 mm instruments, not all instruments offer a wrist-like motion. Nevertheless, the instruments do offer haptic feedback to the surgeon that offers 1:1 force feedback, tissue consistency, and instrument stress information. While 5 mm ports and tactile feedback are a step in the right direction especially for the pediatric world, the limited number of articulating instruments is a significant drawback for this platform.

3.2   Flex Robotic System

This system has mainly been used in transoral robotic surgery (TORS), as it was approved by the FDA for this particular indication in 2015. It is comprised of a single-port operator flexible scope controlled by a joystick. The scope offers a high-definition two-dimensional view. Once the scope is in position, it has two 3 mm ports that allow for the passage of flexible instruments. A variety of instruments have been developed. Several ENT procedures have been performed in adult and teenage subjects, including surgery of the tongue base, the palatine tonsils, the supraglottis, the glottis, the hypopharynx, the oral tongue, and the soft palate [8]. It has recently received approval for other procedures including thoracic, general, and gynecological surgery. While it offers a much smaller footprint, it lacks a three-dimensional view, and while the instruments are flexible, they are similar to laparoscopic instruments.

3.3   ENOS™ Surgical System

This is a single-port robotic platform currently being developed by Titan Medical Inc. It is comprised of a surgeon console that offers a three-dimensional visualization and a patient cart with a single robotic arm controlling the four articulated arms that go through the single port. The incision size needed to place the trocar is similar to the da Vinci SP at 25 mm. Successful nephrectomies via a single site have been described in animal models [9]. Like other single-port platforms, the instruments articulate out first then back in which requires additional working space and maybe a limitation for pediatric application.

3.4   Versius Robotic System

This platform offers multiple configurations with each arm located in an individual cart and up to five arms being controlled by the surgeon cart, three-dimensional visualization with the use of glasses, and wristed instruments with a variety of types available in 5 mm. There is also the advantage of haptic feedback. While not yet approved in the USA, it has been successfully used in Europe.

3.5 Medtronic Robotic Surgery Program (HUGO™)

The main goal of the newer robotic system trying to break into the market is to decrease cost while providing flexibility. This system again provides a surgeon console with the ability for 3D view and a vision cart that connects the console to the arms. Each arm is mounted on an individual cart which is again touted to allow for flexibility of use while minimizing the robot footprint. Thus, the system is currently being developed and is not yet approved in the USA for use.

3.6 SurgiBot™

This is another single-site platform that had the plan to provide a low-cost solution and improve accessibility to the robot. It offers ergonomic controls with 3D vision with the precision of movement. The flexible instruments are placed through a single trocar and triangulate. It has been tried in a porcine model, but it has not received approval in the USA for use in human subjects yet.

3.7 MiroSurge

Developed by the German Institute of Robotics and Mechatronics (DLR), this platform offers an open console with 3D visualization and two controllers with haptic feedback. The console can control up to five individual robotic arms that can each be mounted to the bedside rails in a variety of configurations with one arm dedicated to the camera. Instruments offer a similar seven degrees of freedom with the advantage of haptic feedback. No information is available on when or if this platform will be available.

3.8 NOTES (Natural Orifice Transluminal Endoscopic Surgery) Platforms

Natural orifice transluminal endoscopic surgery is considered the next step on single-site endoscopic surgery. Currently, the following two robotic systems are under development to provide a robot that can be used for NOTE surgery: MASTER and ViaCath System. MASTER stands for Master and Slave Transluminal Endoscopic Robot, and it is comprised of an endoscope and two articulating arms. It allows for the triangulation of instruments to improve dexterity with the availability of haptic feedback and 3D visualization. Successful NOTES animal procedures have been reported [10]. ViaCath is a similar system of a surgeon-controlled standard colonoscope or endoscope with long-shafted instruments running alongside through an articulated flexible overture. While the instruments do offer seven degrees of freedom and a variety of instruments, it lacks appropriate triangulation due to the instrument running along with the endoscope. Nevertheless, as technology evolves, NOTES could become a much more feasible procedure in the future.

3.9 Hominis™ Surgical System

This system's main feature is the fact that it offers 360 degrees of freedom as the robotic arms are designed to simulate a human arm. It can be used as a multiport as well as a single-port approach, and it is the first robotic device approved for transvaginal robotic surgery and a pilot study showed successful hysterectomy done in 30 patients. It claims to offer improved ergonomics with low cost and a small footprint.

3.10 Miniature In Vivo Robot (MIVR)

The idea of developing an even small robot footprint by creating smaller robotic devices that can be deployed into the workspace through a single incision was behind the goal for this platform. Developed by a collaboration of multiple departments at the University of Nebraska, it is comprised of multiple small robots with different functions that can be deployed through a single abdominal incision. One of the robots has a flexible laparoscope to provide the visualization, while a second small robot with two arms was designed to accomplish the procedural tasks. The instrument tips in the two arms can be exchanged to accommodate different instruments according to the procedure needs. Successful colectomies in porcine models, as well as prostatectomy in canine models, have been described [11].

4 Training and Simulation

Training the next generation of pediatric surgeons to become robotic surgeons is no easy task. Given the limited number of cases in the field of pediatric subspecialties, it has become very difficult to appropriately prepare a trainee during the current constraints of time of a residency and fellowship. Thus, as the simulation continues to evolve, it offers the next best thing, which is an opportunity to not only become familiar with the machine functionality but also practice in a safe environment many of the maneuvers required to perform intracorporeal surgery. The current simulator associated with the da Vinci robot provides the trainee the opportunity to perform a variety of procedures including cholecystectomy and prostatectomy in a completely virtual environment. While not perfect, it does allow the trainee to familiarize themselves with the equipment and with the many important maneuvers required to master intracorporeal dissection and suturing. It also provides expert surgeons the opportunity to warm up before any case. This warm-up concept continues to grow in popularity among surgeons as it has shown potential to benefit outcomes [12].

Finally, one of the advantages of laparoscopic surgery is the fact that most procedures can be recorded. Watching videos of previous procedures can be helpful not only to trainees but also to expert surgeons looking to further improve their skills. Unfortunately, while this is often not done by either trainee or surgeon, it should become the routine as it is in many other fields such as sports. Surgeons looking to provide the best care to their patients should involve the entire robotic team in reviewing cases and try to figure out areas for improvement.

5   Conclusion

Robotic surgery in pediatrics is here to stay as it offers the next step in the evolution of laparoscopic surgery. New robotic platforms continue to be developed, and this provides the opportunity to reduce cost and improve accessibility to technology around the world. The authors hope that the industry will consider the application of their technologies on pediatric patients and their procedures. This competition will hopefully decrease cost as well as provide further diversity and specificity in instrumentation that may be further tailored to pediatric procedures. The next evolution appears to be on the horizon with the potential integration of artificial intelligence, machine learning, and the development of true self-guided operating robots.

References

1. Varda BK, et al. Has the robot caught up? National trends in utilization, perioperative outcomes, and cost for open, laparoscopic, and robotic pediatric pyeloplasty in the United States from 2003 to 2015. J Pediatr Urol. 2018;14(4):336 e1–8.
2. Meehan JJ. Robotic surgery in small children: is there room for this? J Laparoendosc Adv Surg Tech A. 2009;19(5):707–12.
3. Rague JT, et al. Robot-assisted laparoscopic urologic surgery in infants weighing </=10 kg: a weight stratified analysis. J Pediatr Urol. 2021;17(6):857.e1–7.
4. Carsel AJ, et al. Robotic upper tract surgery in infants 6 months or less: is there enough space? J Robot Surg. 2021;16:193.
5. Li P, et al. Early robotic-assisted laparoscopic pyeloplasty for infants under 3 months with severe ureteropelvic junction obstruction. Front Pediatr. 2021;9:590865.
6. Kang SK, et al. Comparison of intraoperative and short-term postoperative outcomes between robot-assisted laparoscopic multi-port pyeloplasty using the da Vinci Si system and single-port pyeloplasty using the da Vinci SP system in children. Investig Clin Urol. 2021;62(5):592–9.

7. Bozzini G, Gidaro S, Taverna G. Robot-assisted laparoscopic partial nephrectomy with the ALF-X robot on pig models. Eur Urol. 2016;69(2):376–7.
8. Persky MJ, et al. Transoral surgery using the Flex Robotic System: initial experience in the United States. Head Neck. 2018;40(11):2482–6.
9. Rassweiler JJ, et al. Future of robotic surgery in urology. BJU Int. 2017;120(6):822–41.
10. Lomanto D, et al. Flexible endoscopic robot. Minim Invasive Ther Allied Technol. 2015;24(1):37–44.
11. Shah BC, et al. Miniature in vivo robotics and novel robotic surgical platforms. Urol Clin North Am. 2009;36(2):251–63, x.
12. Lendvay TS, et al. Virtual reality robotic surgery warm-up improves task performance in a dry laboratory environment: a prospective randomized controlled study. J Am Coll Surg. 2013;216(6):1181–92.

Robotic Devices in Knee Orthopedic Surgery

Marco Kawamura Demange and Camila Maftoum Cavalheiro

1 Introduction

Total knee arthroplasty (TKA) surgery is performed to treat advanced painful osteoarthritic knee in order to improve function and decrease pain. Total condylar knee replacement has been successfully performed since 1974, proposed by John Insall. Joint replacement surgery is a treatment consideration for patients who are nonresponsive to initial therapy and who continue to experience continuing joint symptoms and pain. Several technological and surgical improvements have been added to this surgery, including implant design, surgical technique, and instrumentation improvement.

Worldwide the demand for knee and hip procedures is on the rise. According to a study evaluating historical procedure rates and population projections using the National Inpatient Sample, primary total hip arthroplasty (THA) in the USA is projected to increase by 71%, 635,000 procedures, by 2030, and primary TKA in the USA is projected to increase by 85%, 1.26 million procedures, by 2030 [1, 2].

As the short-term and long-term success of TKA depends on adequate restoration of knee stability and alignment, improvements in surgery precision and reliability are important goals. In this way, robotic assistance in total knee surgery, especially regarding positioning cutting tools and performing bone cuts, increases precision and reproducibility in the placement of knee replacements.

M. K. Demange (✉)
Orthopedic Surgery, University of, São Paulo, Brazil
e-mail: demange@usp.br

C. M. Cavalheiro
University of São Paulo, São Paulo, Brazil

J. P. Manzano, L. M. Ferreira (eds.), *Robotic Surgery Devices in Surgical Specialties*, https://doi.org/10.1007/978-3-031-35102-0_9

2　Robotic System Evolution

The level of involvement of the robotics can vary and we may didactically divide knee replacement robotic surgical systems in three categories: autonomous (or active), semi-active, and passive. In autonomous systems, the robot executes the pre-planned surgical procedure without physical guidance from the surgeon. Semi-active systems provide intraoperative feedback in order to assist the surgeon during bone cuts. They are tactile feedback systems that augment the surgeon's ability to control and manipulate the robotic tool, typically by restricting the resection volume by haptic constraint or by controlling the cutting tool motion or exposure. In passive systems, also known as computer-assisted navigation systems, they provide the surgeon with perioperative recommendations for guiding positioning, but this and bone resection are all done under direct control of the surgeon without true robotic assistance [3].

Robotic surgery has been under development for knee replacement surgery for almost three decades. The first systems for total knee replacement were autonomous robotic systems. To execute surgery with these systems, the surgeon performs the planning, surgical approach, and setup. After that, the autonomous system has the capability of completing an operation without a surgeon moving the robotic arm.

One of the first systems introduced for total knee and total hip arthroplasty was ROBODOC (Integrated Surgical Systems, Delaware, US). This system was an automated milling robotic arm for hip and knee arthroplasty. Preoperative planning was performed before surgery. The main goal of using ROBODOC focused on improving and decreasing the variability in the mechanical axis of the leg during TKA. Implant alignment and positioning has been demonstrated to be within 1° of error. On the other hand, one of the most significant limitations of this system is that it does not allow surgeon to perform adjustments during surgery in order to improve ligament balancing. Even though many studies have demonstrated less outliers to the mechanical axis, there was limited data regarding the clinical benefits of the ROBODOC system [4].

Historically, there were also other active robotic systems such as CASPAR (Ortho-Maquet/URS Ortho Rastatt, Germany) and Acrobot with limited published clinical data. Both are image-based and are no longer available for clinical use.

Currently, the robotic-assisted systems for total knee replacement are based on robotic devices that assist surgeons during the procedure (semi-active or passive). As modern systems are more adaptable during the procedure, newer robotic systems allow more accurate soft tissue balance (Table 1).

Table 1 Robotic systems used for total knee arthroplasty

Robotic system	Resection type	Preop imaging	Control	FDA approval date
MAKO	Semi-active	Preop CT	Haptic feedback	Aug. 2015
NAVIO	Semi-active	Imageless	Robotic assisted non-haptic	Jun. 2017
ROSA	Semi-active	Preop radiograph or imageless	Manual (robotically positioned cutting guide)	Jun. 2019
ROBODOC	Active	Preop CT	Autonomous control	Oct. 2019
CORI	Semi-active	Imageless	Robotic assisted non-haptic	Jul. 2020
VELYS	Semi-active	Preop radiograph or imageless	Haptic feedback	Jan. 2021

3 Basic Surgery Concepts

The steps performed during a robotically assisted surgery typically involve (1) creating a patient-specific model preoperatively (in image-based systems), (2) tracker positioning and intraoperatively registering the patient to create a final model and developing a plan based on the patient's anatomy, (3) soft tissue balancing and intraoperative adjustments, and (4) using robotic assistance to make bone cuts and carry out the procedure.

3.1 Preoperative Planning

Some robotic systems need a preoperative image ("image-based" systems) and others do not ("imageless"). Preoperative images may be obtained by CT scan or panoramic X-rays to upload a 3-D model of the bone anatomy before surgery to the system. During surgery, information regarding bone surface and anatomy of the femur and tibia is uploaded to the system using several anatomic landmarks.

Having preoperative images and a preoperative plan to approve allows the surgeon to devise the entire surgical resection plan, implant sizing, and implant positioning and alignment before even entering the operating room. Potential disadvantages of image-based systems include the increased cost of the imaging study, patient inconvenience and additional travel to obtain the study, and risk of radiation exposure during the CT scan.

Imageless systems rely solely on the surgeon's accuracy of inputting data points at the time of surgery. Advantages to imageless systems include decreased cost of the procedure, increased convenience to the patient, and no preoperative radiation exposure. Potential disadvantages include lack of true preoperative planning and inability to verify the anatomic registration points at the time of surgery against a more detailed three-dimensional imaging set.

3.2 Tracker Positioning and Landmark Registration

In the operation room the cart containing the robotic arm and monitor is positioned next to the operating table. The robotic assistant system is always on the same side as the surgeon, but it can be on the contralateral side from the knee to be replaced.

After incision, tracking arrays are attached to both the femur and the tibia using a two-pin bi-cortical fixation system. On the tibia, the pins are placed percutaneously inferior to the tibial tubercle on the medial side of the tibial crest. On the femur, the screws are placed superior to the patella.

A landmark registration is then performed either to confirm previously defined points in image-based systems or to create a 3D virtual model of a patient's anatomy intraoperatively in imageless systems. Mapping points must be registered in both system types so that the robot knows where the cutting tools are in space in relation to the anatomy. In image-based systems, this registration is directly tied to the preoperative imaging.

The landmarks are collected using a point probe, which contains a tip that is tracked using the infrared cameras. The surgeon is guided to collect points on distal femur, proximal tibia, and ankle, additionally to a leg rotation about the hip to calculate the hip center. Based on the registered points, the robotic system determines (or confirms) soft tissue boundaries and mechanical axis of the limb, including femur and tibia individual axis, femoral rotation, tibial slope, and estimated bone cut.

The user then takes the knee through a full range of motion and a varus or valgus stress is applied to tension the soft tissues on the sides of the knee to plan the desired soft tissue laxity. This helps the surgeon plan for implant positioning and volume bone resections, taking into account virtual soft tissue laxity prior to making any cuts.

3.3 Soft Tissue Balancing and Intraoperative Adjustments

Prior to bone cut, all peripheral osteophytes are removed so that joint stability can be adequately assessed. The removal of anterior cruciate and posterior cruciate (if wished to) should also be performed before stability evaluation. The maintenance of these structures affects the planning and final balance of the TKA as they can tension the soft tissues and register an unreal tension in one of the compartments.

The robotic software provides the user with the expected laxity balance throughout a range of flexion and extension. The goal is to adjust the implant positions and orientations such that the gaps in extension and flexion are balanced, with roughly 1–2 mm of laxity between the components through a full arc of motion, and avoid over-correction of alignment into the opposite compartment. To achieve adequate balance, adjustments in implant flexion, rotation, translation, varus/valgus, and depth can be made. Once the surgeon is satisfied with the implant positions and soft tissue balance, the next step is preparation of the bone surfaces.

3.4 Bone Cuts with Robotic Assistance

There is variability in how the robotic arm is used to assist bone cuts. Among the available devices, the robotic arm can be used in two main ways: to position the cutting block, in which the surgeon handles the saw itself, or to effectively be the cutting tool, either with a blur or a saw blade. The robotic restraint methods and cutting control are also different from each other; it can be a haptic system or a simple boundary delimitation.

The handling of the robotic arm is controlled by the surgeon, usually by a foot pedal. Femoral and tibial cuts are performed as planned using the specific robotic system. The surgeon then manually provisionally inserts the trial components ensuring appropriate alignment and balance through a full range of motion. The system displays the achieved coronal alignment and laxity of the knee and allows a comparison with the initial plan created in the planning stage.

All systems allow adjustments and re-cuts if balance or alignment modifications are considered appropriate. This is done with ease by returning to the planning and bone removal stage and adjusting appropriate parameters. When the surgeon is satisfied with the final results, manual implantation proceeds using the surgeon's standard methods [3, 5–7].

4 Device Types

The main robotic systems available in the USA are MAKO (Stryker), ROSA (Zimmer Biomet), CORI (Smith and Nephew), and VELYS (Depuy Synthes) (Fig. 1).

4.1 MAKO (Stryker)

The Robotic Arm Interactive Orthopedic System (RIO; MAKO Stryker, Fort Lauderdale, Florida) is a haptic system available for partial and total knee replacement and total hip replacement. As an image-based system, a preoperative CT scan of the involved limb from the hip to ankle is obtained preoperatively and it is used in surgical planning to help determine component sizing, positioning, and bone resection. The MAKO cannot be performed without a previous CT scan.

The total knee application utilizes the MAKO Integrated Cutting System (MICS). The MICS powers a saw blade that the surgeon guides according to the cuts programmed in the preoperative software. Several studies have shown that it is a safe and precise system [8–10]. The robotic arm uses AccuStop™ haptic technology to help ensure only the desired bone is resected. The robotic arm will give resistance

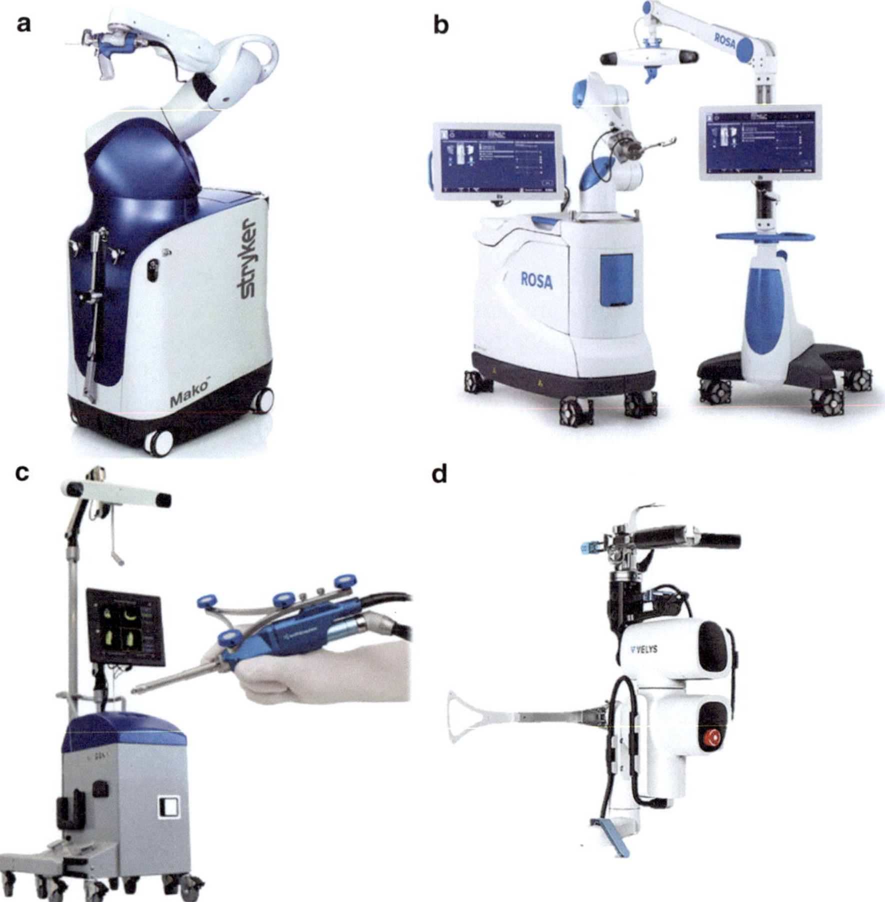

Fig. 1 Robotic arm systems for total knee arthroplasty. (**a**) MAKO (Stryker), (**b**) ROSA (Zimmer Biomet), (**c**) CORI (Smith and Nephew), and (**d**) VELYS (Depuy Synthes)

and an audible warning and ultimately turn off if the surgeon attempts to move the cutting tool on the robotic arm outside the boundaries created in the preoperative plan.

MAKO robotic arm-assisted procedures have been shown to overcome technical challenges associated with manual partial and multicompartmental knee procedures. A series of feasibility studies demonstrated that, as compared with manual techniques, the robotic system has increased accuracy in recreating the posterior tibial slope and coronal tibial alignment [11, 12]. The learning curve of robotic-assisted TKA procedures averaged 6–7 cases, and the learning cases did not present an increased risk to the patient.

4.2   ROSA (Zimmer Biomet)

The ROSA Knee Robot® (Zimmer Biomet, Warsaw, IN) received the FDA approval in 2019. The ROSA Knee Robot system does not require advanced preoperative imaging, such as CT scanning. Optional planning may be performed preoperatively with long-length lower limb X-rays. A computer software program to convert 2D X-ray images into a 3D patient-specific bone model allows virtual planning on implant positioning and ligament balancing before execution. It allows performing imageless cases.

It is a semi-autonomous surgical system that haptically positions bone cutting guide to femoral distal resection and tibial proximal resection and determines femoral rotation guide. This system does not have the saw blade attached to the system. The aim of this collaborative robotic system is to improve the accuracy and reliability of the bone resections and the ligament balancing, without replacing the steps well performed by the surgeon.

This system is exclusive for total knee arthroplasty and despite its recently approval has consistently data for achieving great accuracy when compared to manual techniques both in cadaveric studies [13, 14] and clinical studies [15].

4.3   CORI (Smith and Nephew)

Smith and Nephew has upgraded its robotic system to the CORI Surgical System; previously the main system was the NAVIO System. Essentially it is a semi-autonomous tool that uses handheld miniaturized robotic-assisted instrumentation that the surgeon manipulates in 6° of freedom, but restricts cutting to within the confines of the pre-designated resection area of the patient's bone [3].

It is an imageless portable robotic system for use in total and unicompartmental knee arthroplasty. The system offers image-free mapping of bone geometry, intraoperative planning and gap assessment, and confirmation of alignment and knee balance after the surgery. It does not have an image-based option.

The CORI system has been developed to operate within a smaller footprint than earlier generations of robotic systems in order to increase efficiency of surgical workflow (higher-speed camera technology and higher-speed cutting burrs). The CORI system was approved by the FDA in 2020.

Due to its recent FDA approval it has limited clinical data. But its precursor, NAVIO System, also shows great accuracy consistency [3].

4.4 VELYS (Depuy Synthes)

The most recently approved robotic system, in January 2021, is the VELYS Robotic-Assisted Solution (Depuy Synthes). It is a table-mounted hardware, with an advantage of design that integrates into any operating room.

The VELYS is a semi-autonomous system which has a saw blade arm and uses haptic technology to define the boundaries mechanisms to help surgeons to accurately resect bones that align and position the implant relative to the soft tissue during total knee replacement. It does not need or support preoperative imaging.

It does not have a consistent data, but it has promising expectations [16, 17].

5 Indications and Perspectives

The current motivations behind robotic-assisted TKA are improved surgical implant positioning, alignment accuracy, advancing articular surface design that allows for independent intercompartmental resurfacing, optimizing component positioning based on normal soft tissue balancing and tension, and ultimately improving patient clinical and functional outcomes [18].

In a comparative study, Kayani et al. [19] reported that robotic-assisted TKA was associated with reduced bone and periarticular soft tissue injury compared with conventional TKA. Some cadaveric studies [20, 21] showed that less soft-tissue damage occurs utilizing robotic-assisted TKA, particularly regarding the posterior cruciate ligament [18].

The key findings of this systematic review are reduction of postoperative pain and decreased analgesia requirements during the hospitalization with the robotic-assisted system, and more accurate and reproducible implant positioning with robotic-assisted TKA [18].

Several studies suggested that the implementation of robotic arm-assisted surgery may help to further improve early functional recovery and reduce time to hospital discharge in patients undergoing TKA. However, at 6 months and at 1 year, the functional results are similar for both surgical techniques [22–24].

Operative and cadaveric studies assessed the soft tissue injuries in robotic-assisted TKA and in conventional TKA, with less damage in robotic TKA. This system allowed better soft tissue protection around the knee and facilitated knee exposure.

A few studies assessed implant positioning after robotic-assisted TKA with the MAKO system. All these studies demonstrated the efficacy of robotic-assisted TKA in restoring the mechanical axis alignment in fairly common clinical scenarios where mild deformity was successfully corrected. The technique was also more accurate than the conventional method in restoring mechanical alignment and decreasing the number of outliers [18].

Most of these studies found that there were improvements in pain reduction and functional mobility. These are clinically significant outcomes which may improve the patient's satisfaction levels and quality of life following knee arthroplasty [24].

We use a quad-sparing midvastus approach for TKA. We have found that the amount of exposure, dissection, and length of required incision with TKA are less than in our manual total knee arthroplasty cases due to less need to directly visualize bone cuts [5].

6 Learning Curve and Potential Risks

An improvement of the operative time of robotic arm-assisted TKA was described (89.2 min vs. 66.8 min, $p = 0.01$) and of the surgical team stress levels after seven robotic cases. But there was no learning curve effect of robotic arm-assisted TKA on accuracy of achieving the planned implant position and limb alignment [19]. In a comparative study of 240 robotic-assisted TKAs, a significant difference was found in mean operative times for the first robotic-assisted cohort and the conventional cohort (81 min vs. 68 min, $p < 0.05$). However, no significant differences in mean operative times were found between the last robotic-assisted cohort and the conventional cohort (70 min vs. 68 min, $p > 0.05$) [15].

Kayani et al. [19] reported a minor wound dehiscence over the incision for the proximal tibial registration pins. There were no other specific complications of the image-based robotic-assisted system.

This review of image-based robotic-assisted TKA did not find any specific complications for the robotic-assisted system. The complication and revision rates were low in both robotic-assisted and conventional technique cohorts at short-term follow-up. Other studies of the robotic-assisted system for knee replacements found some specific complications of this system, such as infection or fracture at the pin insertion site or pin breakage [15].

References

1. Sloan M, Premkumar A, Sheth NP. Projected volume of primary total joint arthro-plasty in the U.S., 2014 to 2030. J Bone Joint Surg Am. 2018;100(17):1455–60.
2. CDC. Data and statistics. Atlanta, GA: Centers for Disease Control and Prevention (CDC); n.d.. https://www.cdc.gov/arthritis/data_statistics/index.htm. Accessed 22 Apr 2020.
3. Battenberg A, Netravali NA, Lonner JH. A novel handheld robotic-assisted system for unicompartmental knee arthroplasty: surgical technique and early survivorship. J Robot Surg. 2020;14:55–60.
4. Liow MHL, Goh GSH, Wong MK, Chin PL, Tay DKJ, Yeo SJ. Robotic-assisted total knee arthroplasty may lead to improvement in quality-of-life measures: a 2-year follow-up of a prospective randomized trial. Knee Surg Sports Traumatol Arthrosc. 2017;25:2942–51.
5. Grau L, Ligamfelter M, Ponzio D, Post Z, Ong A, Le D, Orozco F. Robotic arm assisted total knee arthroplasty workflow optimization, operative times and learning curve. Arthroplasty Today. 2019;5:465–70.
6. Bollars P, Boeckxstaens A, Mievis J, Kalaai S, Schotanus MGM, Janssen D. Preliminary experience with an image-free handheld robot for total knee arthroplasty: 77 cases compared with a matched control group. Eur J Orthop Surg Traumatol. 2020;30:723–9.

7. Jacofsky DJ, Allen M. Robotics in arthroplasty: a comprehensive review. J Arthroplast. 2016;31:2353–63.
8. Bhimani SJ, Bhimani R, Smith A, Eccles C, Smith L, Malkani A. Robotic- assisted total knee arthroplasty demonstrates decreased postoperative pain and opioid usage compared to conventional total knee arthroplasty. Bone Joint Open. 2020;1(2):8. https://doi.org/10.1302/2046-3758.12.BJO-2019-0004.R1.
9. Clark G. Australian experience. Mako Robotic TKA. Presented at: Australian Orthopaedic Association (AOA) 77th Annual Scientific Meeting; October 8–12, 2017; Adelaide, Australia.
10. Marchand RC, Sodhi N, Khlopas A, et al. Patient satisfaction outcomes after robotic arm–assisted total knee arthroplasty: a short-term evaluation. J Knee Surg. 2017;30(9):849–53. https://doi.org/10.1055/s-0037-1607450.
11. Lonner JH. Indications for unicompartmental knee arthroplasty and rationale for robotic arm-assisted technology. Am J Orthop. 2009;38(2 Suppl):3. Review.
12. Pearle AD, O'Loughlin PF, Kendoff DO. Robot-assisted unicompartmental knee arthroplasty. J Arthroplast. 2010;25:230.
13. Parratte S, Price AJ, Jeys PLM, Jackson WF, Clarke HD. Accuracy of a new robotically assisted technique for total knee arthroplasty: a cadaveric study. J Arthroplast. 2019;34:2799–803.
14. Seidenstein A, Birmingham M, Foran J, Ogden S. Better accuracy and reproducibility of a new robotically-assisted system for total knee arthroplasty compared to conventional instrumentation: a cadaveric study. Knee Surg Sports Traumatol Arthrosc. 2020;29:859. https://doi.org/10.1007/s00167-020-06038-.
15. Batailler C, Swan J, Marinier ES, Servien E, Lustig S. Current role of intraoperative sensing technology in total knee arthroplasty. Arch Orthop Trauma Surg. 2021;141(12):2255–65. https://doi.org/10.1007/s00402-021-04130-5. Epub 2021 Aug 24. PMID: 34427757.
16. Doan G, Curtis P, Wyss J, Clary C. Resection accuracy improved during robotic-assisted total knee arthroplasty – a cadaveric study. Int Rep:103720852.
17. User experience evaluation of the VELYS robotic-assisted solution for total knee. Int Rep. 2020:103744839.
18. Batailler C, White N, Ranaldi FM, Neyret P, Servien E, Lustig S. Improved implant position and lower revision rate with robotic-assisted unicompartmental knee arthroplasty. Knee Surg Sports Traumatol Arthrosc. 2019;27(4):1232–40. https://doi.org/10.1007/s00167-018-5081-5. Epub 2018 Jul 31.
19. Kayani B, Konan S, Pietrzak JRT, Haddad FS. Iatrogenic bone and soft tissue trauma in robotic-arm assisted total knee arthroplasty compared with conventional jig-based total knee arthroplasty: a prospective cohort study and validation of a new classification system. J Arthroplast. 2018;33:2496–501.
20. Hampp EL, Chughtai M, Scholl LY, Sodhi N, Bhowmik-Stoker M, Jacofsky DJ, et al. Robotic-arm assisted total knee arthroplasty demonstrated greater accuracy and precision to plan compared with manual techniques. J Knee Surg. 2019;32:239–50.
21. Khlopas A, Sodhi N, Hozack WJ, Chen AF, Mahoney OM, Kinsey T, et al. Patient-reported functional and satisfaction out- comes after robotic-arm-assisted total knee arthroplasty: early results of a prospective multicenter investigation. J Knee Surg. 2019;33:685.
22. Khlopas A, Sodhi N, Sultan AA, Chughtai M, Molloy RM, Mont MA. Robotic arm assisted total knee arthroplasty. J Arthroplast. 2018;33:2002–6.
23. Yang HY, Seon JK, Shin YJ, Lim HA, Song EK. Robotic total knee arthroplasty with a cruciate-retaining implant: a 10-year follow-up study. Clin Orthop Surg. 2017;9:169–76.
24. Agarwal N, To K, McDonnell S, Khan W. Clinical and radiological outcomes in robotic-assisted total knee arthroplasty: a systematic review and meta-analysis. J Arthroplast. 2020;35(11):3393–3409.e2. https://doi.org/10.1016/j.arth.2020.03.005.

Robotic Devices in Upper Limb Orthopedic Surgery and Microsurgery

Jose Carlos Garcia Jr

1 Introduction

Robotic upper limb surgery encompasses a wide range of surgical procedures from supermicrosurgery of lymphatic vessels to endoscopies for tendon transfers.

Some procedures were easily adaptable to traditional robotic platforms such as the da Vinci® Robot (Intuitive Sunnyvale-USA), while other procedures required the development of new platforms such as MUSA® (Microsure Eindhoven-Holland) and Symani® (MMI Pisa-Italy).

In our experience the da Vinci® Si and Xi have been less adaptable both for some microsurgical procedures and for supermicrosurgery.

The history of using the robot in microsurgery began in 2007 when Professor Philippe Liverneaux did his training and began his first works demonstrating that robotics could be used in microsurgery using animal models [1]. With the publication of his first papers [2–4], robotic microsurgery began. Manipulation of the brachial plexus [5, 6] and peripheral nerves [7–9] was quickly adapted.

Procedures in cadaveric models combining brachial plexus manipulation and endoscopy were done [5], but in live patients open manipulation was the choice for this procedure [6].

With the release of the ulnar nerve at the elbow, the open experience [7] migrated better to endoscopy in live patients [8]. The axillary nerve was also identified endoscopically with the aid of a robot in cadavers [9], and the release of the quadrangular space was successfully performed in one patient by the author of this chapter (Fig. 1).

J. C. Garcia Jr (✉)
NAEON Institute and Moriah Hospital, São Paulo, SP, Brazil
e-mail: josecarlos@naeon.org.br

© The Author(s), under exclusive license to Springer Nature Switzerland AG 2023
J. P. Manzano, L. M. Ferreira (eds.), *Robotic Surgery Devices in Surgical Specialties*, https://doi.org/10.1007/978-3-031-35102-0_10

Fig. 1 Quadrangular space release and axillary nerve visualization

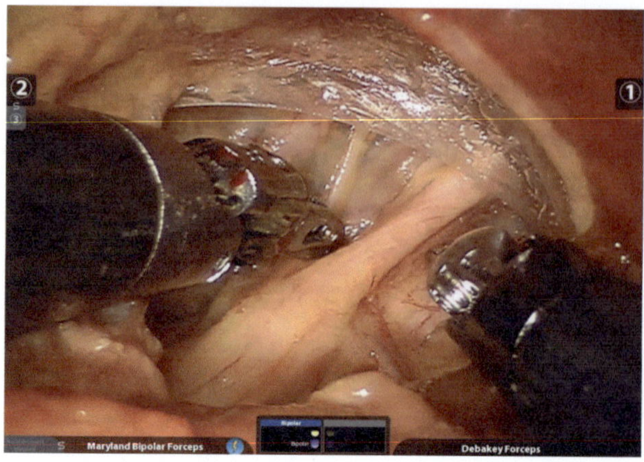

Robotic da Vinci® devices used for endoscopic releases were the Maryland bipolar forceps® and the Hot Shears™ monopolar scissors (Intuitive Sunnyvale-USA).

For microsurgical sutures, Black Diamond micro forceps (Intuitive Sunnyvale-USA) were the most suitable due to their dimensions.

With a better understanding of the posterior shoulder endoscopic anatomy, it was possible for the first time to endoscopically access this region [9]. This meant that new orthopedic procedures in this region of the upper limb could be performed.

The transfer from the origin of the latissimus dorsi to deltoid palsy in axillary nerve injury was performed in a patient [10] with aesthetic improvement, however with poor functional results, possibly because it was not a bipolar transfer, keeping the insertion of the latissimus dorsi intact. Bipolar transfers may have a better effect and be a viable option since the exploration with robotic release of the origin of the latissimus dorsi muscle [10] and the manipulation of its insertion [11] have achieved success, keeping the vascularized graft alive and active.

The transfer of the latissimus dorsi tendon, which until now also required large approaches with cosmetic implications and adhesions, could be performed with a robot in a minimally invasive manner through posterior endoscopic portals [11–13]. However, wide subcutaneous dissection is necessary using the Cadiere forceps®, Maryland bipolar forceps®, and Hot Shears™ monopolar scissors (Intuitive Sunnyvale-USA).

This posterior approach for the transfer of the latissimus dorsi tendon is demanding; it can be more suitable for transfers of this muscle to the scapula or when the transfer of the tendon of the teres major muscle must be associated. For latissimus dorsi tendon isolated transfers, we are currently using the anterior/axillary endoscopic approach. Many applications for this approach such as subscapularis injuries or latissimus dorsi transfer or reinforcement for rotator cuff reconstruction are currently in use (Figs. 2 and 3). For the anterior/axillary approach to the latissimus dorsi, the distances between the portals are smaller with a reduced work space, however visualization of the tendon is much better. When using this approach, the Cadiere forceps® (Intuitive Sunnyvale-USA) does not need to be used. This approach also allowed a significant reduction in costs and surgical time.

Fig. 2 da Vinci® robot. Portals for anterior access to the latissimus dorsi tendon, axillary region

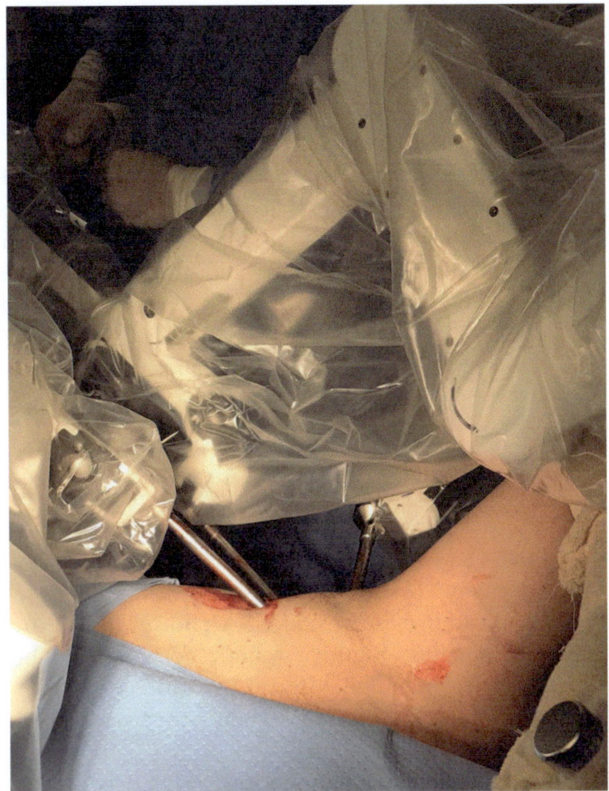

Fig. 3 (A) Radial nerve, (B) long head of the biceps, (C) humerus, (D) latissimus dorsi tendon

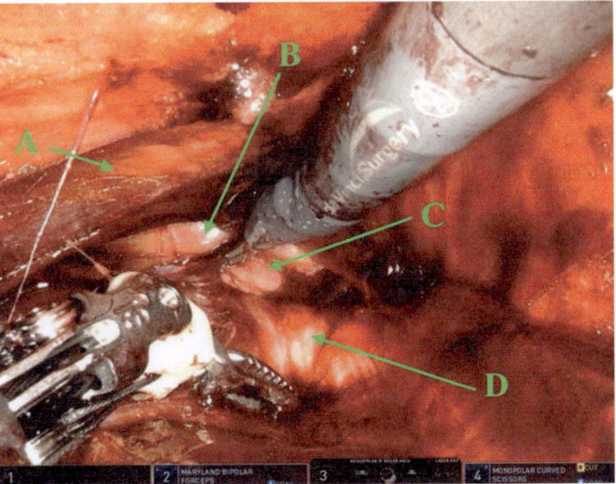

The robotic endoscopic orthopedic surgeries mentioned above are performed in places where there are no natural cavities; therefore, an initial cavity must be created for the dissection to advance to the desired surgical spot. In the anterior/axillary approach to the latissimus dorsi tendon, almost the entire space is previously manually dissected and released.

Regarding microsurgery and supermicrosurgery, endoscopy was not so successful; however, tremor filtration and motion scaling associated with three-dimensional vision were the most important factors for the robotics in these surgical fields.

For microsurgery and supermicrosurgery, the possibility of using smaller, cheaper, and more adapted to open environment robots seems to be the right way to go.

For upper limb micro- and supermicrosurgeries, the surgeons use, by default, only two robotic hands.

In this environment two platforms with different and innovative ideas created more friendly robots.

So the surgeon can enjoy the benefits of robotics without the restrictions imposed by the positioning of the da Vinci® (Intuitive Sunnyvale-USA) for micro- or supermicrosurgery.

The Symani® (MMI Pisa-Italy) features a similar forceps operation mode to the da Vinci® (Intuitive Sunnyvale-USA); however, its extremely delicate micro forceps make the smallest Intuitive robotic forceps look big. As the system is easily attachable to a standard surgical microscope, it does not require the technology involved in the optics and endoscopic part. Its use will depend on specific disposable microforceps.

MUSA® (Microsure Eindhoven-Holland) is a robot also adapted to micro and supermicrosurgeries [14, 15]. With two robotic arms, tremor filtration and scaling of the surgical gesture make it easy to use in microsurgery. An advantage of this robot is that it uses the same forceps regularly used in microsurgeries, making the migration from the manual to the robotic platform even more intuitive and less expensive.

As in the MMI robot, in the MUSA, the system is also easily attached to the operating table and to a standard surgical microscope, eliminating the technology involved in the optics and endoscopy.

Robot-assisted supermicrosurgery of lymphatic vessels [16] is currently only performed using one of the last two platforms, MMI and Microsure, with encouraging results.

Indeed, the Microsure robot has been shown to present superior suturing results to the non-robotic.

2 Surgery

Surgeries using the da Vinci® surgical robot platform are widely publicized and recognized.

As there are major limitations to its endoscopic operation in microsurgery, only the advantages of tremor control and movement scaling show clear superiority to traditional surgery. Costs and the need for training are disadvantages of the method, which, even with a vertical learning curve, does not have specific training.

As for other platforms, Microsure's MUSA® adapts the common microsurgery forceps to the robotic platform, using cheaper materials and possibly easy adaptation by the microsurgeon. The movement occurs through two modules that present the configuration that makes the migration from open surgery to robotics very intuitive with very similar movement but with the advantages of tremor control and movement scaling. The forceps of microsurgery supported by this platform are smaller than those supported by the da Vinci® robot (Figs. 4 and 5).

The author is not very familiar with MMI's Symani® platform; its microforceps are similar to Black Diamond® of the da Vinci® robot but on a much smaller scale. As the MUSA® this robot is specifically targeted for microsurgery.

Indications in upper limb surgery are expanding; currently, they are as follows:

1. Open
    Brachial plexus reconstruction
    Oberlin procedure
    Digital nerve reconstruction
    Scalenectomy for thoracic outlet syndrome [17]
    Lymphatic vessel reconstruction
2. Endoscopic
    Ulnar nerve release (Fig. 6)
    Latissimus dorsi tendon transfers with or without teres minor transfer (Fig. 7)
    Positioning also used in exploration of quadrangular space
    Transfers of the latissimus dorsi
    Surgical flap of the latissimus dorsi muscle
    Rectus abdominis muscle flap

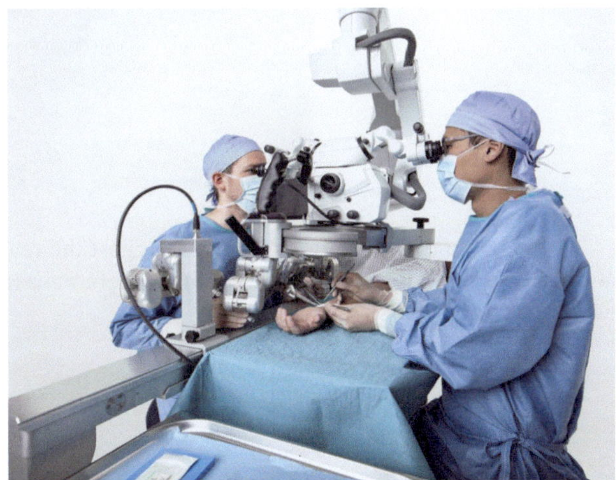

Fig. 4 Robot MUSA in surgery for lymphatic vessel reconstruction. (Courtesy of Microsure®)

Fig. 5 Robot MUSA in surgery for lymphatic vessel reconstruction. (Courtesy of Microsure®)

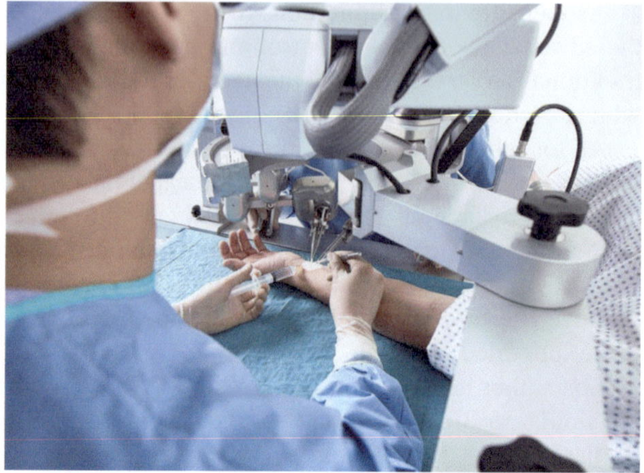

Fig. 6 da Vinci® robot in endoscopic ulnar nerve release

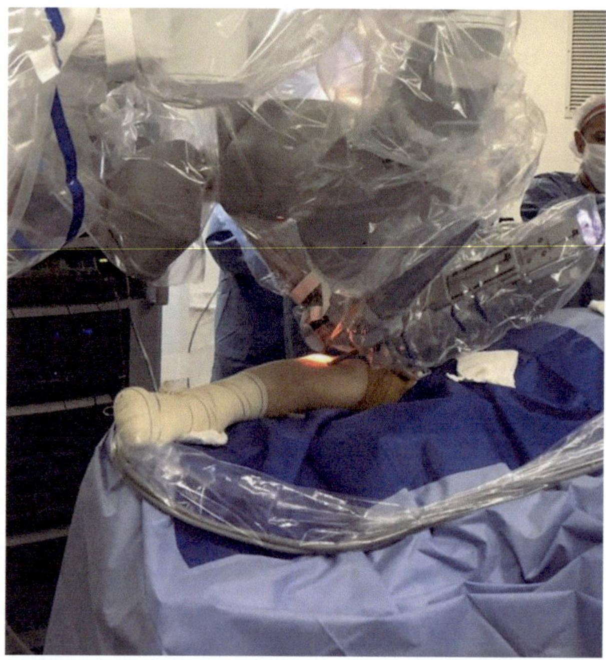

As the range of procedures is wide, I suggest the reader who wants more details about the upper limb to see the works in the References of this chapter and also stay tuned to future papers.

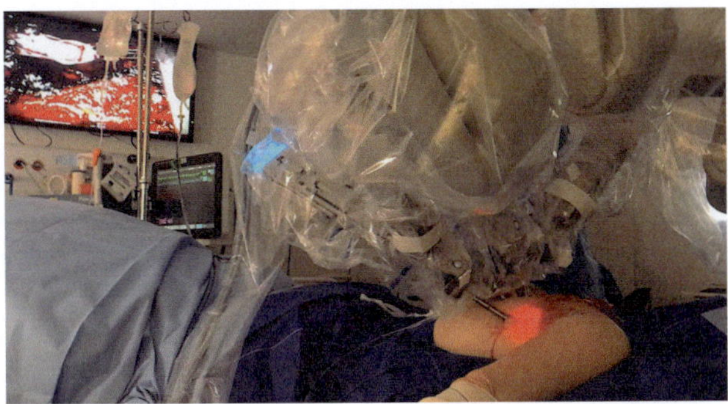

Fig. 7 da Vinci® robot. Posterior approach for latissimus dorsi and teres major

3 Contraindications

Open surgery for tendons is an absolute contraindication at the moment because the surgical trauma is the same and the procedure is not superior. There is only an increase in surgical time and costs, so there is no prospect of adding advantages for the patient with the use of the robot. These procedures have already been performed on cadavers at the Strasbourg IRCAD® with success but without practical applicability. However, endoscopic procedures will present the advantage of minimally invasive surgery.

Microsurgery and upper limb surgery are specialties with expanding indications, so clear limits have not yet been established for the use or not of the robot.

Bone surgeries will need robots with specific materials for the upper limb, still awaiting their launch.

Possibly robots for shoulder arthroplasty will be launched in 2024; however, this robot is very specific.

4 Perspectives

Robotics tends to be increasingly used in the upper limb, especially in shoulder and elbow surgery.

With the evolution of computer technologies, it was possible to better determine the best angles of attack and make adequate planning. The software uses three-dimensional images in order to give the surgeon a previous experience of the surgical procedure, increasing the accuracy significantly.

This previous planning makes the angulation errors go from 11° in the version and 12° in the inclination [18] to values around 6° for the version and inclination [19]. This increased accuracy will potentially improve patient adaptation to the prosthesis, implant longevity, and even final range of motion.

With intraoperative navigation, this accuracy increased even further to only 2° [19].

The next step in arthroplasty will be robotics. With the arrival of the robotic arms of ROSA® from Zimmer-Biomet®, Mako® from Stryker®, and VELYS™ from Johnson & Johnson®, possibly there will be a great advance, the implantation of the glenoid component tends to be even more precise, mainly for the most complex cases, where even navigation may not reach the necessary accuracy.

The problems associated with these platforms in the upper limb are the use of thin-slice computed tomography which will increase the patient's exposure to radiation, costs, and possible surgical time.

Just in the future one will realize how cost-effective or not these technologies will be.

There are also some other soft tissue surgeries that have already been performed on animal models and are still experimental for humans.

One of these procedures is the robotic thoracoscopy to access the intercostal nerves for transfers for brachial plexus injuries [20].

This is a surgery that, when performed open, creates a wide soft tissue lesion with a wide approach, so robotic thoracoscopy may have advantages over traditional surgery. There is already a case report of this procedure in a patient [21].

Surgical procedures that combine soft tissue with bone as a surgical reconstruction of the rotator cuff are in development by the author yet.

References

1. Liverneaux PA, Berner SH, Bednar MS, Parekattil SJ, Ruggiero GM, Selber JC. Telemicrosurgery: robot assisted microsurgery. 1st ed. Paris: Springer; 2013.
2. Nectoux E, Taleb C, Liverneaux P. Nerve repair in telemicrosurgery: an experimental study. J Reconstr Microsurg. 2009;25:261–5.
3. Taleb C, Nectoux E, Liverneaux P. Telemicrosurgery: a feasibility study in a rat model. Chir Main. 2008;28:104–8.
4. Taleb C, Nectoux E, Liverneaux P. Limb replantation with two robots: a feasibility study in a pig model. Microsurgery. 2009;29:232–5.
5. Mantovani G, Liverneaux PA, Garcia JC, Berner SH, Bednar MS, Mohr CJ. Endoscopic exploration and repair of brachial plexus with telerobotic manipulation: a cadaver trial. J Neurosurg. 2011;115(3):659–64.
6. Garcia JC, Lebailly F, Mantovani G, Mendonça LA, Garcia JM, Liverneaux PA. Telerobotic manipulation of the brachial plexus. J Reconstr Microsurg. 2012;28(7):491–4.
7. Garcia JC, Mantovani G, Gouzou S, Liverneaux P. Telerobotic anterior translocation of the ulnar nerve. J Robot Surg. 2011;5(2):153–6.
8. Garcia JC, Montero EFS. Endoscopic robotic decompression of the ulnar nerve at the elbow. Arthrosc Techn. 2014;3:383–7.
9. Melo PMP, Garcia JC, Montero EFS, Atik T, Robert EG, Facca S, et al. Feasibility of an endoscopic approach to the axillary nerve and the nerve to the long head of the triceps brachii with the help of the Da Vinci Robot. Chirurgie de la Main. 2013;32:206–9.
10. Ichihara S, Bodin F, Pedersen JC, Melo PP, Garcia JC, Sybille F, et al. Robotically assisted harvest of the latissimus dorsi muscle: a cadaver feasibility study and clinical test case. Hand Surg Rehabil. 2016;35:81–4.

11. Garcia JC, Gomes RVF, Kozonara ME, Steffen AM. Posterior endoscopy of the shoulder with the aid of the Da Vinci SI robot – a cadaveric feasibility study. Acta Shoulder Elbow Surg. 2017;2(1):36–9.
12. Garcia JC, Cordeiro EF, Raffaelli MP, Mello MBD, Kozonara ME, Cardoso AM, Torres MC. Robotic transfer of the latissimus dorsi. Arthrosc Techn. 2020;9(6):e769–73.
13. Garcia JC Jr, Torres MC, Fadel MS, Bader D, Lutfi H, Kozonara ME. Robotic transfer of the latissimus dorsi associated with levator scapulae and rhomboid minor mini-open transfers for trapezium palsy. Arthrosc Tech. 2020;9(11):e1721–6.
14. van Mulken TJM, Scharmg AMJ, Wilkens B, Cau R, Schoenmakers FBF, et al. The journey of creating the first dedicated platform for robot-assisted (super)microsurgery in reconstructive surgery. Eur J Plast Surg. 2020;43:1–6.
15. van Mulken TJM, Schols RM, Quiu SS, Brouwers K, Hoekstra LT, Booi DI, et al. Robotic (super) microsurgery: feasibility of a new master-slave platform in an in vivo animal model and future directions. J Surg Oncol. 2018;118:826–31.
16. van Mulken TJM, Schol RM, Scharmg AMJ, Schols RM, Cau R, Jonis Y, et al. First-in-human robotic supermicrosurgery using a dedicated microsurgical robot for treating breast cancer-related lymphedema: a randomized pilot trial. Nat Commun. 2020;11:757.
17. Garcia JC. Nerve entrapment. In: Liverneaux P, Berner S, Bednar M, Parekattil S, Mantovani Ruggiero G, Selber J, editors. Telemicrosurgery. Springer: Paris; 2013. p. 109–17.
18. Iannotti J, et al. Three-dimensional preoperative planning software and a novel information transfer technology improve glenoid component positioning. J Bone Joint Surg. 2014;96:e71.1–8.
19. Greene A, Hamilton M, Polakovic S, Mohajer N, Youderian A, Wright T, et al. Navigated versus non-navigated results of a CT-based computer assisted shoulder arthroplasty system in 30 cadavers. Orth Proc. 2019;101-B(Suppl 5):23. https://online.boneandjoint.org.uk/doi/abs/1 0.1302/1358-992X.2019.5.023
20. Miyamoto H, Serradori T, Mikami Y, Selber J, Santelmo N, Facca S, Liverneaux PA. Robotic intercostal nerve harvest: a feasibility study in a pig model. J Neurosurg. 2016;124(1):264–8.
21. Naito K, Imashimizu K, Nagura N, et al. Robot-assisted intercostal nerve harvesting: a technical note about the first case in Japan. Plast Reconstr Surg Glob Open. 2020;8(6):e2888.

Robotic Devices in Hip Orthopedic Surgery

Marco Aurelio Silverio Neves, Fabio Zego, and Osvaldo Guilherme Nunes Pires

1 Introduction

Total hip arthroplasty is one of the most successful surgical procedures performed in orthopedics, with excellent functional and clinical results, when indicated in patients experiencing advanced-stage arthrosis of the hip joint, helping to reduce pain, restore function, and increase the quality of life [1]. The procedure's success results from its consistent technical evolution since being introduced approximately six decades ago [2]. The short and long terms outcomes of THA may be influenced by several factors.

We can therefore highlight the following key topics since the advent of this technique: in the 1970s, tribological pairings of joints were discussed; in the 1980s, a debate was initiated that continues today regarding the use of cemented or cementless prostheses; in the 1990s, new tribological pairings were introduced, such as metal-metal and ceramic-ceramic surfaces, in addition to the use of resurfacing arthroplasty in order to preserve bone stock. Throughout the last two decades, attention was focused on the early failure of implants using a metal-to-metal surface and the use of minimally invasive techniques in hip arthroplasty surgery, in addition to the emergence of alternative surgical approaches. It is

M. A. S. Neves (✉)
Orthopedic Surgery Department, Moriah Hospital, São Paulo, Brazil

Department of Clinical Medicine, Laboratory of Experimental Therapeutics (LIM-20), School of Medicine, University of Sao Paulo, São Paulo, Brazil
e-mail: marcoaurelio@arthron.med.br

F. Zego
Orthopedic Surgery Department, Moriah Hospital, São Paulo, Brazil

O. G. N. Pires
Hip Surgery Department, Alvorada Hospital, São Paulo, Brazil

© The Author(s), under exclusive license to Springer Nature Switzerland AG 2023
J. P. Manzano, L. M. Ferreira (eds.), *Robotic Surgery Devices in Surgical Specialties*, https://doi.org/10.1007/978-3-031-35102-0_11

believed that the main theme over the course of the next decade with regard to hip surgery will be the use of new technologies and robotic surgery [3].

In addition to a series of variables such as patient characteristics, the surgical techniques implemented, the presence of previous surgeries, and the types of implants, technologies, and robotic surgery also influence the outcome of the surgery. Part of these variables are related to the preoperative planning performed by the surgeon as well as their ability to reproduce these conditions during the surgical procedure, since the properties of the materials, the porosity of the interface, and the geometry of the implant play a fundamental role in the stability of the prosthesis, its positioning, and osseointegration [4–6].

One of the surgeon controlled factor is the proper positioning of implants and the restoration of biomechanics. This is one of the most important factors in the success of hip arthroplasty procedures and continue to present a significant challenge for surgeons. Complications such as dislocation, impingement, and accelerated wear of the acetabular liner [7–9] as well as changes in gait, lower limb discrepancy, and early loosening of the implant [10, 11] are all related to the accuracy of implant positioning. Robotic surgery has therefore garnered interest by contributing to improved positioning of the components in recommended zones, seeking to place the acetabular component in the Lewinnek target zone [12], improving positioning of the stem, and contributing to a lower displacement rate when compared to conventional surgery [13].

This chapter describes the development of robotic surgery in hip arthroplasty and its respective principles, in addition to the advantages and disadvantages described in the literature to date.

2 Robots in Total Hip Arthroplasty

2.1 History

The first active robotic system used in hip arthroplasty was ROBODOC (THINK Surgical; Fremont, California, United States). Its development began in the 1980s after cementless stem models were introduced on the market. However, it was only in 1992 that a system was adapted for application in humans through a viability study involving ten patients. The system operates using images generated through computed tomography assisted by a robotic device capable of preparing the femoral canal and implanting the cementless stem [14].

A new multicenter study was carried out between 1994 and 1998 on 136 different hips, demonstrating an improvement in implantation of the femoral stem in terms of alignment, adjustment, and filling of the femoral canal, in addition to the absence of intraoperative fractures with the use of ROBODOC in relation to conventional surgery, with no differences in relation to the functional "Harris Hip Score" seen over the course of a 2-year follow-up. The following sequence was used in the procedure: preoperative preparation, including implantation of locator pins, computed tomography, preoperative planning, surgical configuration of the workstation in the operating room, surgical steps with sequential anatomical exposure, pin location, registration, and robotic preparation of the femoral cavity [14].

Certain issues were reported as increasing surgical time due to the respective learning curve and operational errors in the recovery system, which caused the robot to interrupt operation if the monitoring system detected any failures, such as a bone movement. These interruptions were followed by a lengthy process required to restart the system. There was also increased blood loss compared to the control group resulting from the abovementioned operational issues. Additionally, the fact that a previous surgical procedure was necessary in installing locator pins prior to the carrying out of computed tomography for use as a parameter may present an additional potential risk [14].

Much like ROBODOC, the CASPAR System (Universal Robot Systems; Rastatt, Germany) also uses preoperative computed tomography and robot assistance to provide support during milling and positioning of the femoral stem in the canal. However, certain studies presented divergences in results. A study comparing contact between the femoral stem and bone in surgeries performed using the CASPER system and the conventional method showed a mean contact in the nail-bone interface of 93.2% in procedures assisted by the robot compared to 60.1% using the manual method, which meant that robotic surgery provided 33% more contact [15].

Another study, however, demonstrated that, in ten patients undergoing total hip arthroplasty assisted by the CASPER system assessed using preoperative and postoperative CT, with values compared with procedures involving preoperative planning, a mean difference of 7.8° in the angles and 1.8 and 1.2 mm in the medial and lateral deviations was found. Researchers therefore concluded that it could not be safely stated that positioning of the implant would be as accurate as claimed by the manufacturer. Another article involving an 18-month follow-up presented a longer mean duration for the CASPAR procedure (CASPAR, 100.6 min; conventional, 51.5 min), above-average hemoglobin loss (CASPAR, 4.5 mg/dL; conventional, 3.3 mg/dL), similar complication rates (CASPAR, two dislocations, one sciatic paresis, one deep infection; conventional, one dislocation, two fractures) with inferior functional scores (Merle d'Aubigné and Postel, CASPAR, 10.1–16.0 points; conventional, 8.3–16.6 points), and inferior function of the hip abductor musculature, with a higher incidence of the postoperative Trendelenburg sign (CASPAR, 61.1%; conventional, 25.7%; $p = 0.0014$); such data led the author to conclude that the presence of significant functional impairment after robotic-assisted arthroplasty should be taken into account before recommending the procedure [16–18]. This illustrates the challenges and concerns that were encountered when robots were first used in total hip arthroplasty. The company representing the CASPER system eventually filed for bankruptcy, and this robot is currently no longer in use.

The robotic system that is most used in THA is the MAKO system (Stryker Ltd, Kalamazoo, Michigan, USA). MAKO Surgical was founded in 2004 for the purpose of providing medical applications, in addition to a wide variety of other computer-assisted surgery technologies. First adapted for partial knee replacement, with the first procedure performed in 2006, development for use of these technologies in the hip was carried out in October 2010. This robotic arm system was cleared by the FDA in 2015.

The latest system available on the market is the ROSA® Hip System (Zimmer Biomet, Warsaw IN, USA), which was cleared by the FDA in August 2021. The following sections will offer a more detailed description of the technologies that are currently in use.

2.2 MAKO

The Interactive Orthopedic System "MAKO Robotic Arm" (Stryker Corporation; Kalamazoo, MI, USA) was used to perform a hip arthroplasty for the first time in 2015 [19]. Preoperative planning is implemented using computed tomography images of the pelvis and lower limbs. The process of scanning and preparing the images is carried out by representatives from the manufacturer. The orientation and depth of the acetabulum must be adjusted as appropriate and computer-simulated results verified along the coronal, sagittal, and transverse planes in order to guarantee that the implant is properly positioned. Surgeons may, as necessary, select the most appropriate component size for restoring hip length and establishing the appropriate offset. Additionally, the femoral osteotomy line must be measured using the MAKO's software in order to determine the femoral neck length during surgical procedures [20]. Orthopedic Surgeons have been using the Lewinnek safe zone as a guide for cup placement for over 40 years. Studies have shown that greater than 50% of total hip arthroplasty dislocators have cups placed within this safe zone. One shortcoming of the Lewinnek safe zone is that it generically applies to all patients, regardless of their individual bone morphology, kinematics, implant choices or placement. Mako Total Hip has integration of features that allow a surgeon to assess a patient's functional pelvic tilt and virtual range-of-motion (vROM) to help achieve functional implant planning [21]. This study shows that the vast majority of THAs planned with standing combined anteversion between 30 to 50° and sitting combined anteversion between 45 to 65° had impingement and concluded functional combined anteversion, which considers both cup and stem position, should be used when identifying an ideal position for impingement-free ROM [22].

The MAKO system operates through a robotic arm that is guided by a patient-specific 3D computer model derived using computed tomography in conjunction with anatomical points collected during surgery. In addition to pelvic tilt, data on femoral anteversion are collected by tomography in order for acetabular and femoral components to be properly adjusted during the surgical procedure. The MAKO system's robotic arm makes use of tactile feedback technology (i.e., the surgeon maintains partial control of the action of the robotic arm during implantation). Therefore, if there are any deviations from the pre-established surgical plan, the robotic arm offers tactile resistance, and, if the deviation persists, an audio alert is triggered and the arm subsequently deactivated. The system was adapted to perform the procedure through posterolateral and anterior approach, and this choice is made by the surgeon.

The first step involves placing three pins in the thicker portion of the iliac crest, at which optical trackers will be connected to locate the pelvis movements that occur during the procedure. In the case of the posterior approach, the patient is placed in lateral decubitus, and the distal reference is placed on the patella prior to preparation and placement of surgical fields. Pins are then positioned on the ipsilateral iliac crest. After surgical access has been made, the femur is registered and verified in the system.

A femoral marker is placed on the large trochanter in order to record the combined offset, as well as the length of the patient's limb prior to the operation. Once the femoral cut has been made, a new reference point is positioned above the acetabulum in the posterosuperior region, in order to allow points to be obtained along the margin of the acetabulum using a calibrated pointer. The acetabulum is then reamed for cup placement using a haptic robotic arm guide acetabular reaming for cup insertion.

Once this step is complete, the femoral stem and the neck cut can be planned and manually performed or the system offers the ability to navigate the femoral osteotomy level and implantation of the stem by a mapping registration of the proximal part of the femur in order to optimize the adjustment of the femoral version. In this case, the femoral mapping will precede acetabular reaming and cup insertion.

One of the advantages of Mako system is you can use it with your prefferd approach, Posterior, Lateral or Anterior approach. In cases in which the direct anterior approach is used, the procedure is performed with the patient in the supine position both with or without the use of a specific traction table. In cases in which a conventional table is used, the lower extremities are prepared separately using bilateral sterile fields, which allows intraoperative lengths to be compared and stability testing to be performed. This field completely covers both legs, leaving the anterior part of the iliac crest and the anterolateral region of the thigh visible on both sides and protected by a transparent adhesive sterile field.

Three reference pins are placed in the contralateral pelvis, and the anterior and inferior part of the greater trochanter are marked on the femur. A single acetabular cutter can be used in accordance with preoperative planning. Acetabular preparation is carried out using the robotic arm, in addition to impaction of the final implant. Navigation is carried out during insertion of the stem, if the option for insertion using the improved technique is chosen, with the objective of adjusting the size of the neck and prosthesis offset and adjusting the limb's dysmetria. The surgical procedure may be adapted as previously demonstrated [23].

Only two or three surgeons should generally participate in the surgery. An instrumentation nurse and a circulating nurse are responsible for preparing the instrument and content. A representative from the manufacturer operates the software and adjusts the pin detector as needed. The Mako System was introduced with a goal of providing more accurate implant positioning and alignment to plan, to help restore anatomy and biomechanics and enhance patient outcomes. In a clinical trial including 110 patients, acetabular cup position was compared between preoperative plan, assessment, and achieved radiographic measure. Results confirmed that intraoperative robotic-arm assistance achieved greater accuracy in preparation and position of the acetabular cup during THA [24]. A study involving six surgeons at a single institute, in which 1,980 THA surgeries were evaluated. Robotic-arm assisted surgery resulted in a significantly greater percentage of components placed in Callanan's safe zones than all other modalities, including navigation- and fluoroscopy-guided approaches [25]. Anaother study has demonstrated robotic-arm assisted surgery is accurate to 1.0 ± 0.7mm for leg length/offset. Compared to manual THA, robotic-arm assisted THA was five times more accurate to plan in cup inclination and 3.4 times more accurate to plan in cup anteversion. A potential benefit of robotic-arm assisted THA is that it has been shown to be significantly more accurate in reproducing COR when compared to manual implantation, which may result in reduced incidence of hip dislocation [26].

2.3   ROSA

Another device used in robot-assisted hip arthroplasty is the "ROSA® Hip System," which consists of the "ROSA® Recon Robotic Unit," an optical unit and touch screen (optional), and the "ROSA® Tablet" (Zimmer Biomet, Warsaw IN, USA). The "ROSA® Hip System," when used in conjunction with the "ROSA® Recon Robotic Unit," supports surgeons in performing total hip arthroplasty by offering resources that assist in impaction of the acetabular prosthesis during the direct anterior approach. The intraoperative workflow and surgical concepts implemented in the system are therefore aligned with the standard for the anterior route as well as in order to assess any discrepancies in limb length and femoral offset [27].

This system does not use computed tomography imaging or optical navigation through means of bone tracking pins. The digital data used during the surgical procedure, in order to restore the biomechanics of the joint and positioning of the components, is generated only provided through fluoroscopy and is able to correlate between the preoperative template and post-procedure data. Fluoroscopic guidance is used during the surgical procedure to obtain an image of a level pelvis and assess bone preparation and the positioning of components, as well as equalize potential limb dysmetria.

Prior to implementing the technique, a fluoroscopic image of the pelvis in anteroposterior (AP) is acquired (offering an image of both teardrops, obturator foramen and symmetric obturator foramen). A photo of this image is then captured using the "ROSA® Tablet," thereby ensuring that the entire fluoroscopic imaging circle is captured. Automatic detection of the fluoroscopy image area is framed within the camera view, and if necessary the region of interest is adjusted on the ROSA Tablet screen while ensuring that the following areas were not excluded: both hip teardrops are visible, both obturator foramen are shown completely, and alignment of the coccyx corresponds to orientations for preoperative radiography if preoperative imaging was carried, as well as whether orientation of the image is representative of an AP X-ray.

During the procedure, it is mandatory that the Robotic Unit is positioned on the side of the hip being operated upon and that the surgeon is on the same side as the Robotic Unit. The surgical technique is therefore implemented with resectioning and milling of the femoral canal. The instrument used to position the acetabular cup is inserted into the articular space and connected to the robotic arm. The robotic arm is then positioned for tilting and implementing of the target acetabular version and its values shown on the screen. Robot assistance is used to impact the acetabular cup. The femoral canal is prepared using manual instrumentation and a test stem is inserted and reduced.

A new hip image is subsequently acquired, and the dissymmetry measurement is displayed on the test and validation panel for the selected components in addition to projections for all compatible implant combinations. Once the femoral component is implanted, a final image is obtained and the reference points reviewed and confirmed on the tablet. A study was carried out to assess radiological results for accuracy of the orientation of the acetabular component and the ability to equalize the limbs between robot-assisted and manual hip arthroplasty in a group of arthroplasty surgeons experiencing a high volume of procedures. The percentage of cases within the Lewinnek and Callanan "safe zones" was significantly higher for the robot-assisted group compared to the manual group (100% vs. 73%, $p = 0.002$), and discrepancy in the lower limbs was not statistically significant between the groups [27].

The advantages offered by the "ROSA® Hip System" include the fact that special imaging is not required (low cost). Additionally bone trackers are not used and there is no change in the surgeon's work routine or respective surgical approach. The ROSA Hip System may not be suitable for use in cases involving hip pathology with significant bone loss, active infections in the hip joint region, revision surgery, presence of undesirable radiopaque elements during intraoperative image acquisition, adverse side effects in implants provided by the implant manufacturer, and implants that are not compatible with the system.

To understand the real benefit of using these robotic-assisted technologies, many factors must be analyzed, since clinical success is multifactorial in nature. Evidence of the advantages and disadvantages of using these systems is provided below.

2.4 Advantages

2.4.1 Length of Stay

The costs over 9 days of post-operations were evaluated following manual versus robot-assisted arthroplasty, including 938 cases of assisted THA and 4670 manual THA. Patients that had received post-assisted THA were significantly less likely to be admitted to certified nursing facilities and required fewer home visits from healthcare workers when compared to patients that received manual arthroplasty [28]. Another analysis performed recorded an average hospital stay of 2.69 days for

758 patients receiving assisted THA, compared to 2.82 days in 758 patients receiving conventional THA [29].

2.4.2 Risk of Dislocation

A retrospective cohort study compared the rate of postoperative dislocation, and a displacement rate of 5% was found during the early postoperative period for manual arthroplasty and 3% in the late postoperative period versus 0% in the cohort of patients receiving robot-assisted arthroplasty in the first 2 years after surgery [30].

Another study was carried out at a single institution between 2016 and 2020 and involves 13,802 primary, unilateral, elective, and posterior-approach arthroplasties, of which 1770 were assisted by robot, 3155 were performed through navigation, and 8877 were performed manually. The robot-assisted group had an odds ratio of 0.3 (95% confidence interval 0.1–0.9, $p = 0.046$) compared to manual THA for reoperation due to dislocation, and surgeries performed through navigation presented an odds ratio of 3.0 for reoperation due to dislocation (95% confidence interval 0.8–11.3, $p = 0.114$) compared to the robot-assisted group. It can therefore be concluded that the THA-RA is associated with a lower risk of review due to dislocation within 1 year of surgery when compared to the manual THA performed using the posterior approach [31].

2.4.3 Acetabular Reaming, Cup Implantation, and Leg Length Discrepancy

Kong et al. [32] assessed whether the laterality of hip arthroplasty would affect the positioning of the acetabular component and whether the robot could reduce the surgeon's impact on implant positioning. Although there was no statistical difference in the functional score for the pre- and postoperative periods, the anteversion of the implant in the left hip was significantly higher than in the right hip in the group for which surgery was performed manually, while statistical differences were not observed in the group receiving robot-assisted THA.

Additionally, the manual surgery group was more likely to present a difference in positioning between the bilateral hips (77% vs. 45%, $p = 0.000$) and positioning outside the target zones than in robot-assisted arthroplasties (70% vs. 48%, $p = 0.001$). It was concluded that the surgeon's laterality tended to influence positioning of the implants and robot-assisted arthroplasties were capable of eliminating this adverse effect. In another study in patients involving a minimum monitoring period of 5 years, functional scores (Harris Hip Score, Forgotten Joint Score-12, Veterans RAND-12 Mental, Veterans RAND-12 Physical, 12-Item Short Form Mental Survey, 12-Item Short Form Physical Survey, visual analog scale and satisfaction) were evaluated, in addition to implant positioning and revision rate comparing a group of 66 patients undergoing manual arthroplasty and 66 patients receiving the robot-assisted technique.

Placement of acetabular implant using robotic THA presented a ninefold and 4.7-fold reduction in risk of placement outside Lewinnek and Callanan "safe zones," respectively (relative risk, 0.11 [95% confidence interval, 0.03–0.46]; $p = 0.002$; relative risk, 0.21 [95% confidence interval, 0.01–0.47]; $p = 0.001$). Additionally, patients receiving assisted surgery presented lower absolute values for discrepancy in lower limb length, global displacement ($p = 0.091$, $p = 0.001$), and significantly higher functional scores [33].

During a meta-analysis that was carried out, 14 different articles were included, which revealed that the robot-assisted group presented fewer intraoperative complications, an improved angle, and higher safe zone placement rate than the group receiving a manual procedure. However, the two groups presented similar functional scores, as well as total number of complications [34].

2.4.4   Bone Preservation

Robotic-arm assisted THA has also been associated with preservation of bone stock. One study that was performed compared the size of the acetabular component in relation to the size of the femoral head in patients undergoing robotic surgery (MAKO) or manual surgery, with 57 representatives included in each group. The size of the acetabular dome in relation to the patient's native femoral head was significantly higher in the robotic surgery group when compared to the manual group, which implies that a reduced amount of bone loss occurs in robotic surgery [35].

2.4.5   Clinical Results

Three groups of 100 consecutive THAs (first 100 manual THAs; last 100 manual THAs; and first 100 Mako Total Hips), were reviewed. Mako Total Hip resulted in significantly higher modified HHSs (92.1 ± 10.5 vs. 86.1 ± 16.2, p = 0.002) and UCLA activity levels (6.3 ± 1.8 vs. 5.8 ± 1.7, p = 0.033) than manual THA at minimum one-year follow-up [36]. Patient satisfaction post-THA is high, where patient satisfaction at a minimum of two-year follow-up was assessed. For the Mako Total Hip cases considered in this study, mean patient satisfaction was a high 9.3 out of 10 [37].

2.4.6   Cost-Effectiveness

A study that was performed looked at the cost-benefit ratio of total hip arthroplasty performed using robotics compared to manual surgery, considering medical costs from the payer's point of view in order to observe the impact of choosing each treatment on the costs incurred. Potential outcomes were categorized as infection, dislocation, revision, or no complications, and their cumulative costs were counted for a period of 1 year over a 5-year study horizon [38].

Results for the cohort indicated a higher profitability of robotic-assisted arthroplasty when compared to the conventional method in terms of costs incurred by the healthcare system and private insurance providers during a 5-year period. Robot-assisted arthroplasty was found, on average, to reduce costs for Medicare and private insurance by $945 and $1810, respectively, when compared to conventional arthroplasty. It was therefore concluded that robot-assisted arthroplasty would be more effective than the traditional method in the public or private system when direct medical costs are considered [38].

A study that compared hospital metrics, including length of stay, discharge, hospital complications, and costs, was carried out, during which robotic-assisted, computer-assisted, and conventional arthroplasty were assessed using a database containing data from 4,699,894 arthroplasty procedures performed between 2008 and 2017. Both robot-assisted and computer-assisted THA presented above-average hospital costs relative to conventional arthroplasty, which suggested that more comprehensive cost analyses in terms of hospital costs and higher index procedures are needed in order to determine the true added value of robot-assisted THA in offering support for healthcare services [39].

Another model was constructed in order to evaluate the cost-effectiveness of robotic and conventional intervention in degenerative hip disease, using a 1-year evaluation cycle with a 5-year follow-up, with robotic surgery found to offer the most effective cost in 99.4% of the evaluated cases [40].

2.5 Disadvantages

2.5.1 Learning Curve

A retrospective study evaluated the cases handled by a single surgeon, analyzing the learning curve in the clinical surgical outcome for three groups: the first 100 patients receiving conventional THA (G1), 100 patients receiving conventional arthroplasty (G2), and the first 100 patients receiving robot-assisted THA (G3). Unlike the other two groups, there were no reported cases of dislocation at the 1-year market in the G3 group [41]. Redmond et al. analyzed the positioning of implants, the duration of surgery, and the rate of complications occurring since the start of their study on robotic procedures. This series assessed results for a single surgeon and also made use of three patient groups: group A with the first 35 patients, group B with the next 35, and group C with the final 35 patients. Given the accuracy of the implant and the time required to complete the operation, the author reported a rapid learning curve and a complete acquisition of the procedure after the first 35 cases [42].

For Kayani et al., a learning curve of 12 cases was observed in positioning of the acetabular dome through robotic assistance. The learning curve did not present a reported effect on accuracy in restoring native hip biomechanics or in obtaining the positioning and orientation of the acetabular implant proposed during preoperative planning [43].

2.5.2 Operative Time

Meta-analysis was used to assess three studies in terms of surgical time, and, although the results presented a shorter surgical time in conventional arthroplasty, the combined analysis of the data showed no statistically significant difference between conventional and robot-assisted groups [13].

Another study evaluated controlled clinical trials published between 1998 and 2018 with regard to the clinical efficacy of the two approaches. Results demonstrated that the conventional group required a shorter operating time when compared to the robot-assisted group (95% CI [7.50–33.94], $p = 0.002$) [34]. Heng et al. evaluated outcomes for surgical time, length of hospital stay, and surgical complications in patients undergoing robotic arthroplasty MAKO vs. manual surgery and surgical time in terms of the required learning curve: an average of 96.7 min was required for the robotic group and 84.9 min for the conventional group. However, the study suggested that each robotic operation was approximately 1 min shorter than the previous operation and the average time for the last ten cases was reduced to 82.9 min. It was therefore concluded that the learning curve involved in reducing operative time totaled 35 cases [44].

3 Complications

Data collected from 162 patients undergoing robotic arthroplasty with a minimum follow-up of 2 years revealed the following intra- and postoperative complications: three trochanteric fractures (1.9%), three calcaneus fractures (1.9%), two deep vein thromboses (1.3%), one infection (0.6%), one aseptic hematoma (0.6%), one foot drop (0.6%), and one case of loosening of the femoral stem (0.6%) [45].

A meta-analysis was carried out that included ten trials comparing the complications observed in robotic and conventional arthroplasty, which were subsequently divided into eight subgroups: intraoperative fracture, nerve paralysis, severe pain, knee pain, dislocation, hcterotopic ossification, revision surgery, and total number of complications. Results suggested that intraoperative complications were less frequent in robot-assisted THA, while fewer cases of dislocation and revision were seen in the conventional THA group. With regard to the total number of complications, there was no statistical difference observed between the methods [34].

4 Limitations

Robotic surgery has evolved over the years and its use in hip arthroplasty has the potential to improve accuracy in implant placement. Limitations, however, arise whenever the respective operation involves dependence on the engineering team and the respective cost-benefit ratio. Additionally, integration of the spinopelvic sagittal balance in the planning carried out by the software should also be taken into consideration during potential development of the systems, which is already underway in MAKO.

5 Conclusion

The use of robot-assisted hip arthroplasty has been increasing in recent years, and it is essential that surgeons familiarize themselves with the main differences between the options present under current systems available on the market, including autonomy, preoperative planning software, and implant options, and follow the most up-to-date literature on the subject. Robotic THA can achieve the same clinical results provided by traditional surgeries and offer fewer intraoperative complications and improved implant positioning. The traditional arthroplasty initially presented a shorter operating time and intraoperative bleeding. Within the current context, long-term performance data would help to better define the role that robotics play in hip arthroplasty and determine whether optimized implant positioning leads to improved implant survival over time.

References

1. Varacallo M, Chakravarty R, Denehy K, Star A. Joint perception and patient perceived satisfaction after total hip and knee arthroplasty in the American population. J Orthop. 2018;15(2):495–9.
2. Charnley J. The long-term results of low-friction arthroplasty of the hip performed as a primary intervention. J Bone Joint Surg (Br). 1972;54:61–76.
3. Subramanian P, et al. Hip Int. 2019;29(3):232–8. https://doi.org/10.1177/1120700019828286.
4. Liu Z, Gao Y, Cai L. Imageless navigation versus traditional method in Total hip arthroplasty (THA): a meta-analysis. Int J Surg. 2015;21:122–7.
5. Banerjee S, Cherian JJ, Elmallah RK, et al. Robot assisted total hip arthroplasty. Expert Rev Med Devices. 2016;13:47–56.
6. Paul HA, Bargar WL, Mittlestadt B, et al. Development of a surgical robot for cementless total hip arthroplasty. Clin Orthop. 1992;285:57–66.
7. Barrack RL. Dislocation after total hip arthroplasty (THA): implant design and orientation. J Am Acad Orthop Surg. 2003;11:89–99.
8. Renkawitz T, Haimerl M, Dohmen L, Gneiting S, Lechler P, Woerner M, Springorum HR, Weber M, Sussmann P, Sendt-ner E, Grifka J. The association between femoral tilt and impingement-free range-of-motion in total hip arthroplasty. BMC Musculoskelet Disord. 2012;13:65.
9. Kennedy JG, Rogers WB, Soffe KE, Sullivan RJ, Griffen DG, Sheehan LJ. Effect of acetabular component orientation on recurrent dislocation, pelvic osteolysis, polyethylene wear, and component migration. J Arthroplast. 1998;13:530–4.
10. El Bitar YF, Stone JC, Jackson TJ, Lindner D, Stake CE, Domb BG. Leg-length discrepancy after total hip arthroplasty (THA): comparison of robot-assisted posterior, fluoroscopy-guided anterior-rior, and conventional posterior approaches. Am J Orthop. 2015;44:265–9.

11. Capón-García D, López-Pardo A, Alves-Pérez MT. Causes for revision surgery in total hip replacement. A retrospective epidemiological analysis. Rev Esp Cir Ortop Traumatol. 2016;60:160–6.

12. Lewinnek GE, Lewis JL, Tarr R, Compere CL, Zimmerman JR. Dislocations after total hip-replacement arthroplasties. J Bone Joint Surg. 1978;60(2):217–20.

13. Chen X, Xiong J, Wang P, et al. Robotic assisted compared with conventional total hip arthroplasty (THA): systematic review and meta-analysis. Postgrad Med J. 2018;94(1112):335–41. https://doi.org/10.1136/postgradmedj-2017-135352.

14. Bargar WL. Robots in orthopaedic surgery past, present, and future. Clin Orthop Relat Res. (463):31–6.

15. Wu L, Hahne HJ, Hassenpflug J. The dimensional accuracy of preparation of femoral cavity in cementless THA. J Zhejiang Univ (Sci). 2004;5:1270–8.

16. Mazoochian F, Pellengahr C, Huber A, et al. Low accuracy of stem implantation in THR using the CASPAR-system: anteversion measurements in 10 hips. Acta Orthop Scand. 2004;75:261–4.

17. Siebel T, Käfer W. Clinical outcome following robotic assisted versus conventional THA: a controlled and prospective study of seventy-one patients. Z Orthop Ihre Grenzgeb. 2005;143:391–8.

18. Perets I, et al. Current topics in robotic-assisted total hip arthroplasty (THA): a review. Hip Int. 2020;30:118. https://doi.org/10.1177/1120700019893636.

19. Kouyoumdjian P, Mansour J, Assi C, Caton J, Lustig S, Coulomb R. Current concepts in robotic total hip arthroplasty. SICOT-J. 2020;6:45.

20. Qin J, Xu Z, Dai J, Chen D, Xu X, Song K, Shi D, Jiang Q. New technique: practical procedure of robotic arm-assisted (MAKO) total hip arthroplasty. Ann Transl Med. 2018;6(18):364. https://doi.org/10.21037/atm.2018.09.30.

21. Callanan MC, Jarrett B, Bragdon CR, et al. The john charnley award: risk factors for cup malpositioning: quality improvement through a joint registry at a tertiary hospital. Clin Orthop Relat Res. 2011;469:319–29.

22. O'Conner P, Thompson M, Esposito C, Poli N, McGree J, Donnelly T, Donnelly W. Change in pelvic position in total hip arthroplasty patients through functional range of motion. Bone Jt Open. 2021;2-10:834–41.

23. Tarwala R, Dorr LD. Robotic assisted THA using the MAKO platform. Curr Rev Musculoskelet Med. 2011;4:151–6.

24. Elson L, Dounchis J, Illgen R, et al. Precision of acetabular cup placement in robotic integrated total hip arthroplasty. Hip Int. 2015;25(6):531–36. https://doi.org/10.5301/hipint.5000289.

25. Domb BG, Redmond JM, Louis SS, et al. Accuracy of component positioning in 1980 total hip arthroplasties: a comparative analysis by surgical technique and mode of guidance. J Arthroplasty. 2015;30(12):2208 18. https://doi.org/10.1016/j.arth.2015.06.059.

26. Nawabi DH, Conditt MA, Ranawat AS, et al. Haptically guided robotic technology in total hip arthroplasty: a cadaveric investigation. Proc Inst Mech Eng H. 2013;227(3):302–09. https://doi.org/10.1177/0954411912468540.

27. Kamath AF, Durbhakula SM, Pickering T, Cafferky NL, Murray TG, Wind MA Jr, Méthot S. Improved accuracy and fewer outliers with a novel CT-free robotic THA system in matched-pair analysis with manual THA. J Robot Surg. 2021;16:905. https://doi.org/10.1007/s11701-021-01315-3. PMID: 34709535.

28. Pierce J, Needham K, Adams C, Coppolecchia A, Lavernia C. Robotic-assisted total hip arthroplasty (THA): an economic analysis. J Comp Eff Res. 2021;10(16):1225–34. https://doi.org/10.2217/cer-2020-0255. Epub 2021 Sep 28. PMID: 34581189.

29. Kirchner GJ, Lieber AM, Haislup B, Kerbel YE, Moretti VM. The cost of robot-assisted total hip arthroplasty (THA): comparing safety and hospital charges to conventional total hip arthroplasty. J Am Acad Orthop Surg. 2021;29(14):609–15. https://doi.org/10.5435/JAAOS-D-20-00715. PMID: 32991384.

30. Nd IRL, Bukowski BR, Abiola R, Anderson P, Chughtai M, Khlopas A, Mont MA. Robotic-assisted total hip arthroplasty (THA): outcomes at minimum two-year follow-up. Surg Technol Int. 2017;30:365–72. PMID: 28537647.

31. Bendich I, Vigdorchik JM, Sharma AK, Mayman DJ, Sculco PK, Anderson C, Della Valle AG, Su EP, Jerabek SA. Robotic assistance for posterior approach total hip arthroplasty is associated with lower risk of revision for dislocation when compared to manual techniques. J Arthroplast. 2022;37(6):1124–9. https://doi.org/10.1016/j.arth.2022.01.085. Epub 2022 Feb 4. PMID: 35124193.

32. Kong X, Yang M, Li X, et al. Impact of surgeon handedness in manual and robot-assisted total hip arthroplasty. J Orthop Surg Res. 2020;15(1):159. https://doi.org/10.1186/s13018-020-01671-0.

33. Domb BG, Chen JW, Lall AC, Perets I, Maldonado DR. Minimum 5-year outcomes of robotic-assisted primary total hip arthroplasty with a nested comparison against manual primary total hip arthroplasty (THA): the propensity score-matched study. J Am Acad Orthop Surg. 2020;28:847. https://doi.org/10.5435/JAAOS-D-19-00328.

34. Han PF, Chen CL, Zhang ZL, et al. Robotics-assisted versus conventional manual approaches for total hip arthroplasty (THA): a systematic review and meta-analysis of comparative studies. Int J Med Robot. 2019;15(3):e1990. https://doi.org/10.1002/rcs.1990.

35. Suarez-Ahedo C, Gui C, Martin TJ, Chandrasekaran S, Lodhia P, Domb BG. Robotic-arm assisted total hip arthroplasty results in smaller acetabular cup size in relation to the femoral head size: a matched-pair controlled study. Hip Int. 2017;27(2):147–52. https://doi.org/10.5301/hipint.5000418.

36. Bukowski BR, Anderson P, Khlopas A, Chughtai M, Mont MA, Illgen RL 2nd. Improved Functional Outcomes with Robotic Compared with Manual Total Hip Arthroplasty. Surg Technol Int. 2016;29:303–08.

37. Perets I, Walsh JP, Mu BH, Mansor Y, Rosinsky PJ, Maldonado DR, Lall AC, Domb BG. Short-term clinical outcomes of robotic-arm assisted total hip arthroplasty: a pair-matched controlled study. Orthopedics. 2021;44(2):e236–e242. https://doi.org/10.3928/01477447-20201119-10.

38. Maldonado DR, Go CC, Kyin C, Rosinsky PJ, Shapira J, Lall AC, Domb BG. Robotic arm-assisted total hip arthroplasty is more cost-effective than manual total hip arthroplasty (THA): a Markov model analysis. J Am Acad Orthop Surg. 2020;29:e168. https://doi.org/10.5435/JAAOS-D-20-00498.

39. Emara AK, Zhou G, Klika AK, Koroukian SM, Schiltz NK, Higuera-Rueda CA, Molloy RM, Piuzzi NS. Is there increased value in robotic arm-assisted total hip arthroplasty?: a nationwide outcomes, trends, and projections analysis of 4,699,894 cases. Bone Joint J. 2021;103-B(9):1488–96. https://doi.org/10.1302/0301-620X.103B9.BJJ-2020-2411.R1. PMID: 34465149.

40. Maldonado DR, Go CC, Kyin C, Rosinsky PJ, Shapira J, Lall AC, Domb BG. Robotic arm-assisted total hip arthroplasty is more cost-effective than manual total hip arthroplasty (THA): a Markov model analysis. J Am Acad Orthop Surg. 2021;29(4):e168–77. https://doi.org/10.5435/JAAOS-D-20-00498. PMID: 32694323.

41. Bukowski BR, Anderson P, Khlopas A, et al. Improved functional outcomes with robotic compared with manual total hip arthroplasty. Surg Technol Int. 2016;29:303–8.

42. Redmond JM, Gupta A, Hammarstedt JE, et al. The learning curve associated with robotic-assisted total hip arthroplasty. J Arthroplast. 2015;30:50–4.

43. Kayani B, Konan S, Huq SS, et al. The learning curve of robotic arm assisted acetabular cup positioning during total hip arthroplasty. Hip Int. 2019;31:311.

44. Heng YY, Gunaratne R, Ironside C, Taheri A. Conventional vs robotic arm assisted total hip arthroplasty (THA) surgical time, transfusion rates, length of stay, complications and learning curve. J Arthritis. 2018;7:272. https://doi.org/10.4172/2167-7921.1000272.

45. Perets I, Walsh JP, Close MR, Mu BH, Yuen LC, Domb BG. Robot-assisted total hip arthroplasty (THA): clinical outcomes and complication rate. Int J Med Robot. 2018;14(4):e1912. https://doi.org/10.1002/rcs.1912.

Robotic Systems in Ophthalmologic Surgery

Marina Roizenblatt, Ali Ebrahini, Iulian Iordachita, and Peter Louis Gehlbach

Abbreviations

FDA	Food and Drug Administration
ILM	Internal limiting membrane
IRISS	Intraocular robotic interventional surgical system
OCT	Optical coherence tomography
SHER	Steady-Hand Eye Robot
t-PA	Tissue plasminogen activators
US	United States

M. Roizenblatt (✉)
Department of Ophthalmology, Universidade Federal de São Paulo, São Paulo, Brazil

A. Ebrahini · I. Iordachita
Mechanical Engineering Department and Laboratory for Computational Sensing and Robotics (LCSR), Johns Hopkins University, Baltimore, MD, USA
e-mail: aebrahi5@jhu.edu; iordachita@jhu.edu

P. L. Gehlbach
Mechanical Engineering Department and Laboratory for Computational Sensing and Robotics (LCSR), Johns Hopkins University, Baltimore, MD, USA

Wilmer Eye Institute, Johns Hopkins Hospital, Baltimore, MD, USA
e-mail: pgelbach@jhmi.edu

© The Author(s), under exclusive license to Springer Nature Switzerland AG 2023
J. P. Manzano, L. M. Ferreira (eds.), *Robotic Surgery Devices in Surgical Specialties*, https://doi.org/10.1007/978-3-031-35102-0_12

1 Introduction

Robot-assisted surgery in a human patient was first reported by Kwoh in 1985 when the PUMA 560 robotic surgical arm was used for a neurosurgical needle biopsy while being guided by computed tomography [1]. Since then, robot-assisted surgery has found a growing niche in medicine, gradually becoming integral to improvements in surgical care, with potential applicability across numerous surgical specialties. Present and emerging robotic systems promise improvements in surgical scope, capability, efficacy, reproducibility, safety, and cost—over manually performed procedures. This is due in part to their increased precision, ability to reproducibly perform repetitive tasks, and the ability to overcome a number of human physiological limitations. Integrating robotics with other support capabilities such as imaging systems and sensors further extends the relevant competence of human-robot cooperation.

The expansion of robotic applications in the field of minimally invasive surgery has been marked by success, with systems such as the da Vinci (Intuitive Surgical Inc., Sunnyvale, CA, USA) being perhaps the most notable to date. Despite rapid implementation in surgery, the near-term intention is not for robots to replace surgeons, but that they function as assistants. Potential roles include but are not limited to working cooperatively directly with the surgeon or in the role of a specialized tool directed by the surgeon. Therefore, the concept of robot-assisted surgery is at present a most fitting framework by which to envision the role of robotics in microsurgery [2].

Ophthalmic microsurgery is a highly specialized microsurgical niche dealing with surgical procedures performed on the eye. Of the various ophthalmic microsurgical subspecialty areas, intraocular vitreoretinal microsurgery remains among the most technically challenging, despite recent advances in the field. The use of robotics offers numerous potential solutions to the challenges of retinal microsurgery, which include, but are not limited to, a confined space, a fragile and nonregenerative surgical target, micron-scale movement requirements, and visualization challenges [3].

Unassisted ophthalmic surgery requires a dexterous, stable, and precise surgical approach that lies at the limits of human motor function to perform [4]. Membrane peeling in vitreoretinal surgery, for instance, is known as one of the most delicate routinely performed surgical tasks, not only in ophthalmology but among all microsurgical disciplines. In this setting, microsurgical force measurement experiments show that typical intraoperative forces applied to retinal tissue by microsurgical instrument tips are routinely less than 7.5 mN. Forces on this order of magnitude are often below the threshold of the surgeon's tactile sensitivity [5–7]. Further complicating retinal membrane peeling is surgeon physiological hand tremor, which can prevent procedure completion and significantly increase the risk of iatrogenic retinal damage from unintentional tool-to-tissue contact [8]. Another challenge to be overcome encompasses the ergonomic aspects of ophthalmologic surgical practice that may predispose ophthalmologists to a high rate of acquired musculoskeletal disorders at a relatively early career age.

With these and other factors in mind, robotic technology has continued to develop with current advancements nearing feasibility for routine clinical use. The barriers of dexterity, visualization, force perception, tremor, and ergonomics in ophthalmic surgery have all been significantly diminished by recent advancements in robotics for microsurgery [9–12]. Despite these and other improvements, vitreoretinal surgery still has many challenges to overcome. As a result, many studies developing robotic applications in ophthalmic surgery focus on vitreoretinal surgery. This chapter presents an overview of potential current vitreoretinal applications and the role of the prevalent robotic platforms developed to date (Fig. 1).

Robotic technology has only recently begun to be integrated into the ocular microsurgery field; therefore, its development, progress, and penetration are in their infancy relative to other surgical disciplines where the role is now better defined. This relative delay in robotic adoption is in part attributed to unique technological challenges present in ocular surgery. Barriers such as the need to operate on the order of millinewton (mN) forces and on single micron-scale surgical targets and others have delayed the full promise of a robotic system for vitreoretinal surgery [13]. Another potential explanation for delayed adoption of robotics into vitreoretinal surgery relates to application-specific challenges inherent in engineering machines that work safely and with micrometer precision, within a fragile and tightly confined anatomic work space. A high cost, intrinsic learning curves, longer surgical times, and patient acceptance present other current challenges to robotics in ophthalmology [14].

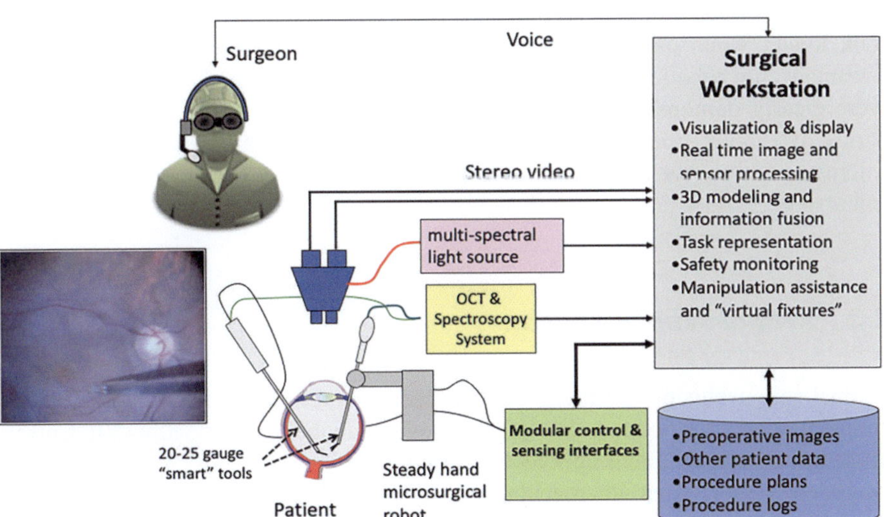

Fig. 1 Flowchart showing possible interactions between the ophthalmic surgeon and the robotic assistant

2 Ophthalmic Diseases That May Benefit from Robot-Assisted Surgery

2.1 Membrane Peeling

In retinal microsurgery, precise manipulation of delicate and often transparent tissues is carried out by applying very small forces, the majority of which are below the surgeons' tactile sensory threshold [15]. Membrane peeling is a common task in vitreoretinal surgery, during which excessive peeling forces or inopportune maneuvers can lead to retinal trauma, hemorrhage, and tears. Iatrogenic operative trauma may be a cause of prolonged surgery times, failure to achieve surgical objectives, and suboptimal visual outcomes [16, 17]. Membrane peeling is among the essential tasks in vitreoretinal surgery and has generally been accepted as a fundamental step in prevalent procedures such as macular hole repair (internal limiting membrane (ILM) peeling) or in epiretinal membrane removal (epiretinal membrane peeling, which can also be associated, or not, with ILM peeling). The ILM is an approximately 2.5 µm thick layer [18] formed by a basement membrane that constitutes the boundary between the retina and vitreous surface. It is adherent to the retinal surface and is transparent, requiring staining to visualize well. The goal of ILM peeling is to delaminate this micron-scale fibrous membrane from the inner retinal surface and relieve pathologic tractional forces from the retinal surface.

With this background, Edwards et al. [19] reported the first-in-human study that used a teleoperated robotic device called Preceyes to perform membrane peeling surgery, in 2018. Twelve patients undergoing dissection of an epiretinal or internal limiting were randomly assigned to either robot-assisted or freehand surgery. Surgical outcomes were not significantly different in either group and the procedure took longer when performed with the robot. Despite no clear measurable early advantage for robotic assistance, high precision and minimal tremor maneuvers were clearly demonstrated in the human eye. As a result, this proof-of-concept series of robotic microsurgical procedures has opened the field of ophthalmic microsurgery to potential next-level improvements and applications in robotic microsurgery.

2.2 Retinal Vein Cannulation

Retinal vein occlusion is among the most prevalent retinal vascular disorders and a frequent cause of vision loss that is second only to diabetic retinopathy [20]. Current standard of care treatment options focus on mitigating downstream sequelae of the occluded vessel, such as macular edema, retinal neovascularization, vitreous hemorrhage, and traction retinal detachment, rather than directly addressing the retinal vascular occlusion. While each of the complications of retinal vein occlusion has management options that are variably effective (laser therapy, intraocular injections of steroid or anti-VEGF drugs, and surgical approaches), none of these definitively addresses the underlying cause (vascular occlusion) and even when successful can leave the patient in chronic therapy and with some level of continued vision loss [20, 21].

Weiss et al. [22] demonstrated the relative safety of performing vitrectomy followed by freehand retinal vein cannulation for infusion of tissue plasminogen activators (t-PA) directly to the thrombus. The hypothesis was that this would improve vision. Twenty-eight patients with central retinal vein occlusion and vision loss were enrolled. However, 25% of this study population experienced procedure-related postoperative vitreous hemorrhages and one patient had a postoperative retinal detachment, demonstrating just some of the technical challenges inherent in this unassisted freehand approach.

Human retinal veins are at their largest most proximally just prior to entering the optic nerve. At this point they measure on the order of 125 μm. By way of comparison the size of one of the smallest structures that vitreoretinal surgeons target for treatment, the ILM, is on the order of 2.5 μm [18]. Human hand tremor is variable but it is not unusual for it to be on the order of 100 μm when translated to the tip of a vitreoretinal instrument [23]. Therefore, for vitreoretinal microsurgery to be performed, human physiological tremor must be overcome. Robotic assistance using fully stabilized robotic tools is a logical potential approach. In the case of treating retinal vein occlusion, a further advantage of robotic assistance is not only the provision of efficient and safe cannulation, but also the intraluminal stabilization of the needle in the vein, allowing for the extended infusion period required for delivery of therapeutic agent to the thrombus [24].

Various robotic assistant modalities have been proposed over the past 20 years [25]. However in 2018 the world's first-in-human robot-assisted retinal vein cannulation study was performed [21]. Four patients diagnosed with retinal vein occlusion were treated using the KU Leuven robot, a co-manipulated robotic assistance device. This investigation demonstrated that it was technically feasible to safely inject an anticoagulant into a 100 μm width retinal vein over a "prolonged period" of 10 min, using robotic assistance.

2.3 Subretinal Injections

The field of gene therapy has made remarkable strides in recent years. The United States (US) Food and Drug Administration (FDA) approval of Luxturna in 2017 (the first US gene therapy for a genetic disease) marked a new cycle of innovation in ophthalmic therapy [26]. Luxturna is an intraocular suspension with a gene transfer vector that employs an adeno-associated viral vector capsid as a delivery vehicle for the human DNA necessary to replace the protein product of the RPE65 gene in the retinal pigment epithelium, via injection into the subretinal space. However, the emerging era of ocular gene therapy extends beyond Luxturna, bringing a broad array of new treatments for inherited retinal disease [27].

In this context, subretinal drug delivery has become increasingly useful and accepted in both scientific research and clinical application due to the more direct effects on the targeted cells in the subretinal space. This provides a new therapeutic method for vitreoretinal diseases, including but not limited to gene therapy [28]. Ideally, subretinal injection would result in the placement of the entire therapeutic solution in the subretinal space in immediate proximity to the targeted photoreceptors and RPE cells [29].

Unlike intravitreal drug delivery, which is relatively simple in practice, subretinal delivery is associated with a number of technical challenges. Moreover, its effectiveness relies on several factors, including the surgical delivery of drug to the subretinal space while minimizing eye trauma and any negative effects on the therapeutic agent. Similar to vein cannulation, subretinal injection not only involves accessing the correct anatomical space but also requires the ability to maintain the needle tip position stably in the correct position for the entire (sometimes prolonged) duration of drug injection. Among the challenges to performing minimally traumatic injections is the ability to form and maintain an injection bleb without drug refluxing throughout the duration of the injection phase. To achieve this, it is essential to minimize surgeon tremor to avoid enlargement of the needle entry point and injury to the associated tissues [30].

Faced with such novel surgical challenges, Ladha et al. [29] recently published a comparison between manual and robotic assistance in simulated subretinal injections in an artificial retina model using Preceyes Surgical System (Preceyes BV, Eindhoven, the Netherlands) as the robotic platform. They showed that the robotic device was associated with improved tremor, diminished retinal entry hole size, prolonged allowable injection times, and a higher rate of bleb formation with a reduction in drug reflux through the injection entry point. Edwards et al. [19] have used the Preceyes teleoperated robot to successfully inject recombinant t-PA beneath the retina to displace sight-threatening hemorrhage in three patients. This work reinforces the concept of robotic assistance for subretinal injections in the setting of retinal gene therapy.

3   Ophthalmic Robotic Devices

The ophthalmic robots can be broadly categorized into three main groups: teleoperated systems, co-manipulated or cooperative platforms, and handheld robots.

3.1   *Teleoperated Robots*

Telerobotic surgery represents a major area of interest and progress over the last decade due in part to the substantial number of potential high impact applications. Telepresence is the presentation of a remote environment in a natural way, thus generating a sense of presence in remote locations. This concept describes the basis of both telemedicine and telerobotics [31]. The increasing acceptance of robot-assisted surgery commensurate with advances in telecommunications has led to progress in related technology and the further development and the use of telemedicine, extending from telepresence to telesurgery [32]. Teleoperated robotic surgical systems now allow a surgeon who is remotely located to provide various levels of training or patient care from a distance [16].

Teleoperated robotic platforms are divided into two main components: a master console, where the surgeon receives visual and tactile feedback, allowing him/her to control the active part of the robot, which is called the follower console and is located in a remote location [33]. The da Vinci Surgical System was the first telemanipulation robot to receive complete FDA approval [34] and has since been widely applied in various types of minimally invasive surgery. However, the microscopic scale of eye surgery and the rotational instability of the globe within the orbit place additional demands on the system that preclude the implementation of da Vinci-like systems in the ophthalmic surgical field [35].

To date, the Preceyes Surgical System is not only the first robotic device to be used in a safety and feasibility study for intraocular robotic surgery but also the first robotic surgery system dedicated to ophthalmology to become commercially available (Fig. 2) [19]. Originated in the Netherlands, the Preceyes robot positions the surgeon at the head of the operating table, where the robot is attached to a headrest. A motion controller positioned in the surgical field records the surgeon's movements, which are filtered in real time and enhanced by a computer before being transmitted to the slave console. In addition, Preceyes utilizes a hybrid approach that allows intraoperative switching from freehand to robot-assisted surgical steps and to simultaneously operate the robot with one hand while manipulating a handheld instrument with the other.

The intraocular robotic interventional surgical system (IRISS) is another example of a teleoperated robot [36]. It was developed through a partnership between the Department of Mechanical and Aerospace Engineering of the University of California and the Jules Stein Eye Institute, motivated by the goal of performing

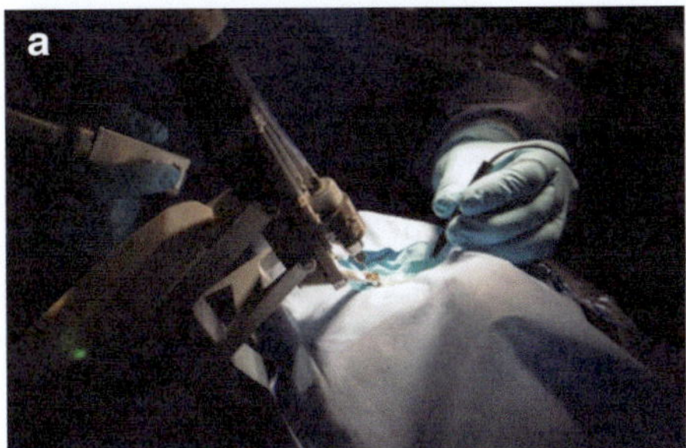
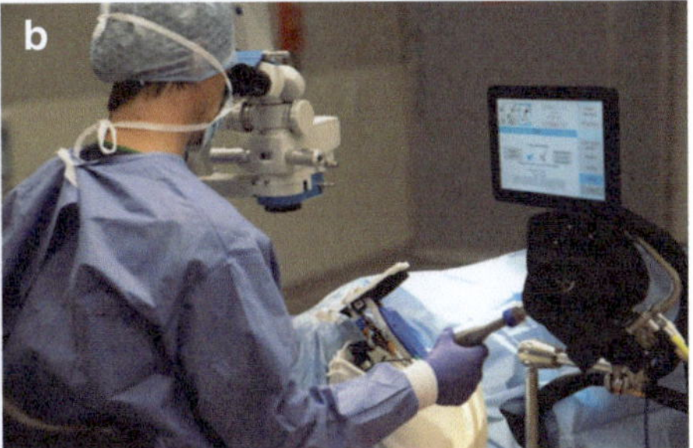

Fig. 2 (**a**) The Preceyes Surgical System developed by the Preceyes BV, Eindhoven, the Netherlands. (**b**) Operating room setup. (Figure kindly provided by Dr. Gerrit Naus, CEO and Co-founder Preceyes BV, Eindhoven, the Netherlands)

complete, multistep, intraocular surgical procedures. The IRISS master console includes two joysticks and the robotic tissue manipulator (slave side) consists of two independently controllable arms, each capable of holding two automatically interchangeable surgical tools. These tools may consist of many types of commercially available microsurgical instruments that have been adapted to fit the surgical manipulator with a large range of motion. The robotic platform is positioned between the patient and surgeon in the surgical setup, in a way that the surgeon works from a surgical cockpit. The IRISS has been shown to be effective in completing many key steps in a variety of intraocular surgical procedures in postmortem porcine eyes, such as capsulorhexis, lens cortex removal, core vitrectomy, and retinal vein cannulation, and is now capable of performing an entire cataract extraction [37]. Therefore, this teleoperated system may eventually be suitable for performing both anterior and posterior segment ocular surgery.

3.2   Co-manipulated/Cooperative Robots

In a co-manipulated, also known as a cooperative robotic, system, the surgeon holds and maintains direct manual control over the motion of the surgical tool, which is simultaneously held by the robotic platform. The robot is then able to provide direct assistive compensation to the surgeon, e.g., physiologic human hand tremor or others, to meet the performance, accuracy, and safety requirements of microsurgery [13, 38–41]. Various surgical instruments, whether conventional or "smart," can be attached to the robotic tool holder [38, 42, 43].

In this setting, the Steady-Hand Eye Robot (SHER) was developed by the Johns Hopkins University research team (Fig. 3) [44, 45]. This device is able to cooperatively guide instruments enabled to sense micro-forces exerted by the

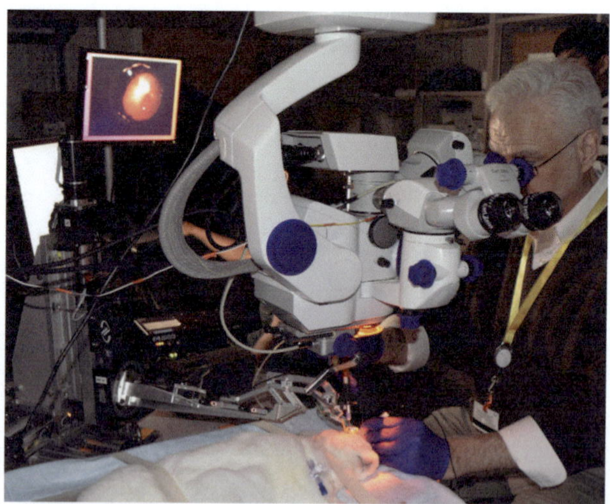

Fig. 3 The Steady-Hand Eye Robot developed by Johns Hopkins University

instrument to the eye, and to filter out any tremor via the robot's stiff mechanical structure, as it follows the user's motion [46–49]. In addition, the SHER is also capable of detecting tool tip micro-forces, in a way that provides effective assistance to perform surgical tasks safely and efficiently [44, 50–55]. Balicki et al. [56] went beyond the force sensing feature and integrated OCT-based distance sensors at the robot tool tip to enable vitreoretinal surgical interventions that utilized the maintenance of a constant distance from the retina, thereby avoiding inadvertent collision with tissue, as well as facilitating the targeting of anatomical structures inside of the eye.

Despite continuing improvements, the American SHER remains in preclinical development. The first, and for now the only one, co-manipulated robotic assistance device that has migrated to the living human eye environment as a clinically applicable robotic platform is a Belgian robot [57] that in 2018 successfully injected an anticoagulant into the retinal veins of four patients with retinal vein occlusion. The injections were carried out over 10 min in a phase 1 clinical trial [21]. This device consists of a parallel arm mechanism with a mechanical remote center of motion controlled through a spherical mechanism that provides motion scaling, tremor compensation, and scaled force feedback [13].

Although more complex than the handheld robots, the co-manipulated robots can still be built at a lower cost than teleoperated platforms due to the non-requirement for separate master and follower consoles [58]. A limitation of co-manipulated robots is their inability to provide variable motion scaling, semi-automation of surgical tasks, or improved ergonomic conditions for surgeons, as compared to teleoperated systems [35].

3.3 Handheld Robots

The handheld robots are manually operated enhanced surgical instruments equipped with a limited distance sensing and servo action capability that allows autonomy. The tools provide the user with real-time information during each surgical maneuver, and a resulting automated response that, depending on the function, can compensate for the surgeon's physiological limits in the challenging surgical environment of the eye [59, 60]. While guided and manipulated by the surgeon's hand, the handheld robots can correct actions, attenuate interaction forces with the target tissue, and augment surgical capabilities to an optimized level during each step of the surgical procedure [61, 62].

An example of such a function is providing real-time force information during tissue manipulation at levels beneath human tactile abilities [63]. Tool action is programmed to respond to various force levels, potentially limiting excess force related to surgical complications. Visual, tactile, and auditory feedback are among the effective ways to communicate intraoperative forces to a surgeon [16, 64]. Similarly, obtaining live intraocular optical coherence tomography (OCT) scans during surgery can direct surgeon decision making based on intraoperative

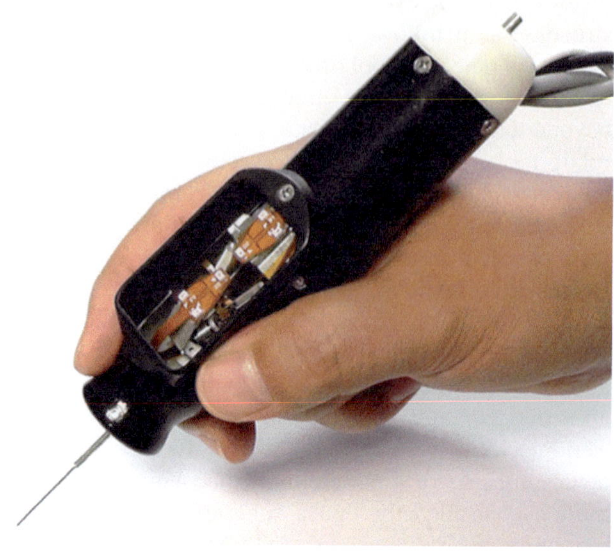

Fig. 4 The Micron handheld micromanipulator from Carnegie Mellon University

information [65]. An active handheld OCT imaging system developed by Yang et al. [66] is capable of canceling hand tremor, as is the Micron [67], which consists of an externally guided portable micromanipulator designed to remove tremor and increase positional accuracy (Fig. 4).

Handheld instruments are intrinsically intuitive for a surgeon to handle, mechanically simpler, and significantly less expensive to produce than large robotic platforms. Moreover, the motion control of the tool remains in the surgeon's hands, which may enhance safety, as the surgeon can manually finish a procedure in the case of robotic failure or unexpected patient movement. Alternatively handheld robots can simply be used to perform the portions of a procedure that are less effectively/efficiently executed freehand [68, 69]. An inherent limitation of handheld robots is the requirement to be continuously held and guided by the surgeon [58].

4 Conclusion

Ophthalmic surgery, and especially vitreoretinal surgery, represents a unique set of opportunities amenable to the potential advantages of robotic surgery. Increasingly widespread use of robotic platforms and a greater number of potential applications in the ophthalmologic surgical field are expected. Now however, the implementation of the full potential of surgical robotics in ophthalmology relies on the further development of technological platforms and integrated robotic systems that add significant value over current manual surgical techniques. Ultimately, the surgeon equipped with a robotic system will be able to perform procedures that are currently impossible in a freehand environment. It is expected that further developments will improve the safety, efficiency, efficacy, and cost of these robot-assisted procedures.

Acknowledgment Dr. Roizenblatt reports receiving research funding from Lemann Foundation, Instituto da Visão, Latinofarma, and Coordination of Improvement of Higher Education Personnel. Dr. Gehlbach reports receiving research funding from Research to Prevent Blindness and gifts from the J. Willard and Alice S Marriott Foundation, the Gale Trust, Herb Ehlers, Bill Wilbur and Rajandre Shaw, Helen Nassif, Mary Ellen Keck, Don and Maggie Feiner, and Ronald Stiff. Dr. Maia and Dr. Belfort Jr. report receiving research funding from the National Council of Scientific and Technological Development. Dr. Iordachita reports receiving funding from US National Institutes of Health under grant numbers of 1R01EB023943-01 and 1R01EB025883-01. Ali Ebrahimi reports receiving funding from Link Foundation. The abovementioned institutions had no role in the design and conduct of the study; collection, management, analysis, and interpretation of the data; preparation; and review.

Conflicts of Interest No conflicting relationship exists for any author.

References

1. Kwoh YS, Hou J, Jonckheere EA, Hayati S. A robot with improved absolute positioning accuracy for CT guided stereotactic brain surgery. IEEE Trans Biomed Eng. 1988;35(2):153–60.
2. Davies B. A review of robotics in surgery. Proc Inst Mech Eng H J Eng Med. 2000;214(1):129–40.
3. Gehlbach PL. Robotic surgery for the eye. Nat Biomed Eng. 2018;2(9):627–8.
4. He B, de Smet MD, Sodhi M, Etminan M, Maberley D. A review of robotic surgical training: establishing a curriculum and credentialing process in ophthalmology. Eye. 2021;35:3192.
5. Gupta PK, Jensen PS, de Juan E. Surgical forces and tactile perception during retinal microsurgery. International conference on medical image computing and computer-assisted intervention. New York, NY: Springer; 1999.
6. Berkelman PJ, Whitcomb LL, Taylor RH, Jensen P. A miniature microsurgical instrument tip force sensor for enhanced force feedback during robot-assisted manipulation. IEEE Trans Robot Autom. 2003;19(5):917–21.
7. He C, Roizenblatt M, Patel N, Ebrahimi A, Yang Y, Gehlbach PL, et al. Towards bimanual robot-assisted retinal surgery: tool-to-sclera force evaluation. Proc IEEE Sens. 2018;2018:1701.
8. Roizenblatt M, Grupenmacher AT, Belfort Junior R, Maia M, Gehlbach PL. Robot-assisted tremor control for performance enhancement of retinal microsurgeons. Br J Ophthalmol. 2019;103(8):1195–200.
9. Ahronovich EZ, Simaan N, Joos KM. A review of robotic and OCT-aided systems for vitreoretinal surgery. Adv Ther. 2021;38(5):2114–29.
10. Roizenblatt M, Edwards TL, Gehlbach PL. Robot-assisted vitreoretinal surgery: current perspectives. Robot Surg. 2018;5:1–11.
11. He C, Yang E, Patel N, Ebrahimi A, Shahbazi M, Gehlbach P, et al. Automatic light pipe actuating system for bimanual robot-assisted retinal surgery. IEEE ASME Trans Mechatron. 2020;25(6):2846–57.
12. Ebrahimi A, Urias M, Patel N, Gehlbach P, Alambeigi F, Iordachita I. FBG-based Kalman filtering and control of tool insertion depth for safe robot-assisted vitrectomy. Int Symp Med Robot. 2020;2020:1.
13. Gerber MJ, Pettenkofer M, Hubschman JP. Advanced robotic surgical systems in ophthalmology. Eye. 2020;34(9):1554–62.

14. Pandey SK, Sharma V. Robotics and ophthalmology: are we there yet? Indian J Ophthalmol. 2019;67(7):988–94.
15. Gonenc B, Chamani A, Handa J, Gehlbach P, Taylor RH, Iordachita I. 3-DOF force-sensing motorized micro-forceps for robot-assisted vitreoretinal surgery. IEEE Sensors J. 2017;17(11):3526–41.
16. Channa R, Iordachita I, Handa JT. Robotic vitreoretinal surgery. Retina. 2017;37(7):1220–8.
17. Gonenc B, Gehlbach P, Taylor RH, Iordachita I. Safe tissue manipulation in retinal microsurgery via motorized instruments with force sensing. Proc IEEE Sens. 2017;2017:1.
18. Rodrigues EB, Meyer CH, Farah ME, Kroll P. Intravitreal staining of the internal limiting membrane using indocyanine green in the treatment of macular holes. Ophthalmologica. 2005;219(5):251–62.
19. Edwards TL, Xue K, Meenink HCM, Beelen MJ, Naus GJL, Simunovic MP, et al. First-in-human study of the safety and viability of intraocular robotic surgery. Nat Biomed Eng. 2018;2:649–56.
20. Rehak J, Rehak M. Branch retinal vein occlusion: pathogenesis, visual prognosis, and treatment modalities. Curr Eye Res. 2008;33(2):111–31.
21. Gijbels A, Smits J, Schoevaerdts L, Willekens K, Vander Poorten EB, Stalmans P, et al. In-human robot-assisted retinal vein cannulation, a world first. Ann Biomed Eng. 2018;46(10):1676–85.
22. Weiss JN, Bynoe LA. Injection of tissue plasminogen activator into a branch retinal vein in eyes with central retinal vein occlusion. Ophthalmology. 2001;108(12):2249–57.
23. Riviere CN, Rader RS, Khosla PK. Characteristics of hand motion of eye surgeons. Proceedings of the 19th Annual International Conference of the IEEE Engineering in Medicine and Biology Society 'Magnificent Milestones and Emerging Opportunities in Medical Engineering' (Cat No 97CH36136); 1997, Washington, DC: IEEE.
24. Sommersperger M, Weiss J, Ali Nasseri M, Gehlbach P, Iordachita I, Navab N. Real-time tool to layer distance estimation for robotic subretinal injection using intraoperative 4D OCT. Biomed Opt Express. 2021;12(2):1085–104.
25. Ebrahimi A, Roizenblatt M, Patel N, Gehlbach P, Iordachita I. Auditory feedback effectiveness for enabling safe sclera force in robot-assisted vitreoretinal surgery: a multi-user study. Rep U S. 2020;2020:3274.
26. Ciulla TA, Hussain RM, Berrocal AM, Nagiel A. Voretigene neparvovec-rzyl for treatment of RPE65-mediated inherited retinal diseases: a model for ocular gene therapy development. Expert Opin Biol Ther. 2020;20(6):565–78.
27. Prado DA, Acosta-Acero M, Maldonado RS. Gene therapy beyond luxturna: a new horizon of the treatment for inherited retinal disease. Curr Opin Ophthalmol. 2020;31(3):147–54.
28. Peng Y, Tang L, Zhou Y. Subretinal injection: a review on the novel route of therapeutic delivery for vitreoretinal diseases. Ophthalmic Res. 2017;58(4):217–26.
29. Ladha R, Meenink T, Smit J, de Smet MD. Advantages of robotic assistance over a manual approach in simulated subretinal injections and its relevance for gene therapy. Gene Ther. 2021;30:264.
30. Xue K, Groppe M, Salvetti AP, MacLaren RE. Technique of retinal gene therapy: delivery of viral vector into the subretinal space. Eye. 2017;31(9):1308–16.
31. Aracil R, Buss M, Cobos S, Ferre M, Hirche S, Kuschel M, et al. The human role in telerobotics. Advances in telerobotics. New York, NY: Springer; 2007. p. 11–24.
32. Evans CR, Medina MG, Dwyer AM. Telemedicine and telerobotics: from science fiction to reality. Updat Surg. 2018;70(3):357–62.
33. Farajiparvar P, Ying H, Pandya A. A brief survey of telerobotic time delay mitigation. Front Robot AI. 2020;7:578805.
34. Himpens J, Leman G, Cadiere GB. Telesurgical laparoscopic cholecystectomy. Surg Endosc. 1998;12(8):1091.
35. Xue K, Edwards T, Meenink H, Beelen M, Naus G, Simunovic M, et al. Robot-assisted retinal surgery: overcoming human limitations. Surgical retina. New York, NY: Springer; 2019. p. 109–14.

36. Rahimy E, Wilson J, Tsao TC, Schwartz S, Hubschman JP. Robot-assisted intraocular surgery: development of the IRISS and feasibility studies in an animal model. Eye. 2013;27(8):972–8.
37. Wilson JT, Gerber MJ, Prince SW, Chen CW, Schwartz SD, Hubschman JP, et al. Intraocular robotic interventional surgical system (IRISS): mechanical design, evaluation, and master-slave manipulation. Int J Med Robot Comput Assist Surg. 2018;14(1):1.
38. Fleming I, Balicki M, Koo J, Iordachita I, Mitchell B, Handa J, et al. Cooperative robot assistant for retinal microsurgery. Med Image Comput Comput Assist Intervent. 2008;11(Pt 2):543–50.
39. Ebrahimi A, Patel N, He C, Gehlbach P, Kobilarov M, Iordachita I. Adaptive control of sclera force and insertion depth for safe robot-assisted retinal surgery. IEEE Int Conf Robot Autom. 2019;2019:9073–9.
40. Ebrahimi A, Urias M, Patel N, He C, Taylor RH, Gehlbach P, et al. Towards securing the sclera against patient involuntary head movement in robotic retinal surgery. Roman. 2019;2019:1.
41. Ebrahimi A, Alambeigi F, Sefati S, Patel N, He C, Gehlbach P, et al. Stochastic force-based insertion depth and tip position estimations of flexible FBG-equipped instruments in robotic retinal surgery. IEEE ASME Trans Mechatron. 2021;26(3):1512–23.
42. Cheon GW, Gonenc B, Taylor RH, Gehlbach PL, Kang JU. Motorized micro-forceps with active motion guidance based on common-path SSOCT for epiretinal membranectomy. IEEE ASME Trans Mechatron. 2017;22(6):2440–8.
43. Zhou M, Wu J, Ebrahimi A, Patel N, He C, Gehlbach P, et al. Spotlight-based 3D instrument guidance for retinal surgery. Int Symp Med Robot. 2020;2020:1.
44. Uneri A, Balicki MA, Handa J, Gehlbach P, Taylor RH, Iordachita I. New steady-hand eye robot with micro-force sensing for vitreoretinal surgery. Proc IEEE/RAS-EMBS Int Conf Biomed Robot Biomechatron. 2010;2010(26–29):814–9.
45. Taylor R, Jensen P, Whitcomb L, Barnes A, Kumar R, Stoianovici D, et al. A steady-hand robotic system for microsurgical augmentation. Int J Robot Res. 1999;18(12):1201–10.
46. He C, Ebrahimi A, Roizenblatt M, Patel N, Yang Y, Gehlbach PL, et al. User behavior evaluation in robot-assisted retinal surgery. Roman. 2018;2018:174–9.
47. He C, Patel N, Shahbazi M, Yang Y, Gehlbach P, Kobilarov M, et al. Toward safe retinal microsurgery: development and evaluation of an RNN-based active interventional control framework. IEEE Trans Biomed Eng. 2020;67(4):966–77.
48. Ebrahimi A, Urias M, Patel N, Taylor RH, Gehlbach PL, Iordachita I. Adaptive control improves sclera force safety in robot-assisted eye surgery: a clinical study. IEEE Trans Biomed Eng. 2021;68:3356.
49. Ebrahimi A, He C, Patel N, Kobilarov M, Gehlbach P, Iordachita I. Sclera force control in robot-assisted eye surgery: adaptive force control vs. auditory feedback. Int Symp Med Robot. 2019;2019:1.
50. Balicki M, Uneri A, Iordachita I, Handa J, Gehlbach P, Taylor R. Micro-force sensing in robot assisted membrane peeling for vitreoretinal surgery. Med Image Comput Comput Assist Intervent. 2010;13(Pt 3):303–10.
51. He C, Ebrahimi A, Yang E, Urias M, Yang Y, Gehlbach P, et al. Towards bimanual vein cannulation: preliminary study of a bimanual robotic system with a dual force constraint controller. IEEE Int Conf Robot Autom. 2020;2020:4441–7.
52. Wu J, He C, Zhou M, Ebrahimi A, Urias M, Patel NA, et al. Force-based safe vein cannulation in robot-assisted retinal surgery: a preliminary study. Int Symp Med Robot. 2020;2020:1.
53. Alamdar A, Patel N, Urias MG, Ebrahimi A, Gehlbach PL, Iordachita I. Force and velocity based puncture detection in robot assisted retinal vein cannulation: in-vivo study. IEEE Trans Biomed Eng. 2021;2021:1.
54. Ebrahimi A, Alambeigi F, Zimmer-Galler IE, Gehlbach P, Taylor RH, Iordachita I. Toward improving patient safety and surgeon comfort in a synergic robot-assisted eye surgery: a comparative study. Rep U S. 2019;2019:7075–82.
55. Patel N, Urias M, Ebrahimi A, Gehlbach P, Iordachita I. Scleral force evaluation during vitreoretinal surgery: in an in vivo rabbit eye model. Annu Int Conf IEEE Eng Med Biol Soc. 2020;2020:6049–53.

56. Balicki M, Han JH, Iordachita I, Gehlbach P, Handa J, Taylor R, et al. Single fiber optical coherence tomography microsurgical instruments for computer and robot-assisted retinal surgery. Med Image Comput Comput Assist Intervent. 2009;12(Pt 1):108–15.
57. Gijbels A, Willekens K, Esteveny L, Stalmans P, Reynaerts D, Vander Poorten EB. Towards a clinically applicable robotic assistance system for retinal vein cannulation. Proc IEEE Ras-Embs Int. 2016:284–91.
58. de Smet MD, Naus GJL, Faridpooya K, Mura M. Robotic-assisted surgery in ophthalmology. Curr Opin Ophthalmol. 2018;29(3):248–53.
59. Gonenc B, Chae J, Gehlbach P, Taylor RH, Iordachita I. Towards robot-assisted retinal vein cannulation: a motorized force-sensing microneedle integrated with a handheld micromanipulator. Sensors. 2017;17(10):2195.
60. Horise Y, He X, Gehlbach P, Taylor R, Iordachita I. FBG-based sensorized light pipe for robotic intraocular illumination facilitates bimanual retinal microsurgery. Annu Int Conf IEEE Eng Med Biol Soc. 2015;2015:13–6.
61. Dario P, Hannaford B, Menciassi A. Smart surgical tools and augmenting devices. IEEE Trans Robot Autom. 2003;19(5):782–92.
62. Gonenc B, Tran N, Gehlbach P, Taylor RH, Iordachita I. Robot-assisted retinal vein cannulation with force-based puncture detection: micron vs. the steady-hand eye robot. Annu Int Conf IEEE Eng Med Biol Soc. 2016;2016:5107–11.
63. Gonenc B, Gehlbach P, Handa J, Taylor RH, Iordachita I. Motorized force-sensing microforceps with tremor cancelling and controlled micro-vibrations for easier membrane peeling. Proc IEEE/RAS-EMBS Int Conf Biomed Robot. 2014;2014:244–51.
64. Sunshine S, Balicki M, He X, Olds K, Kang JU, Gehlbach P, et al. A force-sensing microsurgical instrument that detects forces below human tactile sensation. Retina. 2013;33(1):200–6.
65. Song C, Park DY, Gehlbach PL, Park SJ, Kang JU. Fiber-optic OCT sensor guided "SMART" micro-forceps for microsurgery. Biomed Opt Express. 2013;4(7):1045–50.
66. Yang S, Balicki M, Wells TS, Maclachlan RA, Liu X, Kang JU, et al. Improvement of optical coherence tomography using active handheld micromanipulator in vitreoretinal surgery. Annu Int Conf IEEE Eng Med Biol Soc. 2013;2013:5674–7.
67. Maclachlan RA, Becker BC, Tabarés JC, Podnar GW, Lobes LA Jr, Riviere CN. Micron: an actively stabilized handheld tool for microsurgery. IEEE Trans Robot. 2012;28(1):195–212.
68. Kuru I, Gonenc B, Balicki M, Handa J, Gehlbach P, Taylor RH, et al. Force sensing micro-forceps for robot assisted retinal surgery. Annu Int Conf IEEE Eng Med Biol Soc. 2012;2012:1401–4.
69. Gonenc B, Feldman E, Gehlbach P, Handa J, Taylor RH, Iordachita I. Towards robot-assisted vitreoretinal surgery: force-sensing micro-forceps integrated with a handheld micromanipulator. IEEE Int Conf Robot Autom. 2014;2014:1399–404.

Robotic Devices in Gynecology

Renato Moretti-Marques, Mariana Corinti, Vanessa Alvarenga-Bezerra, Luisa Marcella Martins, and Mariano Tamura Vieira Gomes

1 Introduction: History and Reality of Robotic Surgery in Gynecology

Technology is increasingly ingrained in our daily lives, and, of course, medicine would be no different. In gynecology, the advent of robotic-assisted devices has taken a large role in benign and malignant pelvic disease. What was previously only possible to be seen through large incisions and palpated with the hands is now possible to be seen with magnification through small orifices, with three-dimensional vision, and using instruments that reproduce and enhance human hand movements.

Since 1998, when the first tubal anastomosis was reported using the ZEUS robot [1], the use of robotic surgery in gynecology has not only improved outcomes but also opened the horizons for new perceptions of anatomy and dissection.

In April 2005, the da Vinci Surgical System (Intuitive Surgical, Sunnyvale, CA, USA) gained the Food and Drug Administration (FDA) approval for gynecologic surgery procedures. Since then, robotically assisted hysterectomies had an exponential crescent along with the open abdominal surgery decline in Western countries [2]. As of 2015, over 3400 robotic systems were in use around the world. The da Vinci system remained the main robotic device for over 20 years having released four generations of multi-arm robots and being used in various surgical fields [3, 4]. More recently, in 2018, the da Vinci Single-Port (SP) a single-arm robot was approved for use in urologic surgeries and was also used for hysterectomies. In the same year, approximately 265,000 gynecologic procedures were performed robotically in the world [5–7].

R. Moretti-Marques (✉) · M. Corinti · V. Alvarenga-Bezerra · L. M. Martins · M. T. V. Gomes
Department of Gynecology, Hospital Israelita Albert Einstein, Sao Paulo, Brazil

J. P. Manzano, L. M. Ferreira (eds.), *Robotic Surgery Devices in Surgical Specialties*, https://doi.org/10.1007/978-3-031-35102-0_13

In the last decade, other robotic systems have emerged and have been approved for gynecological use. The Senhance Surgical System (TransEnterix Surgical Inc., Morrisville, NC, USA), a pioneer in providing haptic feedback, received the CE (Conformite Europeenne) mark certification in 2016 and in 2017 became the first new robotic system to receive FDA clearance since 2000 [8]. Also, Versius Surgical System (Cambridge Medical Robotics Ltd., Cambridge, UK) and Avatera system (avateramedical GmbH, DE) received the CE mark in 2019 for use in Europe [9, 10]. In Korean and Japanese markets the robotic systems Revo-I (Meere Company Inc., Yongin, Korea) and Hinotori (Medicaroid Corporation, Kobe, Japan) are available for use [11, 12].

Other large companies compete in the robotic surgery market, such as Medtronic, Johnson & Johnson and Google, Titan Medical Inc., and Stryker Corporation, among others. Unavoidably, each emerging system has to be compared to the existing gold standard da Vinci and generate data evaluating potential effectiveness and safety.

2 Robotic Systems in Gynecology

2.1 Approved

The current robotic systems are summarized in Table 1.

Table 1 The current robotic systems are summarized in Table 1

	Approved (Year)	Patient Interface	Surgeon Console	3D Vision Technology	Camera Diameter	Instrument Diameter / DOF / Uses	Haptic Feedback	Ergonomy and Controllers	Additional Features
Multiport Platforms									
Da Vinci Si **Da Vinci Xi and X** *Intuitive Surgical, Sunnyvale, CA, USA*	FDA (2000) FDA (2014)	Single cart 4 arms	Closed	Stereoscopic	12 mm 8 mm	8 mm / 7° / 10 times 8 mm / 7° / 10 times	No	• Seated, leaning forward • Armrests • Finger loops • Foot pedals	• Multiquadrant surgery • Port hopping camera • Dual console
Senhance *TransEnterix Surgical Inc., Morrisville, NC, USA*	FDA (2017) CE Mark (2014)	Individual carts 4 arms	Open	Flat panel display with 3D glasses	10 mm	10 mm / 7° / unlimited 5 mm / 6° / unlimited 3 mm / 6° / unlimited	Yes	• Seated upright • Hand controllers like laparoscopic instruments • One foot pedal	• Eye-tracking camera control • Head movements to zoom in and out • No port docking
Revo-I *Meere Company Inc., Yongin, Korea*	KMFDS (2017)	Single cart 4 arms	Closed	Stereoscopic	10 mm	7.4 mm / 7° / 20 uses	Yes	• Seated, leaning forward • Armrests • Finger loops • Foot pedals	• Extensive force use warning message
Versius *Cambridge Medical Robotics (CMR) Ltd., Cambridge, UK*	CE Mark (2019)	Individual carts 5 arms	Open	Flat panel display with 3D glasses	10 mm	5 mm / 7° / NA	Yes	• Seated upright or standing • Armrests • Joystick controllers	• No port docking • Portable independent arms
Avatera *avateramedical GmbH, Germany*	CE Mark (2019)	Single cart 4 arms	Semi-closed	Stereoscopic	10 mm	5 mm / 7° / single use	Yes	• Seated, leaning forward • Integrated seat • Armrests • Finger loops • Foot pedals	• Space saving (2 units)
Hinotori *Medicaroid Corporation, Kobe, Japan*	JMHLW (2020)	Single cart 4 arms	Closed	Stereoscopic	NA	NA / 8o / NA	NA	• Seated, leaning forward • Armrests • Finger loops • Foot pedals	• Space saving (2 units) • No port docking
Singleport Platforms									
Da Vinci SP *Intuitive Surgical, Sunnyvale, CA, USA*	FDA / 2018	Single cart Single port/arm 1 camera 3 instruments	Closed	Stereoscopic	12x10 mm	6 mm / 7° / 10 uses	No	• Seated, leaning forward • Armrests • Finger grips • Foot pedals	• Single port • 360° rotating boom • Articulating camera • Multijointed, wristed

DOF degrees of freedom, *FDA* US Food and Drug Administration, *SP* single port, *3D* three-dimensional, *KMFDS* Korean Ministry of Food and Drug Safety, *NA* no available data, *JMHLW* Japanese Ministry of Health, Labour and Welfare [7, 13, 14]

2.1.1 da Vinci Surgical System

The da Vinci Surgical System was FDA cleared for use in gynecologic laparoscopy in 2005; since then, its usefulness has been recognized, expanding the horizons of minimally invasive surgery (MIS) to the detriment of conventional surgery [2]. Publications on robotic surgery grew dramatically and the da Vinci system from Intuitive Surgical, the patent holder up to 2020, was the only platform put to the test.

Robotic technology has improved the ability to perform complex gynecologic surgeries, on either benign or malignant diseases. Initially, owing to the high cost of robotic surgery, it was focused on malignant pathologies whose costs are more easily borne by the healthcare system, but currently, the trend is likely to become a common procedure for the treatment of benign diseases as well [2, 15].

Complex procedures involving patient obesity, lysis of adhesions, abundant suture, nerve-sparing dissection, anastomosis and exploration of the retroperitoneal space benefit from the robotic system use.

The da Vinci Surgical System comprises three components: the surgeon console, the vision cart, and the patient side cart with four robotic arms manipulated by the surgeon. The latest four-arm da Vinci generation is the Xi version (Fig. 1), released in 2014, and its applications include general, cardiac, colorectal, otolaryngology, neurosurgery, thoracic, gynecologic, and urologic surgery. Its features include a three-dimensional (3D) high- definition (HD) camera with a binocular view and up to three instrument arms, which articulate at the wrist of the instrument with seven degrees of freedom (DOF). There are several available series, including the da Vinci S, Si, X, Xi, and SP (Single Port), with the newest versions having haptic feedback for the operator.

Another benefit of the da Vinci Xi and Si system is being able to count on an extra console for teaching cases, in which the main surgeon passes the robot command to the surgeon in training, being able to supervise and correct him during his learning process (Fig. 1).

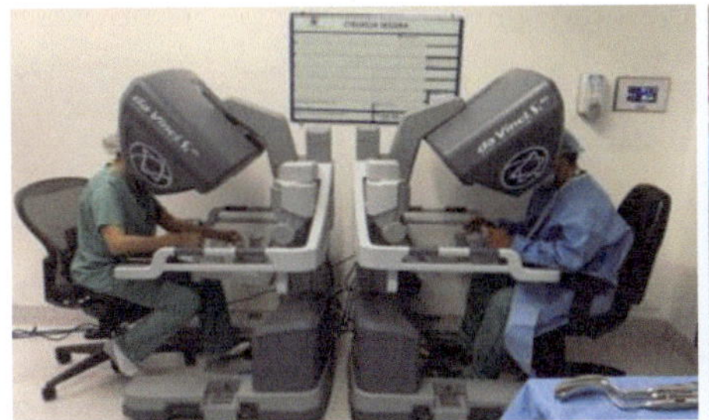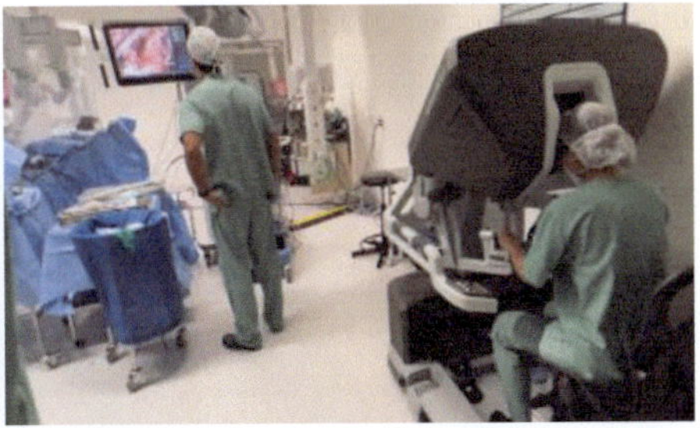

Fig. 1 Top image: picture was taken at Hospital Israelita Albert Einstein operating room, a proctoring case using a double console. Bottom image: surgeon seated on console and proctor pointing out on vision cart touchscreen. (Photos: courtesy of Dr. Renato Moretti-Marques's personal archive)

Advantages and Disadvantages

Robotic surgery still presents controversial results in the medical literature. Some of its advantages are faced with challenges such as oncologic safety, length of surgery, cost, and, even, aesthetic outcomes [16]. However, few studies focus on the concept of surgeon's comfort; most studies take into account the operational outcomes, which undergo an objective rather than a subjective assessment [17]. There are many advantages and a few disadvantages of robotic surgery as shown in Table 2 [18].

Anesthesia and ERAS (Enhanced Recovery After Surgery) Protocol Applied to Gynecology Minimally Invasive Procedures

The anesthesiology team should be aware of the procedure extension and complexity, in particular, changes in physiology brought about by Trendelenburg positioning (around 30°) and CO_2 pneumoperitoneum, essential to ensure patient safety and proficient procedure.

Before inducing general anesthesia, the patient must be properly monitored. This applies to caliber access, pulse oximetry, capnography, electrocardiography (EKG), blood pressure monitoring (invasive if indicated), temperature, level of consciousness, and neuromuscular controls.

The prolonged Trendelenburg position can result in rare but relevant complications in the recovery period that must be known by the anesthesiologist, such as laryngeal edema, postoperative confusion, and delirium presumably secondary to cerebral edema and inadequate clearance of CO_2. Studies suggesting this link have been underpowered due to the small numbers involved [19].

Postoperative pain relief is usually achieved through a multimodal analgesia technique. Intravenous dipyrone and non-steroidal anti-inflammatory drugs are commonly used at our institution, in an attempt to reduce the use of narcotic

Table 2 Advantages and disadvantages of the robotic platform

Advantages	Disadvantages
• The ergonomic position of the surgeon, which reduces fatigue and allows longer focus • Reduced tremor effect, adding precision and finesse to the surgical procedure • Instruments that simulate the wrist anatomy by having seven degrees of freedom • Three-dimensional vision, high definition image and image magnification • Ability to control four surgical instruments, including the camera • Firefly technology, an infrared light source, helps identify lymph nodes and areas of high blood flow when stained with indocyanine green dye • Using the screen, the doctor can write and give instructions to the assistants at any time during the surgery • A dual console system is available, the physician can signal and pass control to the surgeon at the neighbouring console to continue the surgical procedure	• Lack of haptic feedback (in some platforms, da Vinci, for example) • Cost-effectiveness

medication, as recommended by the Enhanced Recovery After Surgery (ERAS) guideline [20]. The use of transversus abdominis plane (TAP) blocks and wound infiltration with local anesthesia has also been described as preemptive anesthesia concepts. The neuraxial blockade is generally not required for postoperative pain relief and thus is rarely used. Nausea and vomiting may persist in the postoperative, principally due to ileus, and anti-emetic medication should be prophylactically prescribed [19].

Patient Positioning, Port Placement, Docking, and Instruments

Patient Positioning

In pelvic gynecological procedures, attention to the patient's positioning is essential in order to ensure safety. The patient should be placed in a dorsal lithotomy position with adequate sacral protection and support, legs placed in stirrups under compression stockings and pneumatic compression devices, and arms should be padded with foam and tucked alongside the body with bedsheets. To avoid cephalad movement in a steep Trendelenburg position, the operating table should have a gel pad to allow friction and molding to the patient's body. When surgery estimating time is over 2 h, it is also recommended to protect bone projections with foam dressings in order to avoid pressure injuries (Fig. 2).

Port Placement

Port placement is vital to a successful procedure. The objectives of port placement are to prevent arm collisions and maximize the range of motion of instruments and endoscope. The port placement should be planned according to the surgical procedure and physical patient characteristics. It should be thoroughly discussed with a senior surgeon to avoid the inadequate port placement and difficulties to carry out the surgery.

In general, the camera port is placed in the umbilical scar and should be at a minimum of 10 to 20 cm to the targeted surgical field. For a successful procedure, determine door placement based on a pattern of parallel lines:

- Inflate before measuring and place the patient in Trendelenburg.
- Use the camera location as the center point (keep it 10–20 cm from the target anatomy).
- Draw parallel lines **8–10 cm** (in the da Vinci Si) or **6–10 cm** (in the da Vinci Xi) apart based on the line from the target anatomy to the chamber door.
- Place da Vinci doors along the lines, keeping a distance of **10–20 cm** from the target anatomy and a distance of 8–10 cm and 6–10 cm from other da Vinci ports.
- Triangulate da Vinci ports so they are closer to or farther from the target anatomy as needed for the procedure.

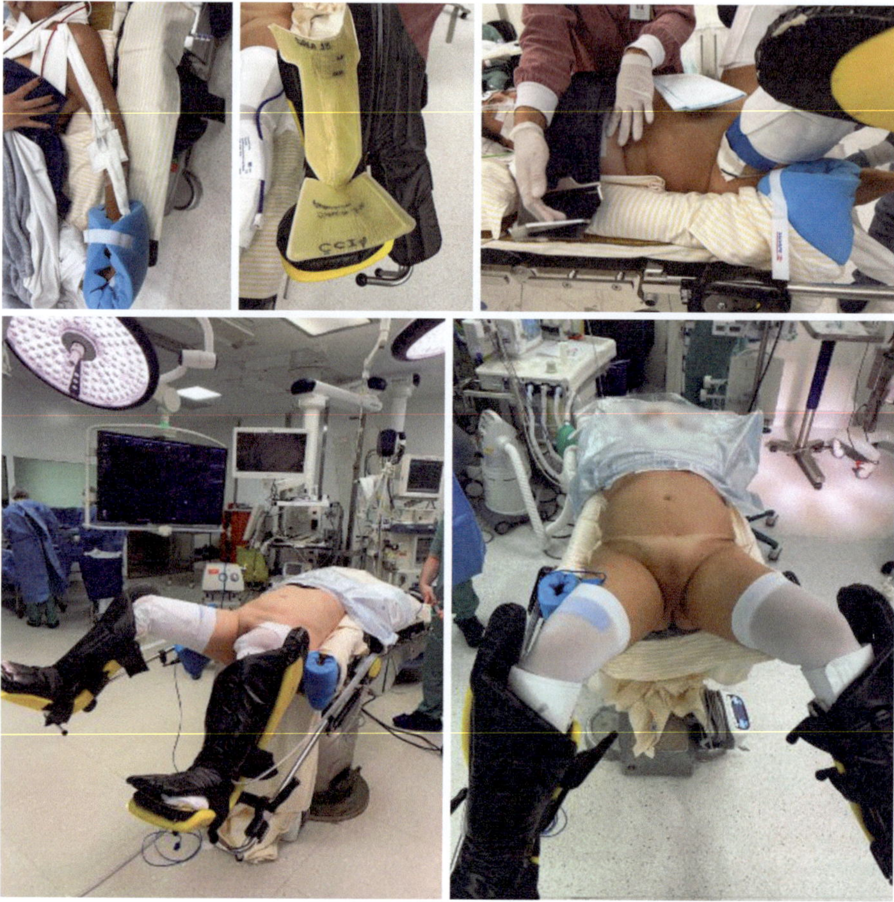

Fig. 2 Patient position before draping. (Photo: courtesy of Dr. Moretti-Marques's personal archive)

- In the case of accessory ports, keep a distance of at least **5 cm** (in the da Vinci Si) and **7 cm** (in the da Vinci Xi) from other ports, with a clear trajectory to the target anatomy.
- Reattach the patient cart (in the da Vinci Si) or set a new target (in the da Vinci Xi) if you are working on more than two quadrants.

In general, ports are placed in an arch or "W" in the da Vinci Si and in line with the da Vinci Xi (Fig. 3).

An example is performing a para-aortic lymphadenectomy in the Si platform. In this case, the surgeon could dock the camera in the umbilical scar or supra-pubic port according to the para-aortic region interested. The other arms should be placed in a "W"-shaped fashion in order to keep the forceps centralized and the optics in an oblique position. The "W" disposal can also be used for sacrocolpopexy once the

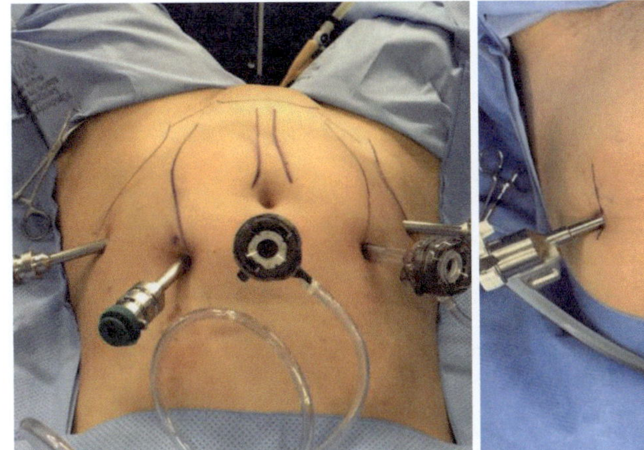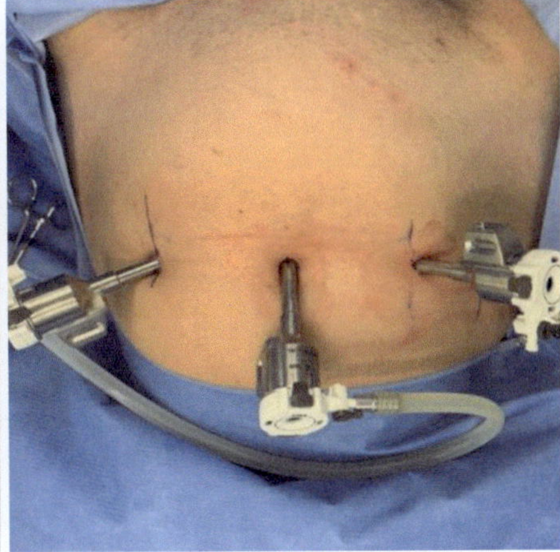

Fig. 3 Examples of port placement in the da Vinci Si (left) and Xi (right). (Photo: courtesy of Dr. Renato Moretti-Marques's personal archive)

pelvic surgical field is deep and narrow, requiring medial arms to avoid restrictions and limitations caused by a pelvic side wall and promontory prominence. In the Xi platform, the ports are placed in line and the boom is rotated for both pelvis and lower abdomen for a para-aortic lymphadenectomy (Fig. 4).

There is a discussion from an aesthetic point of view about robotics being worse than laparoscopy due to the size and location of the incisions. In some cases, we can perform side incisions that promote great satisfaction for the patient because the scars are imperceptible (Fig. 5). Of course, we must always evaluate each case individually, taking into account the anatomical limitation, the type of surgery, and the patient's physical shape.

Docking

The patient cart approximation to the operating table must be done by an unscrubbed trained team and guided by the scrubbed surgeon. For the Si platform, in pelvic gynecological surgery, it is possible to perform central docking between the patient's legs or side docking [21], which is as effective as allowing uterine manipulation and removal of surgical specimens (Fig. 6). To access the upper abdomen, as for para-aortic lymph node dissection or diaphragmatic endometriosis, it is necessary to undock all arms, move the patient cart, and reposition it to the patient's shoulder (Fig. 7).

On the Xi platform, the patient cart is positioned to the patient's left, and the target anatomy can be selected on the display. For multi-quadrant surgeries, it is not necessary to reposition the cart, just uncouple the arms, move the boom, and set a new target (Figs. 8 and 9).

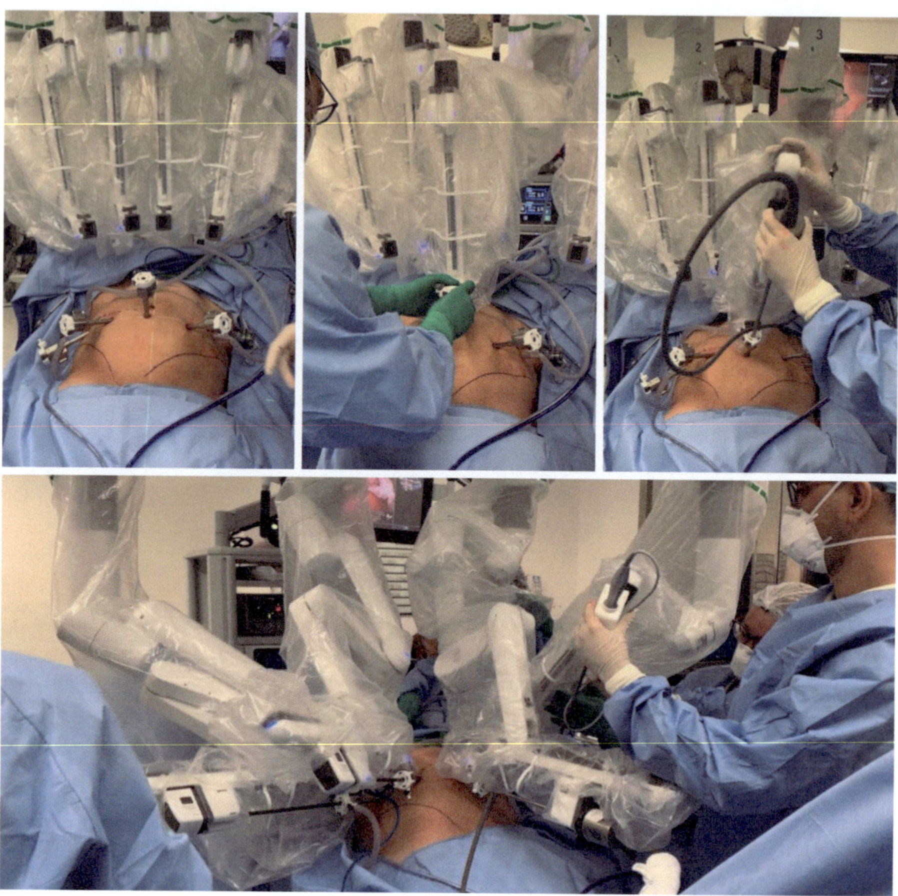

Fig. 4 Robotic hysterectomy and pelvic and para-aortic lymphadenectomy for endometrial cancer using the da Vinci Xi platform. Both four robotic arms were used. Double docking was performed: first pelvic left lateral docking, followed by lower abdominal lateral docking for aortic approach. (Photo: courtesy of Dr. Renato Moretti-Marques's personal archive)

Instruments

The da Vinci platform has an infinity of surgical instruments, most of them with an articulated tip, called EndoWrist, which helps a lot in the range of motion.

These are some examples of 8 mm caliber EndoWrist instruments, among many others better described in the Intuitive catalog [22].

In gynecological surgery we mostly use the monopolar scissors, Maryland or fenestrated bipolar forceps, the large needle, or Mega SutureCut™ needle drivers, and when there is a need for a third arm we use grasping forceps such as the ProGrasp or Cardiere forceps. Eventually, for robotic myomectomies, the tenaculum forceps can be used to traction the leiomyoma.

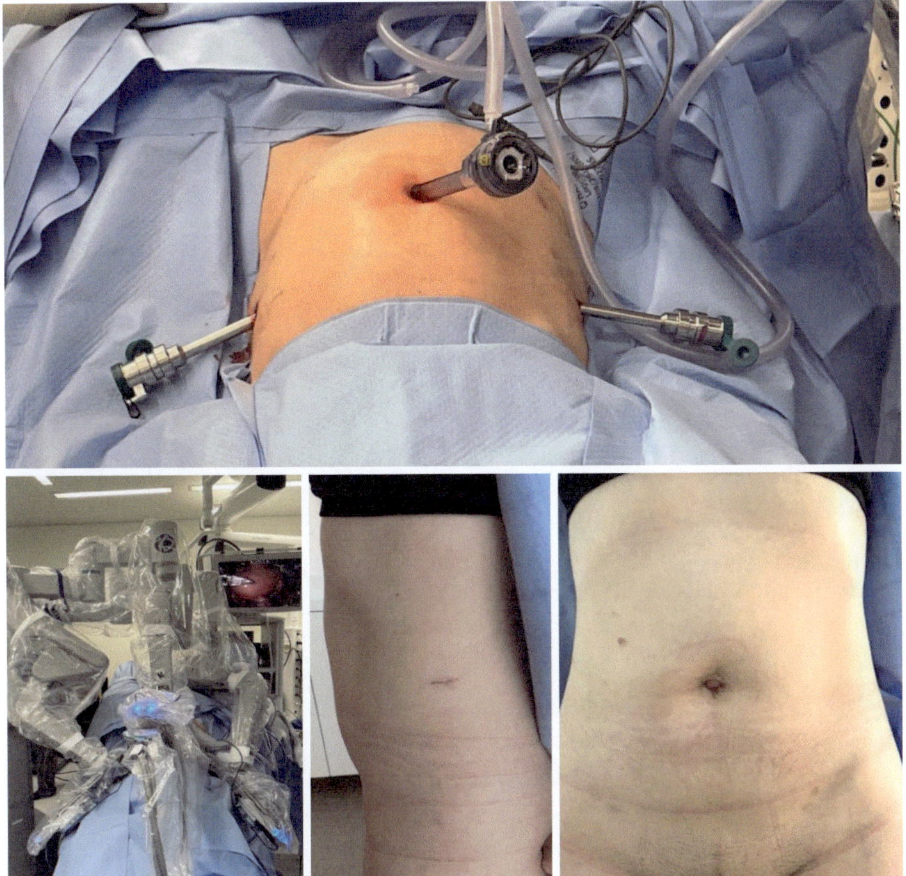

Fig. 5 Robotic treatment of posterior compartment endometriosis using the da Vinci Si platform in a side docking. Ports were placed on both abdominal flanks, plus a 5 mm laparoscopic assistant port, and the patient had a satisfactory esthetic result. (Photo: courtesy of Dr. Renato Moretti-Marques's personal archive)

2.1.2 Hugo™ RAS

The Medtronic Hugo™ robotic-assisted surgery (RAS) system received the CE mark approval for urologic and gynecologic procedures in October 2021 and has already been tested in Europe and Latin America [23]. The system includes high-definition 3D imaging and electromechanical devices for performing minimally invasive surgery. The three main components of the Hugo™ RAS system are the arm carts, the system tower, and the surgeon's console.

The Hugo™ RAS system is compatible with the following devices:

- Medtronic Hugo™ RAS System Multi-Hinged Surgical Instruments

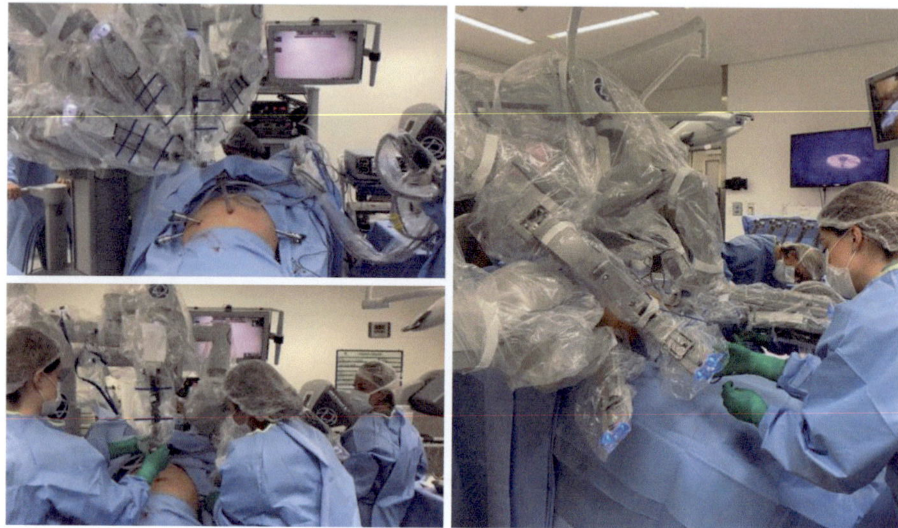

Fig. 6 Side docking for the lower abdomen and pelvis in the Si platform. (Photo: courtesy of Dr. Renato Moretti-Marques's personal archive)

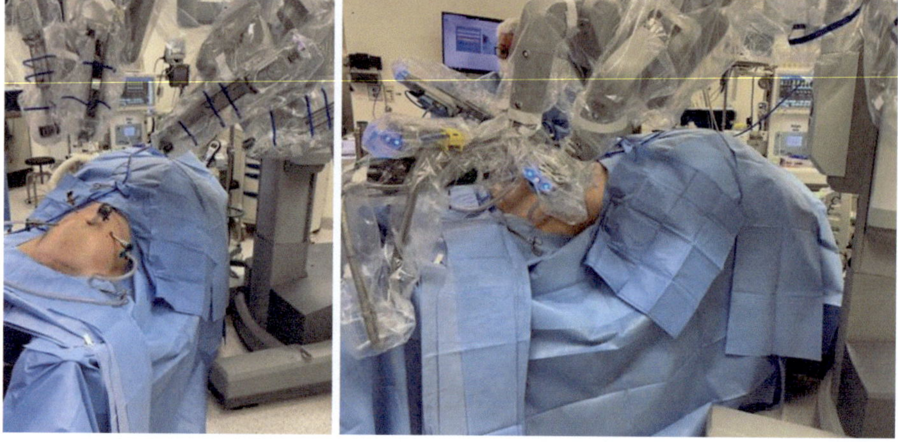

Fig. 7 Side docking for the upper abdomen in the Si platform. (Photo: courtesy of Dr. Renato Moretti-Marques's personal archive)

- The 3D endoscope and Karl Storz imaging system (0° and/or 30° with chip-on-tip technology when used with a designated adapter)
- Covidien Valleylab™ FT10 electrosurgical generator
- VersaOne™ Trocar Placement System and Trocar Placement System reusable VersaOne™

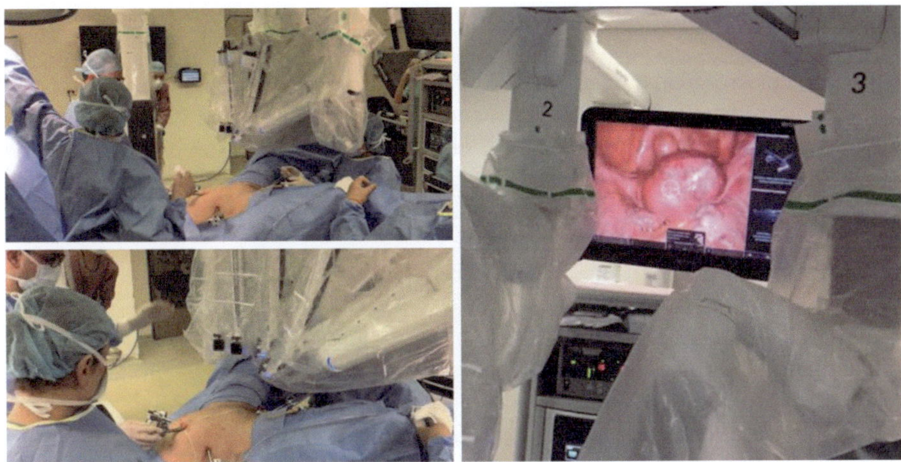

Fig. 8 Patient cart placed on the patient's left side, the boom is rotated to the pelvis, and the target is set on the uterus as observed in the left picture. (Photo: courtesy of Dr. Renato Moretti-Marques's personal archive)

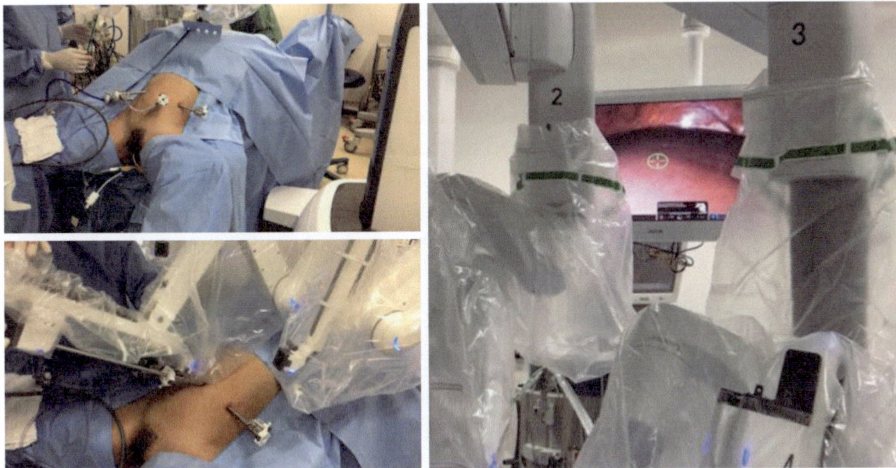

Fig. 9 Patient cart placed on the patient's left side, the boom is rotated to the upper abdomen, and the target is set on the liver as observed in the left picture. (Photo: courtesy of Dr. Renato Moretti-Marques's personal archive)

The system couples permanent materials that the hospital already has, such as the Karl Storz imaging system, trocars, and electrical generator, in order to make the implementation process cheaper and consequently lower surgery costs.

2.1.3 Senhance Surgical System

The Senhance Surgical System (TransEnterix, Morrisville, NC) was FDA cleared in 2017 and introduced to the market at a competitive price by using standard reusable endoscopic instruments. The system is composed of an open surgeon console and up to four detached robotic arms, the same concept as Hugo™ RAS. The platform can use 5 mm instruments, 3 mm instruments for micro-laparoscopy, and fluorescence for enhanced visualization.

Some initial studies have been reported as of initial experience using the Senhance platform in gynecological surgery [24–27]. This was the first system to provide haptic feedback to the surgeon; however, instruments are not wrist-jointed, maintaining the disadvantages of the laparoscopic concept, similar to the laparoscopic platform simulator. Also, criticisms include larger size, restricting space in the operating room, and longer time to dock the robotic arms [28].

2.1.4 Revo-I Surgical System

The Revo-I (Meere Company Inc., Yongin, Korea) received approval for commercial use from the Korean government in August 2017, but it has not received FDA or CE mark to date.

The system, which is quite similar to the da Vinci Si system, consists of a four-arm patient cart, a closed surgeon console, and an HD vision cart. The 3D endoscope is 10 mm in diameter and fully wristed instruments reusable for up to 20 times [11].

Only one study associated with gynecology was published assessing tubal reanastomosis in porcine models. Urology and general surgery already use Revo-I in their procedures, but the fact that it was approved only in Korea may limit further publications [29].

2.1.5 Versius Surgical System

The Versius Surgical System (Cambridge Medical Robotics Ltd., Cambridge, UK) received the European CE mark in March 2019. The system is composed of an operator console and modular wristed robotic arms in individually portable and lightweight carts. Each robotic arm has a shoulder, an elbow, and a wrist joint to mimic human movements. The console has an open design and requires polarized glasses for 3D HD vision (Fig. 10). The surgeon can choose to operate in a sitting or a standing position while controlling the system through joystick handles from which he receives haptic feedback [30]. Like Hugo™, the platform also uses Karl Storz video system and permanent laparoscopic trocars, which could possibly lower costs.

The system has been used in preclinical testing and few, but relevant, studies have been published demonstrating the feasibility of the system in other surgical

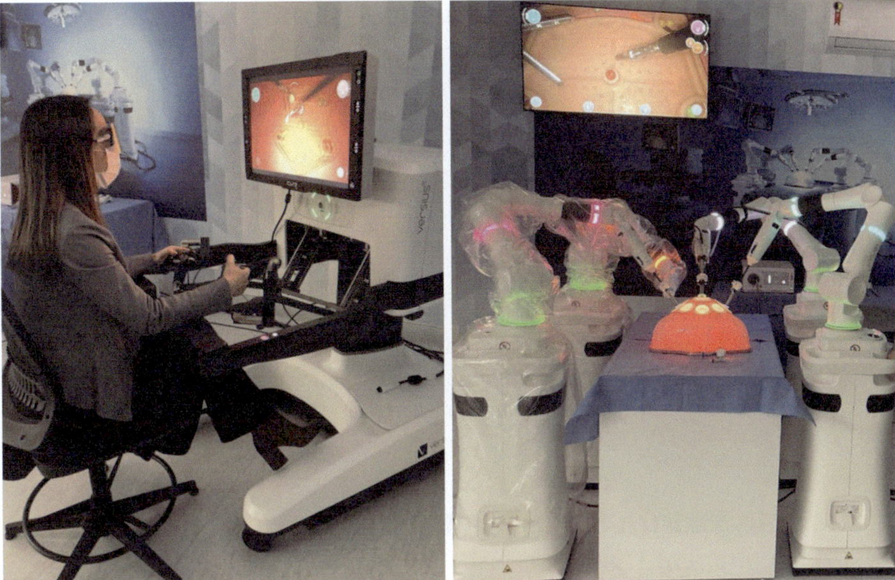

Fig. 10 Versius Surgical System demonstration. (Photo: courtesy of Dr. Mariana Corinti's personal archive)

specialties [31]. The first clinical report of 30 radical hysterectomies has been published in 2021 [32]. More studies are still awaited to possibly prove superiority in terms of cost-benefit face to the dominant da Vinci.

2.1.6 Avatera

The German robot, Avatera system (avateramedical GmbH, Jena, Germany), is another robotic recently cleared device (November 2019) in Europe. It is not commercially available yet, but will focus on gynecology and urology minimally invasive procedures [33]. Avatera is composed of two main units, the patient cart and the surgeon console or the control unit. The patient cart has four robotic arms, three for the 5 mm fully articulating instruments and one for the 10 mm endoscope. All the instruments are single use and disposable.

The surgeon sits in an adjustable chair at the console and a microscope-like eyepiece provides 3D full HD vision without enveloping the entire head of the surgeon for easier communication with the surgical team. Finally, the instruments are controlled by loop-like handles. To date, there is no published data describing the use of the Avatera system, and the publication of clinical studies is awaited.

2.2 Other Robotic Systems: Awaiting Approval

There are some new robotic platforms to be launched in the market. Medtronic's greatest competitor Johnson & Johnson had postponed the **Ottava** robotic system. They offer unrivaled flexibility and control compared to the rest of the market, with six arms to provide more control and flexibility in surgery, while its arms will be integrated into the operating table. Additionally, at the time of its unveiling, the company said the platform has a zero-footprint design to enable patient access, increase space in the operating room, and improve workflow [34].

The **Enos** (previously known as SPORT) robotic system from Titan Medical will mainly act as a single site platform, aiming to focus the surgical procedure through just one orifice in the human body. The platform is composed of a single cart, with a 25 mm single port arm with one camera and two articulated instruments.

3 Robotic-Assisted Surgery in Benign Gynecological Diseases

In this topic, the robotic-assisted surgery (RAS) will be discussed with a focus on the da Vinci system and the current clinical studies available in the body of literature.

3.1 Hysterectomy

Hysterectomy is the second most common gynecological procedure in the USA, with approximately 433,000 cases a year. It can be done in several ways: vaginal, laparoscopic, or abdominal. Although more than half of the cases are performed as abdominal surgery since 2010 the trend is increasing towards minimally invasive surgery [2].

Since the first case series reported in 2002, robotic-assisted hysterectomy has continued to grow [35]. A recent Cochrane Review was published in 2019 [16], which included a total of 12 randomized control trials (RCTs) conducted after 2007. Eight of these studies examined laparoscopic hysterectomy, two of which included hysterectomy for malignant disease.

Low-certainty evidence suggests there might be little or no difference in intra/ postoperative complications and blood transfusions rates between robotic-assisted and conventional laparoscopic surgery. However, other authors have also found that once the learning curve has been done, there is a reduced operative time, reduced blood loss, and a reduced hospital stay in patients treated robotically [36].

Performing a hysterectomy for benign causes (Fig. 11) should be approached primarily by vaginal or conventional laparoscopic approach. Rationally, robotic

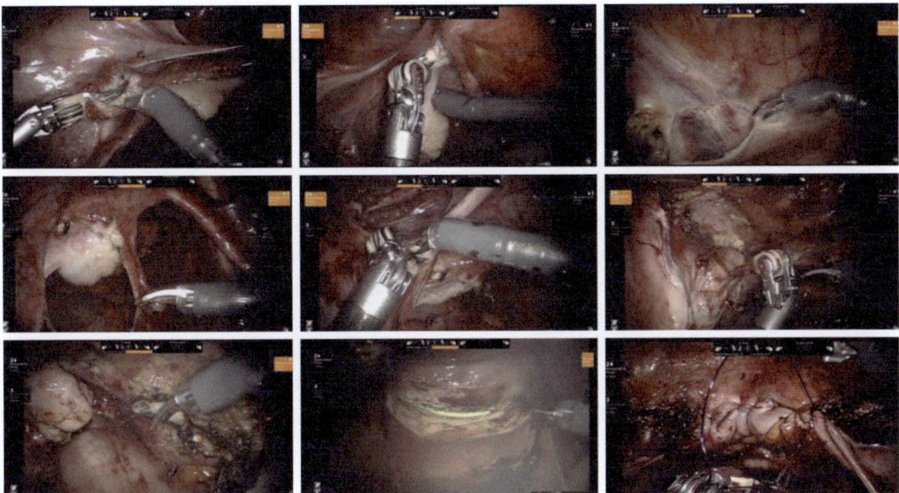

Fig. 11 Steps of a robotic hysterectomy for abnormal uterine bleeding using three robotic instruments: monopolar curved scissors, Maryland bipolar forceps, and large needle driver, helped by the use of a disposable uterine manipulator. (Photo: courtesy of Dr. Renato Moretti-Marques's personal archive)

surgery could be reserved for difficult cases, such as large uteri, or when significant anatomic distortions are suspected. Deep endometriosis, difficult and multiple myomectomies, pelvic inflammatory disease or abscesses, and previous uterine artery embolization suggest that robotic technology could offer some advantages mainly due to the fine dissection required [37, 38].

3.1.1 Costs

Clinical value is calculated by dividing the clinical outcome by the cost necessary to deliver it. Differences in clinical outcomes and cost differentials across the various routes of hysterectomies lead to different clinical values. Vaginal hysterectomy has the highest value, and traditional laparoscopic hysterectomy has an intermediate value, whereas some may argue that robotic hysterectomy (given the high costs with essentially equivalent outcomes) and abdominal approaches (given the less favorable clinical outcomes) have less value. This analysis does not take in surgeon comfort or proficiency with any given approach. Future considerations should be given to improving surgical training in the various methods of hysterectomy as most surgeons are not highly proficient in all routes of hysterectomy, including robotic, conventional laparoscopic, open, and vaginal hysterectomy.

3.2 Myomectomy

Myomectomy is indicated for patients of childbearing age with abnormal uterine bleeding, bulky symptoms, and a desire to preserve fertility. Prior to the surgical approach, the number, size, and location of the fibroids must be evaluated. In more complex cases, in which bleeding control and agility in the suture are required, robotic surgery plays a sensitive role (Fig. 12) [39]. It is one of the most commonly performed benign robotic procedures. Studies show blood loss, postoperative pain, and transfusion requirements similar to laparoscopic myomectomy [40]. An advantage observed with the robotic procedure was a greater mass of removed fibroids suggesting that, for complex cases such as large fibroids, this modality could be a reasonable option [39, 41]. A meta-analysis published in 2019 corroborates a lower incidence of intra- and postoperative complications with the robotic platform [16].

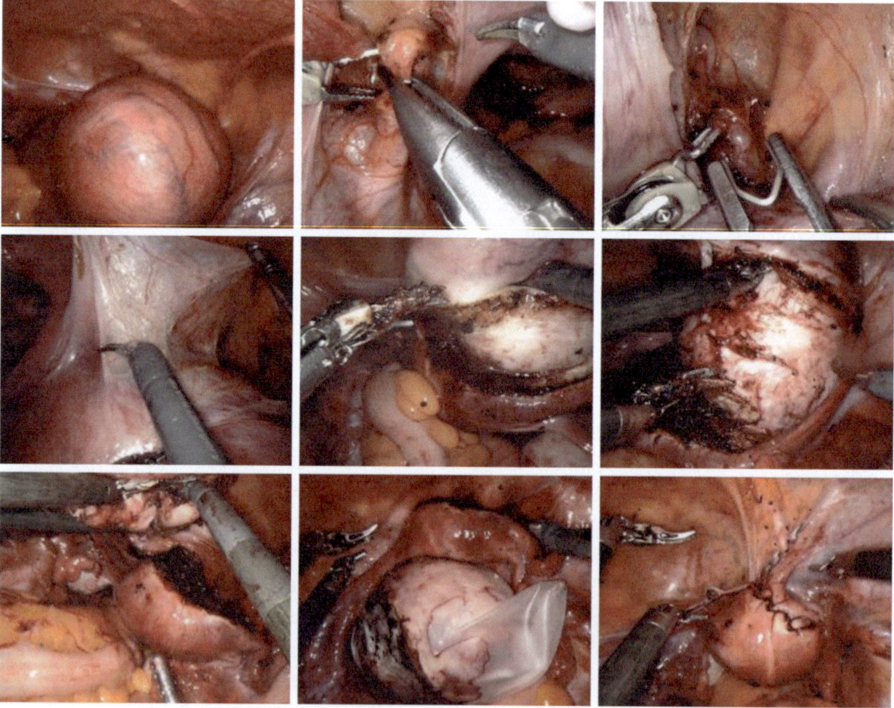

Fig. 12 Steps of a robotic myomectomy using three robotic instruments: monopolar curved scissors, Maryland bipolar forceps, and a large needle driver. Uterine arteries were temporarily clipped to minimize bleeding, and a 7 cm fibroid was enucleated, protected, and removed through posterior vaginal fornix. (Photo: courtesy of Dr. Renato Moretti-Marques's personal archive)

3.3 Deep Endometriosis

Endometriosis is an estrogen-dependent chronic inflammatory condition that affects up to 10% of women in their reproductive period. It is associated with pelvic pain and infertility [42]. This disease can be asymptomatic or be associated with dysmenorrhea, chronic pelvic pain, dyspareunia, as well as cyclic urinary and intestinal symptoms according to the disease topography [43].

The indication for surgery in endometriosis depends on the site of involvement, on the refractoriness of the clinical treatment, or on infertility (Fig. 13).

A meta-analysis published in 2020 [44] confirmed that robotic surgery is safe and feasible in patients affected by endometriosis, mainly in specific severe cases, not being inferior to laparoscopy techniques. Thanks to depth perception with the freedom of movement of robotic instruments and increased dexterity, RAS allows obtaining higher surgical precision on dissection and lesion excision [45].

In special cases such as diaphragmatic endometriosis the robotic pathway allows for an easier approach due to articulated robotic arms in a hard-to-reach region [46]. Diaphragm full-thickness excision was already reported in the literature [47].

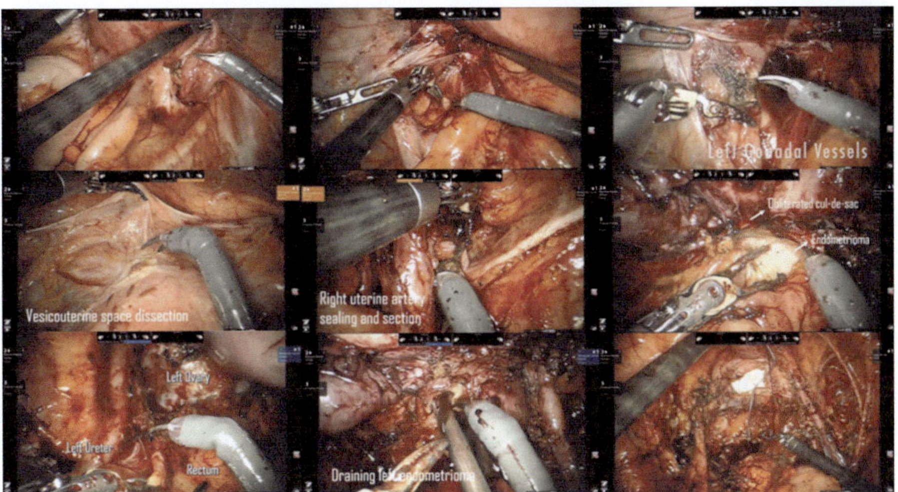

Fig. 13 Complete cul-de-sac obliteration due to left ovary cystic endometrioma, compromising ureters, uterine torus, lateral parametria, rectum anterior aspect, and recto-vaginal septum. Fine dissection for structure identification was necessary, taking care to avoid injuries. A total hysterectomy, left adnexectomy, and complete endometriotic lesion excision were performed. (Photo: courtesy of Dr. Renato Moretti-Marques's personal archive)

3.4 Adnexal Masses

Robotics is seldom used exclusively for approaching adnexal masses, except for challenging cases, such as the presence of multiple adhesions and the need for delicate dissection of structures (Fig. 14).

It is important to emphasize good planning of the surgical strategy, calculation of the risk of malignancy through tumor markers, and imaging tests performed by a qualified professional.

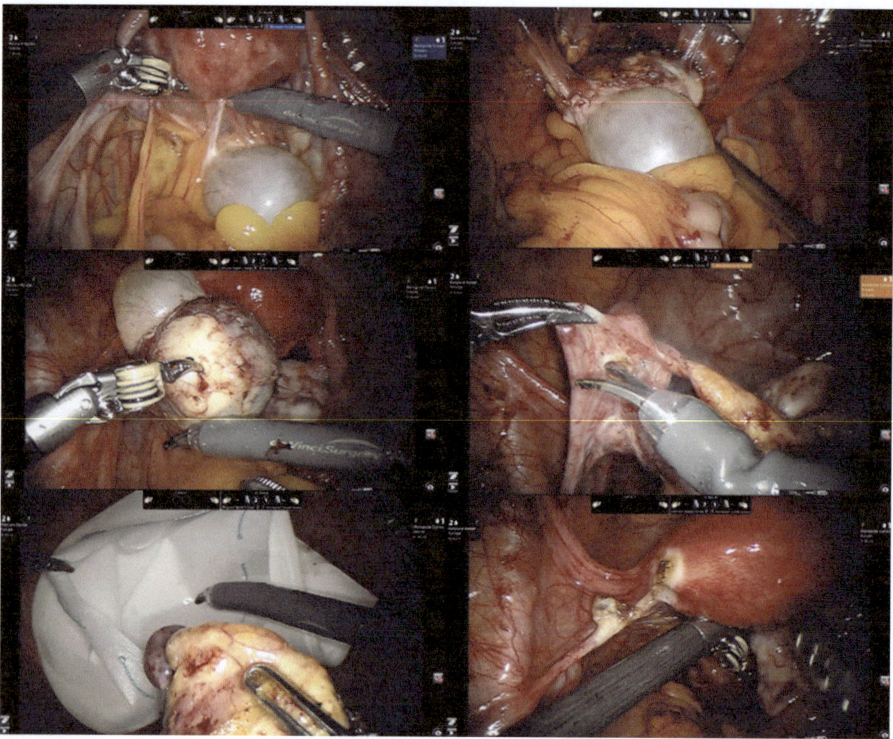

Fig. 14 The picture demonstrates the pelvic blockage by multiple adhesions due to dermoid adnexal torsion in a late diagnosis. After complete anatomic reestablishment, the complete torsion is identified and the salpingo-oophorectomy is done. The bag protective surgical specimen is retrieved through the umbilical scar. (Photo: courtesy of Dr. Renato Moretti-Marques's personal archive)

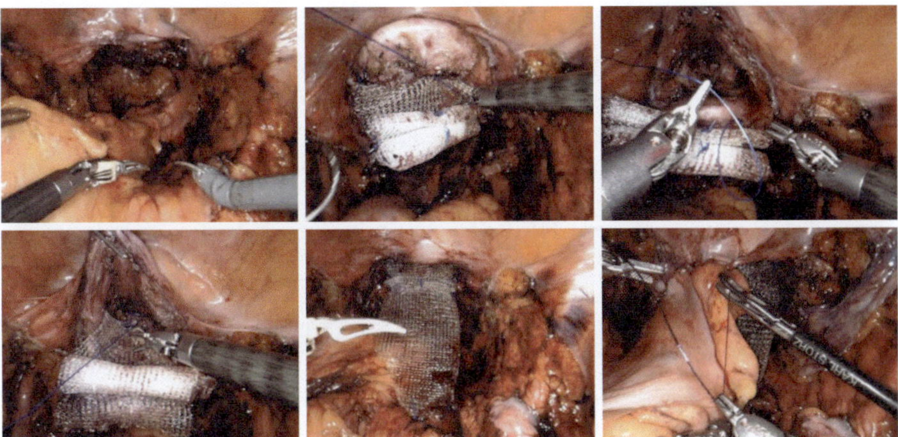

Fig. 15 Steps of a sacrocolpopexy in a post-total hysterectomy patient. A "Y"-shaped polipropilene mesh is attached over the posterior and anterior vaginal aspects and cranially tractioned for fixation into the sacral promontory anterior longitudinal ligament. (Photo: courtesy of Dr. Renato Moretti-Marques's personal archive)

3.5 Pelvic Organ Prolapse

Abdominal sacrocolpopexy is the gold standard in the treatment of apical prolapses (Fig. 15). When compared to transvaginal approaches, it showed a lower rate of recurrence and less postoperative dyspareunia [48].

4 Robotics in Malignant Gynecological Diseases

4.1 Cervical Cancer

The Laparoscopic Approach to Cervical Cancer (LACC) trial results and other complementary studies show worse recurrence rates and overall survival in minimally invasive surgery compared to open surgery in radical hysterectomy for early-stage cervical cancer [49]. On the other hand, there are many arguments that suggest the oncological principles were unfollowed in those studies. New studies are coming to elucidate this issue. The international multi-center, open-label randomized controlled trial Robot-Assisted Approach to Cervical Cancer (RACC) and A Trial of Robotic Versus Open Hysterectomy Surgery in Cervix Cancer (ROCC) are ongoing and aim to answer whether robotic surgery has an effect on cancer outcomes [50].

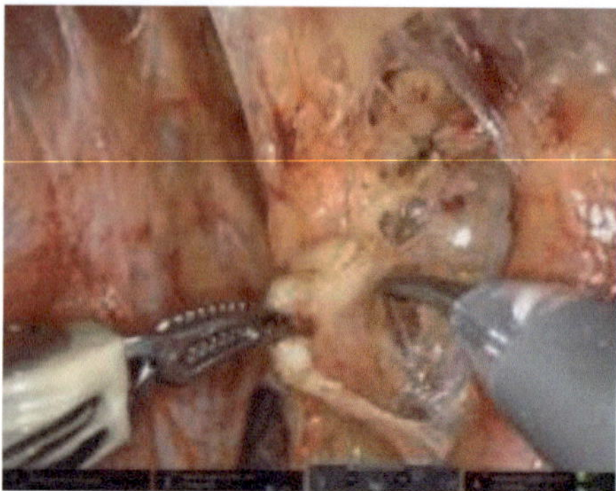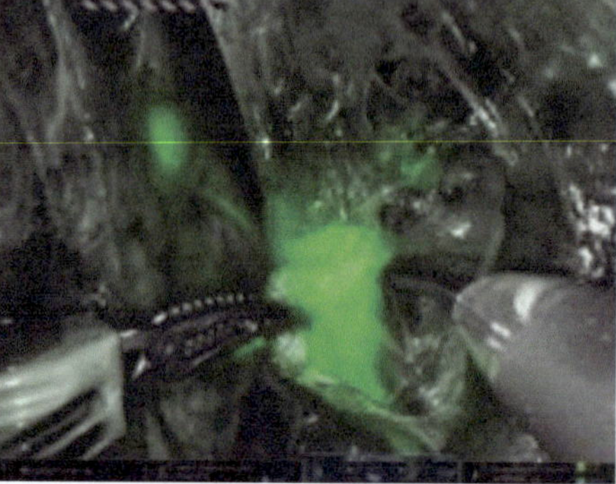

Fig. 16 Right pelvic sentinel lymph node excision during a radical trachelectomy for FIGO IB1 squamous cell cervical carcinoma. (Photo: courtesy of Dr. Renato Moretti-Marques's personal archive)

What we do know is that minimally invasive surgery is superior to open surgery in short-term perioperative outcomes such as blood loss, length of hospital stay, and complications in patients with early-stage cervical cancer treated with radical hysterectomy [51, 52].

For fertility-sparing surgery in early-stage cervical cancer cases, radical trachelectomy is performed. The literature and ongoing studies failed to prove worse oncological results in minimally invasive surgeries in up to 2.0 cm cervical tumors, mostly in non-residual lesions in surgical specimens. The robotic surgery is useful not only for avascular space dissection but also in the identification of sentinel lymph nodes, by the use of near-infrared light on indocyanine green available on da Vinci platforms (Fig. 16), and the tailoring nerve-sparing parametrectomy.

There is no data based on randomized controlled trials (RCTs) to affirm the MIS could not be applied to radical trachelectomy. The most extensive experience in this field comes from laparoscopic-vaginal-assisted surgery, the Dargent's procedure [53, 54].

There is no doubt that once performing minimally invasive surgery on cervical cancer, the LACC trial results should be known and discussed with the multidisciplinary team and the patient. There are no more excuses to not prevent the malignant cell spillage before and during the surgery. The vaginal flap envelopes and covers the cervix, and the non-uterine manipulation procedure and the non-touch tumor surgery are oncological concepts that should be strictly followed.

4.2　Uterine Cancer

The history of robotic surgery in gynecology overlaps the decrease of open surgery in gynecologic oncology since 2005. Two feasibility studies regarding initial endometrial cancers were published. The well-known risk factors and comorbidities

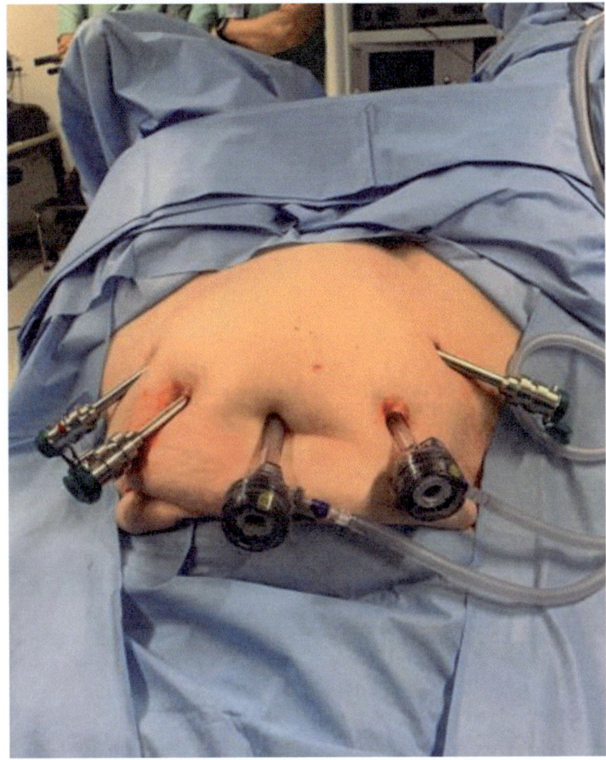

Fig. 17 Robotic treatment of early-stage endometrial cancer using the da Vinci Si platform. (Photo: courtesy of Dr. Renato Moretti-Marques's personal archive)

of endometrial cancer-associated indicate the high risk of perioperative complications rates in surgical staging for this neoplasm. Robotic-assisted surgery (RAS) was proved successful especially for staging early endometrial cancer (stages I and II), due to the lower complication rates (wound infection, evisceration, and urinary fistula) compared to open surgery and conventional laparoscopy [52–54]. Obesity, a condition commonly found among endometrial cancer patients, is one of the most challenging barriers to performing MIS. The choice of robotics in these cases seems to have an important benefit over laparoscopy and laparotomy (Figs. 17, 18, and 19). Years later, the LAP2 trial demonstrated that there were no worse oncological outcomes compared to open surgery. Since then, the MIS, mostly by robotic assistance, became the standard of care [55].

4.3 Ovarian Cancer

Ovarian cancer is one of the most lethal gynecological cancers. The majority of patients are diagnosed in advanced stages and high mortality rates are found. The minimally invasive surgery is used in ovarian cancer patients for a long time, and the

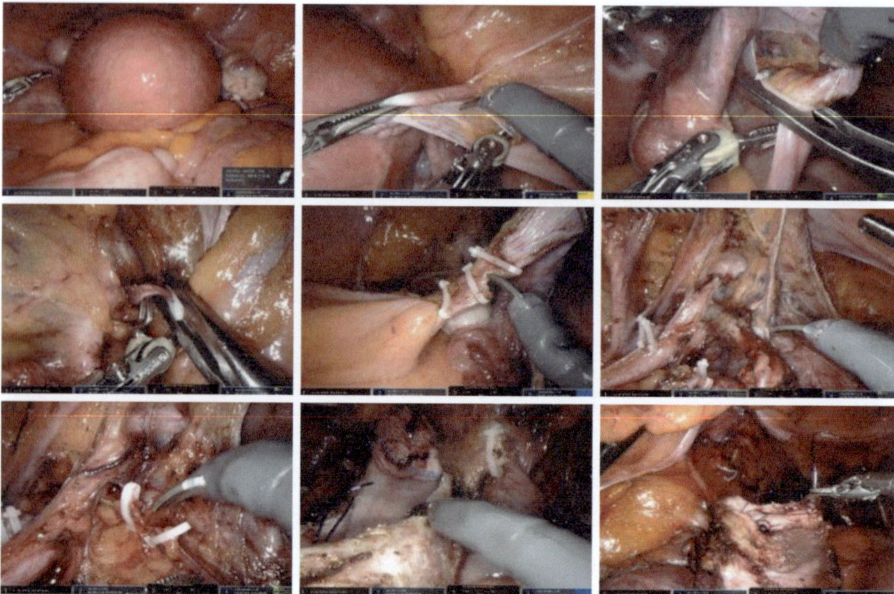

Fig. 18 Robotic treatment of early-stage FIGO IA2 endometrioid endometrial cancer using the da Vinci Xi platform. The camera port was placed cephalad to umbilical scar due to high uterine volume (960 cm^3). The robot was very useful for fine dissection and safe exposure of noble structures. Hysterectomy was performed by clipping the uterine artery at the origin, dissecting avascular spaces, such as medial paravesical, medial pararectal, vesicouterine, and vesicocervical for safe identification of the ureter and dissection of the tunnel to the bladder. Minimal energy use was employed, prioritizing plastic clips. Before the beginning of the surgery, the cervix was enveloped, and at the end the vagina was closed for specimen abdominal removal, through Pfannenstiel incision. (Photo: courtesy of Dr. Renato Moretti-Marques's personal archive)

Fig. 19 Structure identification on the case above. (Photo: courtesy of Dr. Renato Moretti-Marques's personal archive)

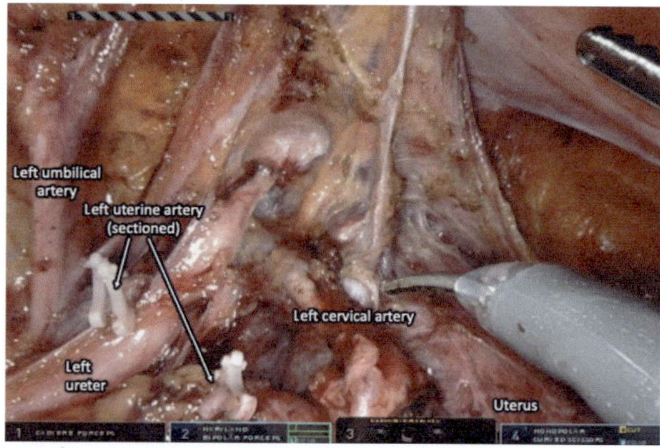

laparoscopy for histological study and to evaluate the extension of carcinomatosis is used until the current days. The management of suspicious adnexal masses requires the surgeon's skills to perform the hysterectomy, the full pelvic and para-aortic lymphadenectomy, and omentectomy. The laparoscopic technique requires a long learning curve for younger surgeons and the robotic surgery indications find room in some of those situations.

4.3.1 Staging of Early Ovarian Carcinoma

The recommended treatment by the International Federation of Gynecology and Obstetrics (FIGO) for apparently early-stage ovarian carcinoma consists of surgical staging based on hysterectomy, bilateral adnexectomy, omentectomy, pelvic and aortic lymphadenectomy, multiple peritoneal biopsies, and appendectomy (for mucinous histology). A multi-quadrant surgery is needed; thus, the best surgical strategy should be considered [56].

Some studies show that, in terms of operative time, robotic surgery is shorter compared to laparoscopy and both are longer compared to open surgery [57, 58]. However, estimated blood loss (EBL) and length of stay (LOS) were higher in laparotomy compared to laparoscopy and robotics. Besides, there was no impairment in surgical staging, there was no increase in the number of complications, and oncological outcomes were similar [58, 59]. Despite the worldwide growth of robotic surgery and probable access so more patients benefit from this technology, data still needs improvement. Most of the studies are retrospective, with a small number of patients, and were carried out in centers whose surgeons had extensive robotic training.

4.3.2 Debulking Advanced Ovarian Carcinoma

The role of robotic surgery in the treatment of patients with advanced-stage or recurrent ovarian cancer is still debated, and the literature is again based on case series and case-control studies. The standard treatment for advanced epithelial ovarian cancer (AEOC) patients includes primary open cytoreductive surgery, with maximal effort to achieve complete tumor resection, followed by platinum-based chemotherapy.

Even with the old robot platforms S and Si, when faced with neoplastic involvement of the upper abdomen, it is up to the surgeon to choose the alternatives: conversion to conventional surgery, conversion to laparoscopy, or redocking to access the upper abdomen, prolonging the surgical time.

The fourth generation of the da Vinci® robots, the Xi model, seems to have solved this dilemma. The greater flexibility for choosing the entrance of the optics and instruments allows easy and agile access to the upper floor, in addition to the possibility of changing the position during surgery [60].

In a study with 76 patients with peritoneal carcinomatosis due to ovarian cancer, they were divided into 3 groups according to the surgical access route and subdivided according to the degree of complexity of the procedure. The expected results of lower blood loss and length of hospital stay were observed in the minimally invasive surgery groups (robot or laparoscopy). As the surgical complexity increased, a significant increase in surgical time was observed among robot-assisted patients.

Despite this, the survival time was similar in the three evaluated groups and the disease-free time was longer in the robot group, probably due to patient selection bias [57, 61].

As for the trocar implant, a fearsome complication due to the use of the technique, a systematic review published in 2015 by Lavazzo identified 20 cases of metastasis at the portal site in robotic surgery (11 cases of endometrial cancer and 9 cases of cervical cancer); however, approaches for ovarian cancer were not included [62]. Another review with 115 robot-operated cases did not identify any metastases from the trocar puncture site [62, 63]. To avoid this event, the tissues should be resected under protection and the trocars must be removed only after the pneumoperitoneum deflation to avoid the so-called chimney effect.

With no significant differences in terms of operative time, RAS had less blood loss and a lower conversion rate to laparotomy [55, 56]. Also, the introduction of robotic surgery for endometrial cancer has reduced costs due to reduced patient stay and complications in morbidity obese patients [57].

5   Robotic-Assisted Surgery in Special Cases

5.1   *Uterine Transposition*

Other procedures performed successfully with robot assistance are ovarian transposition and uterine transposition (Fig. 20) [64–67].

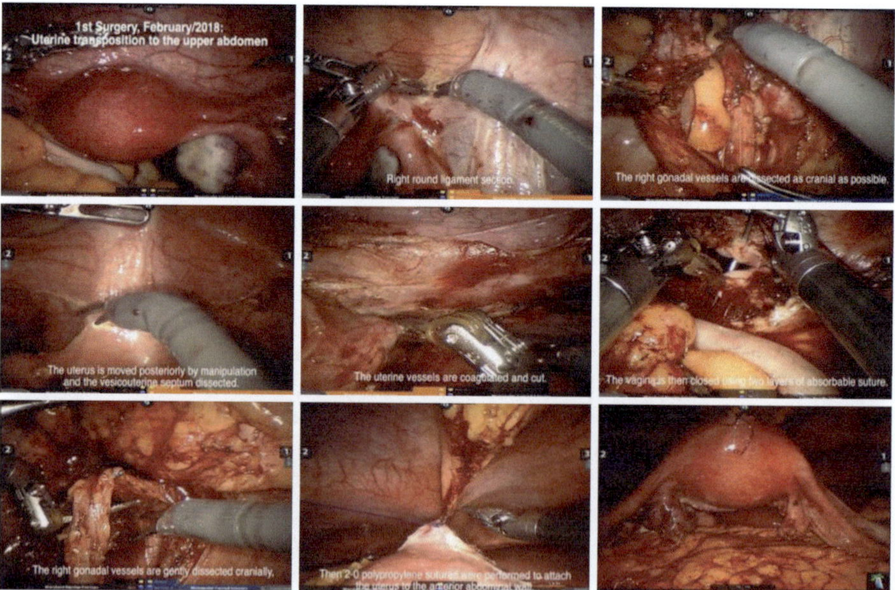

Fig. 20 Surgical steps of the robotic uterine transposition. (Photo: courtesy of Dr. Renato Moretti-Marques's et al. published article [67])

5.2 Abdominal Cerclage in Pregnancy

A recent innovative and promising application is abdominal cerclage for cervical insufficiency for either idiopathic cause or after radical trachelectomy [68, 69].

5.3 Robotics in Mastology

There are reports in the medical literature on nipple-sparing robotic mastectomy; however, the FDA warns patients and health professionals that the safety and effectiveness of robotic-assisted surgery (RAS) devices for use in mastectomy procedures or in the prevention or treatment of breast cancer has not been established.

6 Perspectives

In conclusion, robotic surgery, also called robot-assisted laparoscopic surgery, is a surgical modality that demands structure, availability of materials, and a well-trained multidisciplinary team.

The known benefits of minimally invasive surgery and the additional benefits of robotic surgery already mentioned above encourage us to recommend this surgical modality even more. Ergonomics, precision of movements, articulated movements, and the efficiency of mono- and bipolar energy provide surgical efficiency and safer access to difficult anatomic regions compared to conventional laparoscopy or open surgery. The fact that the trocars are practically fixed avoids the well-known "chimney factor" with the trocars that come out and are replaced in the abdominal wall. It is believed that robotic surgery can be of great value when properly used, respecting the exclusion criteria of minimally invasive surgery in the treatment of gynecological diseases.

References

1. Margossian H, Garcia-Ruiz A, Falcone T, Goldberg JM, Attaran M, Miller JH, Gagner M. Robotically assisted laparoscopic tubal anastomosis in a porcine model: a pilot study. J Laparoendosc Adv Surg Tech A. 1998;8:69–73.
2. Alkatout I, Mettler L, Maass N, Ackermann J. Robotic surgery in gynecology. J Turk Ger Gynecol Assoc. 2016;17:224–32.
3. Oleynikov D. Robotic surgery. Surg Clin N Am. 2008;88:1121–30.
4. Freschi C, Ferrari V, Melfi F, Ferrari M, Mosca F, Cuschieri A. Technical review of the da Vinci surgical telemanipulator. Int J Med Robot Comput Assist Surg. 2013;9:396–406.
5. Gosrisirikul C, Don Chang K, Raheem AA, Rha KH. New era of robotic surgical systems. Asian J Endosc Surg. 2018;11:291–9.

6. Gomes MTV, Machado AMN, Podgaec S, Barison GAS. Initial experience with single-port robotic hysterectomy. Einstein. 2017;15:476–80.
7. Han ES, Advincula AP. Robotic surgery: advancements and inflection points in the field of gynecology. Obstet Gynecol Clin North Am. 2021;48:759–76.
8. Rao PP. Robotic surgery: new robots and finally some real competition! World J Urol. 2018;36:537–41.
9. Peters BS, Armijo PR, Krause C, Choudhury SA, Oleynikov D. Review of emerging surgical robotic technology. Surg Endosc. 2018;32:1636–55.
10. Jena A-K-T. Home—avateramedical. www.avatera.eu/en/avatera-system. 2020. Accessed 5 Jan 2022.
11. Chang KD, Raheem AA, Choi YD, Chung BH, Rha KH. Retzius-sparing robot-assisted radical prostatectomy using the Revo-i robotic surgical system: surgical technique and results of the first human trial. BJU Int. 2018;122:441–8.
12. Profile V. Medicaroid's hinotori surgical robot system approved in Japan. 2020.
13. Koukourikis P, Rha KH. Robotic surgical systems in urology: what is currently available? Investig Clin Urol. 2021;62:14–22.
14. Millan B, Nagpal S, Ding M, Lee JY, Kapoor A. A scoping review of emerging and established surgical robotic platforms with applications in urologic surgery. SIUJ. 2021;2:300–10.
15. Moon AS, Garofalo J, Koirala P, Vu M-LT, Chuang L. Robotic surgery in gynecology. Surg Clin North Am. 2020;100:445–60.
16. Lawrie TA, Liu H, Lu D, Dowswell T, Song H, Wang L, Shi G. Robot-assisted surgery in gynaecology. Cochrane Database Syst Rev. 2019;4:CD011422.
17. Giacomoni A, Concone G, Di Sandro S, Lauterio A, De Carlis L. The meaning of surgeon's comfort in robotic surgery. Am J Surg. 2014;208:871–2.
18. Visco AG, Advincula AP. Robotic gynecologic surgery. Obstet Gynecol. 2008;112:1369–84.
19. White S, Agarwal S, Ratnayake A. Anaesthesia for robotic gynaecological surgery. In: Textbook of gynecologic robotic surgery; 2018. p. 9–12.
20. Website.
21. Einarsson JI, Hibner M, Advincula AP. Side docking: an alternative docking method for gynecologic robotic surgery. Rev Obstet Gynecol. 2011;4:123–5.
22. [No title]. https://www.intuitive.com/en-us/-/media/ISI/Intuitive/Pdf/xi-x-ina-catalog-no-pricing-us-1052082.pdf. Accessed 4 Apr 2022.
23. Monterossi G, Pedone Anchora L, Gueli Alletti S, Fagotti A, Fanfani F, Scambia G. The first European gynaecological procedure with the new surgical robot Hugo™ RAS. A total hysterectomy and salpingo-oophorectomy in a woman affected by BRCA-1 mutation. Facts Views Vis ObGyn. 2022;14:91–4.
24. McCarus SD. Senhance robotic platform system for gynecological surgery. JSLS. 2021;25:e2020.00075. https://doi.org/10.4293/JSLS.2020.00075.
25. Montlouis-Calixte J, Ripamonti B, Barabino G, Corsini T, Chauleur C. Senhance 3-mm robot-assisted surgery: experience on first 14 patients in France. J Robot Surg. 2019;13:643–7.
26. Panico G, Campagna G, Vacca L, Caramazza D, Pizzacalla S, Rumolo V, Scambia G, Ercoli A. The Senhance ® assisted laparoscopy in urogynaecology: case report of sacral colpopexy with subtotal hysterectomy with bilateral salpingo-oophorectomy for pelvic organ prolapse : video article, to see the video use this link: https://qrco.de/bbdi3G. Facts Views Vis Obgyn. 2020;12:245–8.
27. Siaulys R, Klimasauskiene V, Janusonis V, Ezerskiene V, Dulskas A, Samalavicius NE. Robotic gynaecological surgery using Senhance® robotic platform: single Centre experience with 100 cases. J Gynecol Obstet Hum Reprod. 2021;50:102031.
28. Falavolti C, Gidaro S, Ruiz E, Altobelli E, Stark M, Ravasio G, Ravasio G, Lazzaretti SS, Buscarini M. Experimental nephrectomies using a novel Telesurgical system: (the Telelap ALF-X)-a pilot study. Surg Technol Int. 2014;25:37–41.

29. Raheem AA, Troya IS, Kim DK, Kim SH, Won PD, Joon PS, Hyun GS, Rha KH. Robot-assisted fallopian tube transection and anastomosis using the new REVO-I robotic surgical system: feasibility in a chronic porcine model. BJU Int. 2016;118:604–9.

30. Morton J, Hardwick RH, Tilney HS, Gudgeon AM, Jah A, Stevens L, Marecik S, Slack M. Preclinical evaluation of the versius surgical system, a new robot-assisted surgical device for use in minimal access general and colorectal procedures. Surg Endosc. 2021;35:2169–77.

31. Thomas BC, Slack M, Hussain M, Barber N, Pradhan A, Dinneen E, Stewart GD. Preclinical evaluation of the Versius surgical system, a new robot-assisted surgical device for use in minimal access renal and prostate surgery. Eur Urol Focus. 2021;7:444–52.

32. Puntambekar SP, Goel A, Chandak S, Chitale M, Hivre M, Chahal H, Rajesh KN, Manerikar K. Feasibility of robotic radical hysterectomy (RRH) with a new robotic system. Experience at galaxy care laparoscopy institute. J Robot Surg. 2021;15:451–6.

33. Jena A-K-T. Made in Germany—avateramedical. https://www.avatera.eu/en/company/made-in-germany. Accessed 9 Jan 2022.

34. Whooley S. Johnson & Johnson discloses two-year delay for ottava robot. In: MassDevice; 2021. https://www.massdevice.com/johnson-johnson-hits-snag-in-ottava-surgical-robot-development/. Accessed 4 Apr 2022.

35. Diaz-Arrastia C, Jurnalov C, Gomez G, Townsend C Jr. Laparoscopic hysterectomy using a computer-enhanced surgical robot. Surg Endosc. 2002;16:1271–3.

36. Payne TN, Dauterive FR. A comparison of total laparoscopic hysterectomy to robotically assisted hysterectomy: surgical outcomes in a community practice. J Minim Invasive Gynecol. 2008;15:286–91.

37. Pitter MC, Gargiulo AR, Bonaventura LM, Lehman JS, Srouji SS. Pregnancy outcomes following robot-assisted myomectomy. Hum Reprod. 2013;28:99–108.

38. Rivas-López R, Sandoval-García-Travesí FA. Robotic surgery in gynecology: review of literature. Cir Cir. 2020;88:107–16.

39. Truong M, Kim JH, Scheib S, Patzkowsky K. Advantages of robotics in benign gynecologic surgery. Curr Opin Obstet Gynecol. 2016;28:304–10.

40. Gomes MTV, Costa Porto BT, Parise Filho JP, Vasconcelos AL, Bottura BF, Marques RM. Safety model for the introduction of robotic surgery in gynecology. Rev Bras Ginecol Obstet. 2018;40:397–402.

41. Barakat EE, Bedaiwy MA, Zimberg S, Nutter B, Nosseir M, Falcone T. Robotic-assisted, laparoscopic, and abdominal myomectomy: a comparison of surgical outcomes. Obstet Gynecol. 2011;117:256–66.

42. Giudice LC. Clinical practice. Endometriosis. N Engl J Med. 2010;362:2389–98.

43. Kho RM, Andres MP, Borrelli GM, Neto JS, Zanluchi A, Abrão MS. Surgical treatment of different types of endometriosis: comparison of major society guidelines and preferred clinical algorithms. Best Pract Res Clin Obstet Gynaecol. 2018;51:102–10.

44. Restaino S, Mereu L, Finelli A, et al. Robotic surgery vs laparoscopic surgery in patients with diagnosis of endometriosis: a systematic review and meta-analysis. J Robot Surg. 2020;14:687–94.

45. Luu THA, Jean Uy-Kroh M. New developments in surgery for endometriosis and pelvic pain. Clin Obstet Gynecol. 2017;60:245–51.

46. Soares T, Oliveira MA, Panisset K, Habib N, Rahman S, Klebanoff JS, Moawad GN. Diaphragmatic endometriosis and thoracic endometriosis syndrome: a review on diagnosis and treatment. Horm Mol Biol Clin Invest. 2021;43:137. https://doi.org/10.1515/hmbci-2020-0066.

47. Delara R, Suárez-Salvador E, Magrina J, Magtibay P. Robotic excision of full-thickness diaphragmatic endometriosis. J Minim Invasive Gynecol. 2020;27:815.

48. Ko KJ, Lee K-S. Robotic Sacrocolpopexy for treatment of apical compartment prolapse. Int Neurourol J. 2020;24:97–110.

49. Ramirez PT, Frumovitz M, Pareja R, et al. Minimally invasive versus abdominal radical hysterectomy for cervical cancer. N Engl J Med. 2018;379:1895–904.

50. Falconer H, Palsdottir K, Stalberg K, et al. Robot-assisted approach to cervical cancer (RACC): an international multi-center, open-label randomized controlled trial. Int J Gynecol Cancer. 2019;29:1072–6.

51. Nitecki R, Ramirez PT, Frumovitz M, Krause KJ, Tergas AI, Wright JD, Rauh-Hain JA, Melamed A. Survival after minimally invasive vs open radical hysterectomy for early-stage cervical cancer: a systematic review and meta-analysis. JAMA Oncol. 2020;6:1019–27.

52. Obermair A, Asher R, Pareja R, et al. Incidence of adverse events in minimally invasive vs open radical hysterectomy in early cervical cancer: results of a randomized controlled trial. Am J Obstet Gynecol. 2020;222:249.e1–249.e10.

53. Salvo G, Pareja R, Ramirez PT. Minimally invasive radical trachelectomy: considerations on surgical approach. Best Pract Res Clin Obstet Gynaecol. 2021;75:113–22.

54. Dargent D, Martin X, Sacchetoni A, Mathevet P. Laparoscopic vaginal radical trachelectomy. Cancer. 2000;88:1877–82.

55. Walker JL, Piedmonte MR, Spirtos NM, Eisenkop SM, Schlaerth JB, Mannel RS, Spiegel G, Barakat R, Pearl ML, Sharma SK. Laparoscopy compared with laparotomy for comprehensive surgical staging of uterine cancer: gynecologic oncology group study LAP2. J Clin Oncol. 2009;27:5331–6.

56. Lucidi A, Chiantera V, Gallotta V, Ercoli A, Scambia G, Fagotti A. Role of robotic surgery in ovarian malignancy. Best Pract Res Clin Obstet Gynaecol. 2017;45:74–82.

57. Magrina JF, Zanagnolo V, Noble BN, Kho RM, Magtibay P. Robotic approach for ovarian cancer: perioperative and survival results and comparison with laparoscopy and laparotomy. Gynecol Oncol. 2011;121:100–5.

58. Gallotta V, Cicero C, Conte C, Vizzielli G, Petrillo M, Fagotti A, Chiantera V, Costantini B, Scambia G, Ferrandina G. Robotic versus laparoscopic staging for early ovarian cancer: a case-matched control study. J Minim Invasive Gynecol. 2017;24:293–8.

59. Nezhat FR, Finger TN, Vetere P, Radjabi AR, Vega M, Averbuch L, Khalil S, Altinbas SK, Lax D. Comparison of perioperative outcomes and complication rates between conventional versus robotic-assisted laparoscopy in the evaluation and management of early, advanced, and recurrent stage ovarian, fallopian tube, and primary peritoneal cancer. Int J Gynecol Cancer. 2014;24:600–7.

60. Bush SH, Apte SM. Robotic-assisted surgery in gynecological oncology. Cancer Control. 2015;22:307–13.

61. Minig L, Iserte PP, Zorrero C, Zanagnolo V. Robotic surgery in women with ovarian cancer: surgical technique and evidence of clinical outcomes. J Minim Invasive Gynecol. 2016;23:309–16.

62. Iavazzo C, Gkegkes ID. Port-site metastases in patients with gynecological cancer after robot-assisted operations. Arch Gynecol Obstet. 2015;292:263–9.

63. Seror J, Bats A-S, Bensaïd C, Douay-Hauser N, Ngo C, Lécuru F. Risk of port-site metastases in pelvic cancers after robotic surgery. Eur J Surg Oncol. 2015;41:599–603.

64. Molpus KL, Wedergren JS, Carlson MA. Robotically assisted endoscopic ovarian transposition. JSLS. 2003;7:59–62.

65. Baiocchi G, Vieira M, Moretti-Marques R, Mantoan H, Faloppa C, Damasceno RCF, Paula SOC, Tsunoda AT, Ribeiro R. Uterine transposition for gynecological cancers. Int J Gynecol Cancer. 2021;31:442–6.

66. Odetto D, Saadi JM, Chacon CB, Wernicke A, Ribeiro R. Uterine transposition after radical trachelectomy. Int J Gynecol Cancer. 2021;31:1374–9.

67. Marques RM, Tsunoda AT, Dias RS, Pimenta JM, Linhares JC, Ribeiro R. Robotic uterine transposition for a cervical cancer patient with pelvic micrometastases after conization and pelvic lymphadenectomy. Int J Gynecol Cancer. 2020;30:898–9.

68. Corinti M, Ramos GGF, Bezerra VA, Barison GA, Moretti-Marques R, Vieira Gomes MT. Robotic-assisted laparoscopy for abdominal cerclage and correction of amniotic fistula. J Minim Invasive Gynecol. 2021;28:S139.

69. Barmat L, Glaser G, Davis G, Craparo F. Da Vinci-assisted abdominal cerclage. Fertil Steril. 2007;88:1437.e1–3.

Robotic Devices in Neurosurgery

Paulo Porto de Melo

1 Introduction

Neurosurgery is the medical specialty that most requires absolute precision. We, neurosurgeons, face daily the fear of unintended lesions due to errors related to the proximity of critical structures or to the limits of human dexterity to manipulate microsurgical instruments when operating on deep, narrow, and eloquent corridors.

In some cases, for example, one has to insert a screw inside an osseous corridor, called pedicle, surrounded by the dural sac with the medulla inside and exiting nerve roots above and below this corridor, in a total area of about 10 mm. In other cases, as a brainstem tumor, the neurosurgeon operates and removes tumors inside an area which has, in a cylindrical section, no more than 16 mm and carries inside all the body information (including sensory, motor, autonomic, and vegetative pathways).

Because of the inherent architecture of the central and peripheral nervous system, the neurosurgeon almost always operates with the aid of microsurgical devices such as loupes or surgical microscopes, with high magnification and special lights, trying to eliminate shadows and enhance visualization of critical structures.

Allied with all the abovementioned characteristics, the central nervous system is usually protected by thick bones, which makes the surgery last long due to the access route. The longer the surgery, more tired the surgeon gets, with an increase in tremor occurrence and decrease on performance, increasing the risk of unintended surgical damage.

When you present neurosurgeons with a system which is capable of providing magnification, tremor filtering, and motion scaling (providing more precise operation in the tiniest corridors), you are actually giving them a potential solution

P. P. de Melo (✉)
Department of Neurosurgery, Brazilian Army, Sao Paulo, SP, Brazil
e-mail: portodemelo@alumni.harvard.edu

J. P. Manzano, L. M. Ferreira (eds.), *Robotic Surgery Devices in Surgical Specialties*, https://doi.org/10.1007/978-3-031-35102-0_14

to their biggest adversaries and, ultimately, increasing the safety and chances of good outcomes.

2   History in Neurosurgery

The need for improved outcomes, visualization, dexterity, precision and reduced costs, invasion, and tremor points out to robotic assistance as a promising field in neurosurgery.

As a matter of fact, since 1988, there have been reports of the use of robotic assistance to obtain this, as the paper published by Kwoh et al. [1], where an ancient robotic system, called PUMA, was interfaced with a computed tomography (CT) scanner to perform brain tumor biopsies, resulting in not only faster but also more accurate procedures.

Automation, per se, is an old concept in humanity and has been brought to life as early as in the *Iliad*, where Homer described automatons built by Hephaestus (Vulcan), the god of metallurgy. Homer elaborated instruments that followed programming, being automatic by definition. Automation, as a concept, is widely acknowledged as soon as in the fourth century BC, being described in the also classic *The Politics*, by Aristotle. Aristotle described the concept of a society where each instrument would be able to do its own work, "obeying or anticipating the will of others" which is, long story short, the core principle of all the master-slave robotic systems employed nowadays in medical specialties.

Centuries later, in 1898, after the fantastic contributions made by early scientists as Leonardo da Vinci, Nikola Tesla [2] described the concept of *teleautomaton*, a method of controlling automations from a certain distance, an advancement that was received, as almost everything in science, with skepticism and surprise.

It took yet another century for mankind to testify the use of remote manipulation in the surface of Mars, via the Sojourner Mars rover, or in the operating rooms across the planet with the multiple robotic platforms nowadays available.

In the following decades, automation met computer science, and the use of robotics is always at the cutting edge of human endeavors, with systems designed to perform highly dangerous and precise tasks in this planet or at remote locations such as the moon and Mars. They are widespread now on a huge variety of fields of our modern society, from the assembly of automobiles to the manipulation of nuclear reactors and from the assembly of tiny micro-components of a cell phone to the highest precision stitches placed by a neurosurgeon on a brain vascular anastomosis, reaching nanometers.

As stated above, robotics began to pave its way in neurosurgery in the 1980s, with the development of computer-assisted stereotactic guidance. Arteriovenous malformations that were on difficult access regions, were successfully treated by the State University of New York, at Buffalo, by Kelly et al. [3–6].

A seminal paper published by Drake et al. [7], in 1991, showed deep-seated benign tumors, previously considered beyond therapeutic possibilities without significant morbidity-mortality, were successfully removed on six children without mortality or morbidity.

Robotics was also soon adopted on the most revolutionary aid for neurosurgery, the surgical microscope. Focus and magnification are no longer manual but robotically administered and automated, along with laser precision distance estimation on the most recent systems, which gives modern neurosurgeons superb visualization when compared to the practice of heroes as Harvey Cushing, who had no magnification or special lights at all, leading to better outcomes, safer procedures, and inclusion of patients previously considered as beyond surgical possibilities.

The inability of the current robotic systems on providing haptic feedback was one of the main critics and theoretical drawbacks for the widespread adoption of robotic aid in super-microsurgical procedures. Liverneaux et al. [8], in a paper published in 2011, demonstrated that haptic feedback is not useful on micro sutures using 9-0 and 10-0 suture lines since long before the brain realizes that the knot is tied, the force applied will produce its rupture, making the surgeon to rely on his/her vision and dexterity instead of haptics.

Sutherland et al. [9–11], from the University of Calgary, developed a robotic system compatible with magnetic resonance imaging (MRI) machines and specific for neurosurgery, called NeuroArm. The system has the advantage of being capable of using real-time data obtained by an intraoperative MRI, for example, enhancing even more the precision of the surgeon, but its main obstacle to wide acceptance is the high cost involved on an MRI-compatible operating room to be used only with neurosurgery, making it difficult to convince hospital directors to invest a lot of money in a system that will pay itself only on the long term.

There are several other specific neurosurgical robotic systems that were developed during the last decades trying to introduce new features such as haptic feedback or a greater number of robotic arms.

Davies et al. [12], from the Imperial College, developed the Neurobot, for example, which is a specially designed robotic platform for neurosurgery in which the system compensates the brain shift that occurs due to the intraoperative drainage of CSF with real-time ultrasound that, once fused with preoperative MRI, adjust the position of structures in real time.

De Momi et al. [13], from Italy, described in a paper published in 2010 the ROBOCAST, a robotic system which has not only haptic feedback but also artificial intelligence and path-planning integration and is suited for keyhole neurosurgery.

In a similar path, 2004 has witnessed the launch of a robot designed only to aid in complex spine surgery. The platform, called SpineAssist and developed by Israeli company Mazor, intends to provide optimal trajectory for the implant of transpedicular screws by means of positioning a working channel, robotically, based on preoperative CT scan and MRI, with real-time intraoperative navigation and rigid stereotaxy, reducing the need for X-ray checks [13] during surgery, reducing the exposure of the patient and surgical team to radiation with at least the same accuracy with conventional surgery, but requiring less operative time and promising a lower rate of complications. Retrospective data of 3271 pedicle screws in 635 cases demonstrated a 98.3% accuracy rate with this robotic system as reported by Devito et al. [14].

3 Current Robotic Devices in Neurosurgery

The problem with the above mentioned systems and other systems developed for neurosurgery remains the same: they generate an initial high investment for a robotic platform to be used solely by neurosurgery, which makes the return of investment long, in a field where the advances are speedlight. In other words, it would be very likely that new and better systems appeared before the initial investment paid itself.

This is the main reason that drives hospital managers to invest in robotic platforms that can be shared by multiple specialties, as is the case of da Vinci, by Intuitive Surgical. The system, initially developed by DARPA, an agency linked to the Department of Defense of the United States of America, was sold to Intuitive Surgical, who made some enhancements. It provides motion scaling, based on pantographic movements, high magnification, optimal illumination, and tremor filter, besides having an available training platform. Its main advantage is that it already has a vast amount of papers describing its successful use in diverse fields such as urology, gynecology, vascular and plastic surgery, orthopedics, and, of course, neurosurgery.

A diverse array of procedures have already been published as odontoidectomy, intrauterine myelomeningocele repair, paraspinal schwannoma resection, and anterior lumbar interbody fusion [15–20]. The author, himself, has published some papers regarding nerve harvesting and brachial plexus surgery [21–23], with good results regarding dexterity and minimally invasive access for surgeries of the brachial plexus.

Robotics has also got into alternative methods of treatment of neurosurgical diseases, as is the case with radiosurgery and CyberKnife.

Radiosurgery, introduced by Lars Leksell in 1951, consists of a frame-based system that provides localization and treatment for neurosurgical lesions without performing a craniotomy. This is obtained after the placement of a stereotactic frame on the patients' skull and application of multiple beams of ionizing radiation focused on a single point in a three-dimensional space. The radiation originates from Cobalt, and each beam has itself a low radiation dose, thus avoiding injury to the normal tissue, but when the multiple beams combine at intersection point, the energy is destructive and achieves treatment therapy doses. Automated positioning of the patient soon was incorporated, providing higher accuracy rates (within 0.1 mm in any direction of the 3 main axes). The robotic control of collimator size and position allows effective and exact control of complex targets near critical structures [24, 25].

CyberKnife, from Accuray, consists of a major advance with the association between radiation therapy and robotics. It features real-time image guidance achieved through diagnostic X-rays and robotic integration [26–28]. The system is composed of a compact x-band linear accelerator mounted on a robotic arm, orthogonal diagnostic X-ray cameras with amorphous silicon detectors for real-time tracking, and an automated robotic couch.

The robotic arm provides six degrees of freedom and compensates for any possible patient or lesion movement during treatment to deliver accurate and efficient therapeutic radiation at any accessible direction.

4   Conclusion

Despite the numerous and notorious advances in robotic surgery, there are still some limitations on existing platforms such as high diameter of current cameras, preventing its use for endonasal neurosurgery, for example, and the lack of specially designed microsurgical instruments for neurosurgery, still not available for systems as da Vinci, for example.

The development of instruments and minimization of existing cameras will provide broader use of robotic platforms in neurosurgery, keeping in mind that these systems are designed to enhance human capabilities, as in any other tool that was incorporated into medical practice such as laparoscopy, endoscopy, surgical microscope, loupes, or even microsurgical instruments.

References

1. Kwoh YS, Hou J, Jonckheere EA, Hayati S. A robot with improved absolute positioning accuracy for CT guided stereotactic brain surgery. IEEE Trans Biomed Eng. 1988;35:153–60.
2. Roguin A. Nikola tesla: the man behind the magnetic field unit. J Magn Reson Imaging. 2004;19:369–74.
3. Alker G, Kelly PJ, Kall B, Goerss S. Stereotaxic laser ablation of intracranial lesions. AJNR Am J Neuroradiol. 1983;4:727–30.
4. Goerss S, Kelly PJ, Kall B, Alker GJ Jr. A computed tomographic stereotactic adaptation system. Neurosurgery. 1982;10:375–9.
5. Kelly PJ, Kall B, Goerss S, Alker GJ Jr. Precision resection of intra-axial CNS lesions by CTbased stereotactic craniotomy and computer monitored CO2 laser. Acta Neurochir. 1983;68:1–9.
6. Kelly PJ, Kall BA, Goerss S. Computer simulation for the stereotactic placement of interstitial radionuclide sources into computed tomography-defined tumor volumes. Neurosurgery. 1984;14:442–8.
7. Drake JM, Joy M, Goldenberg A, Kreindler D. Computer- and robot-assisted resection of thalamic astrocytomas in children. Neurosurgery. 1991;29:27–33.
8. Panchulidze I, Berner S, Mantovani G, Liverneaux P. Is haptic feedback necessary to microsurgical suturing? Comparative study of 9/0 and 10/0 knot tying operated by 24 surgeons. Hand Surg. 2011;16(1):1–3. https://doi.org/10.1142/S0218810411004984.
9. Sutherland GR, Lama S, Gan LS, Wolfsberger S, Zareinia K. Merging machines with microsurgery: clinical experience with neuroArm. J Neurosurg. 2013;118:521–9.

10. Sutherland GR, Latour I, Greer AD, Fielding T, Feil G, Newhook P. An image-guided magnetic resonance-compatible surgical robot. Neurosurgery. 2008;62:286–92. [discussion 292–293].
11. Sutherland GR, Wolfsberger S, Lama S, Zareinia K. The evolution of neuroArm. Neurosurgery. 2013;72(Suppl 1):27–32.
12. De Momi E, Ferrigno G. Robotic and artificial intelligence for keyhole neurosurgery: the ROBOCAST project, a multi-modal autonomous path planner. Proc Inst Mech Eng H. 2010;224:715–27.
13. Shoham M, Lieberman IH, Benzel EC, Togawa D, Zehavi E, Zilberstein B, Roffman M, Bruskin A, Fridlander A, Joskowicz L, Brink-Danan S, Knoller N. Robotic assisted spinal surgery—from concept to clinical practice. Comput Aided Surg. 2007;12:105–15.
14. Devito DP, Kaplan L, Dietl R, Pfeiffer M, Horne D, Silberstein B, Hardenbrook M, Kiriyanthan G, Barzilay Y, Bruskin A, Sackerer D, Alexandrovsky V, Stuer C, Burger R, Maeurer J, Donald GD, Schoenmayr R, Friedlander A, Knoller N, Schmieder K, Pechlivanis I, Kim IS, Meyer B, Shoham M. Clinical acceptance and accuracy assessment of spinal implants guided with SpineAssist surgical robot: retrospective study. Spine (Phila Pa 1976). 2010;35:2109–15.
15. Lee JY, Lega B, Bhowmick D, Newman JG, O'Malley BW Jr, Weinstein GS, Grady MS, Welch WC. Da Vinci robot-assisted transoral odontoidectomy for basilar invagination. ORL J Otorhinolaryngol Relat Spec. 2010;72:91–5.
16. Yang MS, Kim KN, Yoon DH, Pennant W, Ha Y. Robot-assisted resection of paraspinal schwannoma. J Korean Med Sci. 2011;26:150–3.
17. Yang MS, Yoon DH, Kim KN, Kim H, Yang JW, Yi S, Lee JY, Jung WJ, Rha KH, Ha Y. Robot assisted anterior lumbar interbody fusion in a swine model in vivo test of the da vinci surgical assisted spinal surgery system. Spine (Phila Pa 1976). 2011;36:E139–43.
18. Yang MS, Yoon TH, Yoon DH, Kim KN, Pennant W, Ha Y. Robot-assisted transoral odontoidectomy: experiment in new minimally invasive technology, a cadaveric study. J Korean Neurosurg Soc. 2011;49:248–51.
19. Aaronson OS, Tulipan NB, Cywes R, Sundell HW, Davis GH, Bruner JP, Richards WO. Robot-assisted endoscopic intrauterine myelomeningocele repair: a feasibility study. Pediatr Neurosurg. 2002;36:85–9.
20. Hong WC, Tsai JC, Chang SD, Sorger JM. Robotic skull base surgery via supraorbital keyhole approach a cadaveric study. Neurosurgery. 2013;72(Suppl 1):33–8.
21. Ichihara S, Bodin F, Pedersen JC, Porto de Melo P, Garcia JC, Facca S, Liverneaux PA. Robotically assisted harvest of the latissimus dorsi muscle: a cadaver feasibility study and clinical test case. Hand Surg Rehabil. 2016;35:81–4.
22. Porto de Melo P, Miyamoto H, Serradori T, Mantovani GR, Selber JC, Facca S, Xu WD, Santelmo N, Liverneaux PA. Robotic phrenic nerve harvest: a feasibility study in a pig model. Chir Main. 2014;33:356–60.
23. Porto de Melo PM, Garcia JC, De Souza Montero EF, Atik T, Robert EG, Facca S, Liverneaux PA. Feasibility of an endoscopic approach to the axillary nerve and the nerve to the long head of the triceps brachii with the help of the Da Vinci robot. Chir Main. 2013;32:206–9.
24. Lindquist C, Paddick I. The Leksell gamma knife Perfexion and comparisons with its predecessors. Neurosurgery. 2008;62(Suppl 2):721–32.
25. Yomo S, Tamura M, Carron R, Porcheron D, Regis J. A quantitative comparison of radiosurgical treatment parameters in vestibular schwannomas: the Leksell gamma knife Perfexion versus model 4C. Acta Neurochir. 2010;152:47–55.
26. Adler JR Jr. The future of robotics in radiosurgery. Neurosurgery. 2013;72(Suppl 1):8–11.
27. Adler JR Jr, Chang SD, Murphy MJ, Doty J, Geis P, Hancock SL. The Cyberknife: a frameless robotic system for radiosurgery. Stereotact Funct Neurosurg. 1997;69(1–4 Pt 2):124–8.
28. Chang SD, Murphy M, Geis P, Martin DP, Hancock SL, Doty JR, Adler JR Jr. Clinical experience with image-guided robotic radiosurgery (the Cyberknife) in the treatment of brain and spinal cord tumors. Neurol Med Chir (Tokyo). 1998;38:780–3.

Robotic Microsurgery

Onuralp Ergun, Ahmet Gudeloglu, and Sijo J. Parekattil

1 Introduction

From its early beginnings, microsurgery has been a challenging field so multiple attempts have been made to ameliorate the technique. Robotic platforms made a huge impact on the field providing the ease of microsurgery-specific instrumentation, increased optical magnification, improved surgical efficiency, and absent tremor. In this chapter, we present the current and novel robotic platforms, emerging technologies, and optimization for robotic systems.

2 Current and Novel Robotic Platforms

Although it is controversial to define the first robotic surgery in literature, many honor Kwoh et al. [1] who used the PUMA 560 (Unimation, Danbury, CT, USA) robotic system for neurosurgical biopsies in 1985. The dominating robotic platform of the modern era, da Vinci® (Intuitive Surgical Inc., Sunnyvale, CA, USA) was first utilized in 1997 during a cholecystectomy case performed by Jacques Himpens [2]. This platform came with the ability to provide high-definition optical magnification up to 12–15 times, better control over the endoscope, wider range of motion of the

O. Ergun
Cleveland Clinic, Cleveland, OH, USA

A. Gudeloglu
Hacettepe University, Ankara, Turkey

S. J. Parekattil (✉)
Avant Concierge Urology, University of Central Florida, Winter Garden, FL, USA
e-mail: sijo@avantconciergeurol.com

© The Author(s), under exclusive license to Springer Nature
Switzerland AG 2023
J. P. Manzano, L. M. Ferreira (eds.), *Robotic Surgery Devices in Surgical Specialties*, https://doi.org/10.1007/978-3-031-35102-0_15

Fig. 1 Symani Surgical System

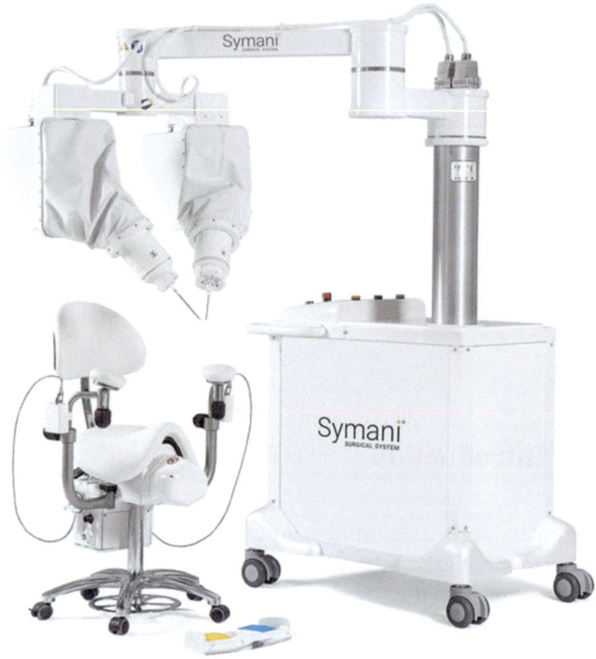

instruments, elimination of tremor, and decreased surgeon fatigue [3]. Robotic-assisted microsurgery is becoming the standard of care in many settings, promoting further interest in the development of adjunctive instruments and novel platforms.

Symani Surgical System (Medical Microinstruments Inc. [MMI], Calci, Italy) is one of these newer platforms (Fig. 1). Despite having limited human studies, the preliminary studies show promising results for this system. Lindenblatt et al. reported successful utilization of this novel platform in humans undergoing lymphatic surgery in early 2022. 100% patency rate was achieved in a total of 10 anastomoses including robotic lymphovenous, robotic lympho-lymphatic, and robotic arterial anastomoses under the size of 1 mm done on 5 patients [4]. Advantages to this system could be the following: wristed micro instruments allowing for movement in 7 planes, lower cost than other widely used platforms, and high accuracy of the robotic arms, whereas the limitations might be the lack of an internal optical unit making the system dependent on complementary surgical setup, lack of high evidence studies with more patients, and having only two robotic arms that can be used at once.

MUSA (Microsure, Eindhoven, the Netherlands), another robot, was introduced in 2021 (Fig. 2). Early studies showed propitious results indicating the platform is as successful in treating breast cancer-related lymphedema as the standard manual lymphatic drainage therapy conducted in a randomized manner [5]. Longer follow-up in this cohort still suggests the robot is feasible and comparable to standard care [6]. To our understanding, this platform has advantages like being more feasible for super microsurgical procedures, being easily maneuverable, and being compatible with standard surgical microscopes and microsurgical instruments. The limitation of this platform could be the lack of cost-related information available to the public.

Fig. 2 MUSA Surgical System

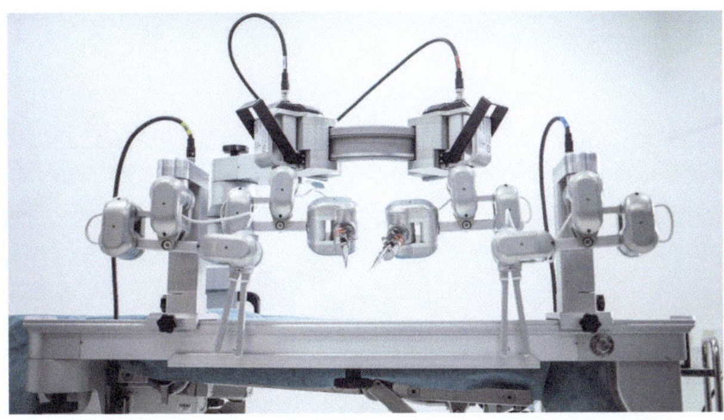

Furthermore, a short time ago, another robotic platform named KangDuo (Suzhou Kangduo Robot Co., Ltd., Jiangsu, China) emerged supported by human studies in urological cases [7–9]. The evidence so far suggests the robot is safe and feasible in a microsurgical setting. In a prospective manner, this robotic platform is the only one providing a study comparing its efficacy and safety to another robot, the da Vinci® [10]. We also want to state that there is no reported data for the cost of this platform too which might be considered a limitation. On the other hand, the cost is expected to be groundbreaking in the robotic field based on the expenses of development reported by the manufacturer (25–30% of expenses for the development of the da Vinci® robot [9]).

3 Robotic Microsurgical Instrumentation

Despite the newly launched robotic systems, da Vinci systems are still the most commercially available robotic system approved by the FDA. Currently, there are more than 5500 da Vinci robots worldwide [11]. The da Vinci systems typically have three components: the surgeon console, a patient cart with one camera arm providing three-dimensional (3D) high-definition vision and three instrument arms that provide a wide range of motion, and an imaging tower. The system supports more than 40 types of robotic EndoWrist instruments. Black Diamond microforceps, micro bipolar forceps, Potts scissors, and curved monopolar scissors are the most commonly used EndoWrist instruments in robotic microsurgical practice (Fig. 3) [12]. These instruments are docked into the robotic arms controlled by the surgeon through the console. The system also grants the surgeon 10–15 times digital magnification and motion scaling.

Robotic arms are attached to 8 mm trocars, and the instruments are passed through. This also applies to ex vivo surgeries for stability purposes. Robotic instruments are advanced 2–3 inches beyond the trocar tip for maximum range of motion. The Black Diamond microforceps are generally used for microdissection, retraction, and as a needle driver for sutures even smaller than 10-0. The bipolar microforceps are mostly utilized for microdissection and retraction in addition to hemostasis by fine cauterization. Furthermore, they can be used as a needle driver

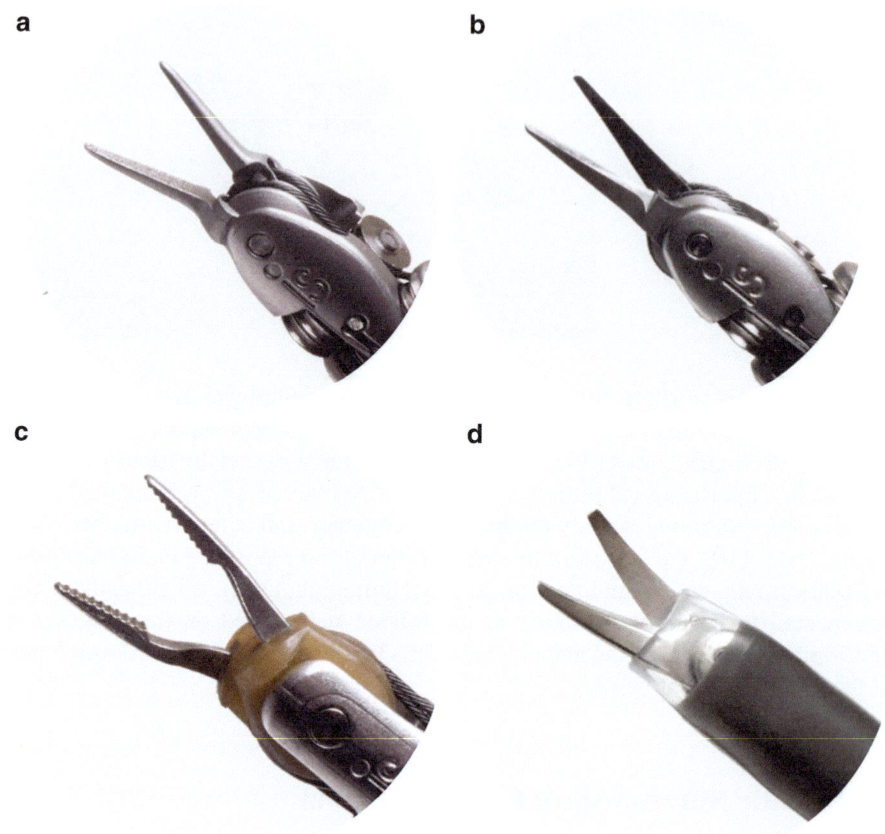

Fig. 3 da Vinci Robotic Platform Microsurgical Instruments. (**a**) Black Diamond microforceps. (**b**) Microbipolar forceps. (**c**) Potts scissors. (**d**) Curved monopolar scissors

for sutures that are larger in size (6-0). Both instruments can be used with supplementary microsurgical tools that will be covered later in this chapter.

Although similar in many ways, the da Vinci had three devices historically. Their latest Xi system has some upgrades to its predecessor, the Si system, including thinner robotic arms with increased joint numbers, better accuracy, and shorter docking times.

4 Optical Magnification

Microsurgery needs enhanced optical view usually up to 20 to 25 times magnification. The da Vinci optical units can only support magnification up to 15 times and may cause pixelation at that level. This could be a limitation for microsurgery and could

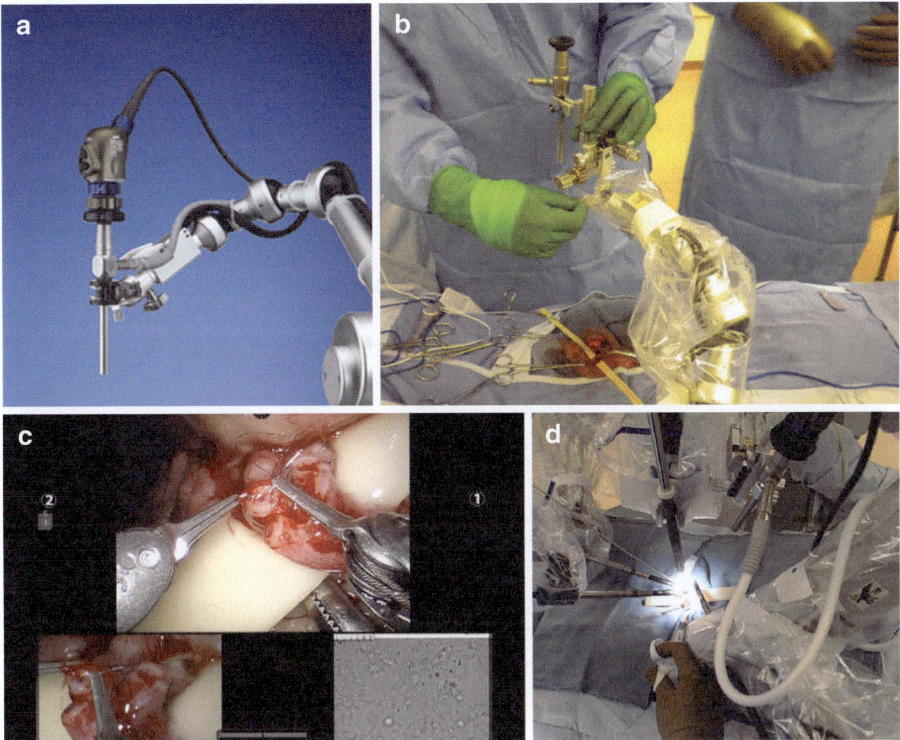

Fig. 4 VITOM Magnification System. (**a**) Camera and its holder. (**b**) Its setup before docking. (**c**) The view in the surgeon console (lower left-hand side view from VITOM camera). (**d**) Its position during the procedure

be overcome by adjunctive optical systems. In our practice, we utilized a new technique with a fifth nitrogen-powered robotic arm that has a video lens system named VITOM (Karl Storz, Tuttlingen, Germany). This system offers up to 25 times magnification without compromising the HD quality. It can also be integrated into the TilePro system (Intuitive Surgical Inc.) of the surgeon console which creates a multi-tab view on the screen of the surgeon resembling a cockpit field (Fig. 4). This allows the surgeon to simultaneously view the image in multiple magnification levels (regular robotic camera and the VITOM camera views) in addition to the surgical systems that are connected to the tower (i.e., real-time microscope view for intra-op semen analysis). We use VITOM in our robot-assisted vasovasostomy and vasoepididymostomy cases routinely applied to TilePro. The authors believe this improves efficiency in many ways: allows two-angle view of complex structures in the microsurgical environment which allows a better understanding of the anatomy, eliminates the need to zoom in and zoom out by providing differently magnified images at the same time, and allows the surgeon to handle semen analysis in real time without leaving the console. Further information on our procedures promoting these devices and their results will be assessed later in this chapter.

5 Assisting Intraoperative Devices

Despite the superiorities of robotic systems in microsurgery, there's still the issue of tactile feedback that is crucial in all means of surgery. Without the tactile feedback, dissecting anatomical structures, feeling tumors, and adjusting strength when tying sutures become harder. Although there is evidence that visual perception over time can result in almost similar error rates with tactile feedback [13], attempts have been made to help the surgeon with certain tasks during the microsurgical procedure. These include but are not limited to Firefly fluorescence imaging (Intuitive Surgical Inc.), micro-Doppler imaging, and VeinViewer (Christie Digital Systems, Cypress, CA). Additional sensory navigation is contributed by these technologies.

6 Firefly Fluorescence Imaging

Firefly technology is a da Vinci integrated imaging system that allows the surgeon to assess vascular perfusion. This imaging system can be thought of as a special near-infrared filter that emits a certain wavelength of light when there is a special chemical (indocyanine green [ICG]) in the field. ICG when given IV binds to plasma proteins and accumulates in tissues that are well vascularized. There are numerous studies in various surgical departments [14–16] wielding ICG for challenging anatomy, but to our understanding, it is mostly used in urological procedures with unexpected anatomy, in distinction of tumor vs. normal tissue, and in ureteral surgery [17–19]. Also, this integrated technology allows better identification of spermatic arteries during robotic microsurgical varicocelectomy (Fig. 5).

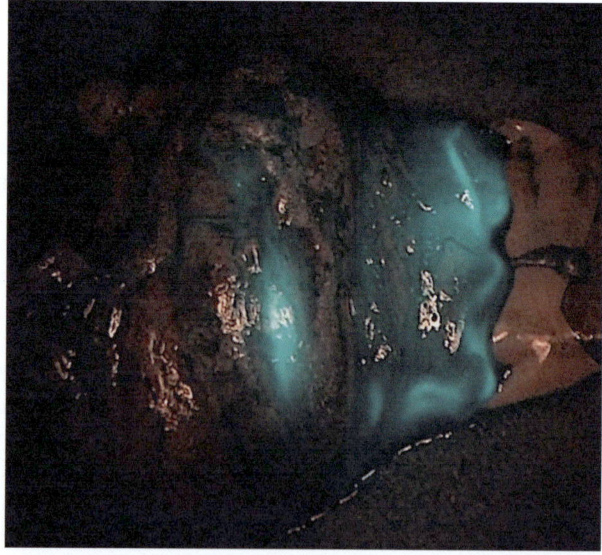

Fig. 5 ICG application during robotic microsurgical varicocelectomy

7   Micro-Doppler Sensing and Ultrasound

A flexible, open, or laparoscopic drop-in micro-Doppler (Vascular Technology Inc., Nashua, NH) probe emerged around 2010. The system works on the same principle as a Doppler setting during ultrasound imaging but comes with special sterile disposable probes that can be easily set up for robotic surgery. The system uses auditory output to help identify blood flow (Fig. 6). There are two distinct types depending on the wavelength/frequency of the sound produced by the device. 8 MHz probe is used to detect larger vessels (4–5 mm) and 20 MHz is used for vessels that are smaller than 2 mm. One limitation of this device is that it has no imaging and solely gives auditory feedback. On the other hand, it is very easy to recognize blood flow and estimate the location of the vessel without the need for any imaging.

Another novel device has been developed by Hitachi (Hitachi Aloka, Wallingford, CT). This probe provides up to 6 cm depth imaging with Doppler flow imaging option. The images can be synched with TilePro as mentioned before for surgeon comfort and efficiency. Robotic platform is excellent for utilizing these additional devices in the surgical field as it has steady arms that can be used to hold the probes without the need for a qualified assistant. It allows the surgeon to keep operating with two arms while using the additional arm for holding the device in place and has real-time images/sounds (Fig. 7).

Fig. 6 Micro-Doppler probe during robotic microsurgical varicocelectomy

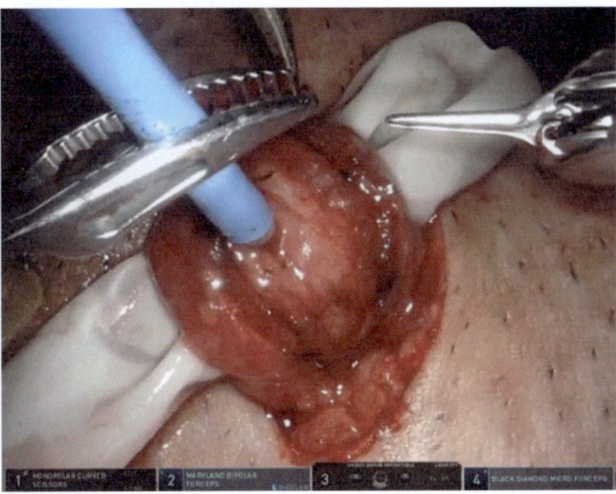

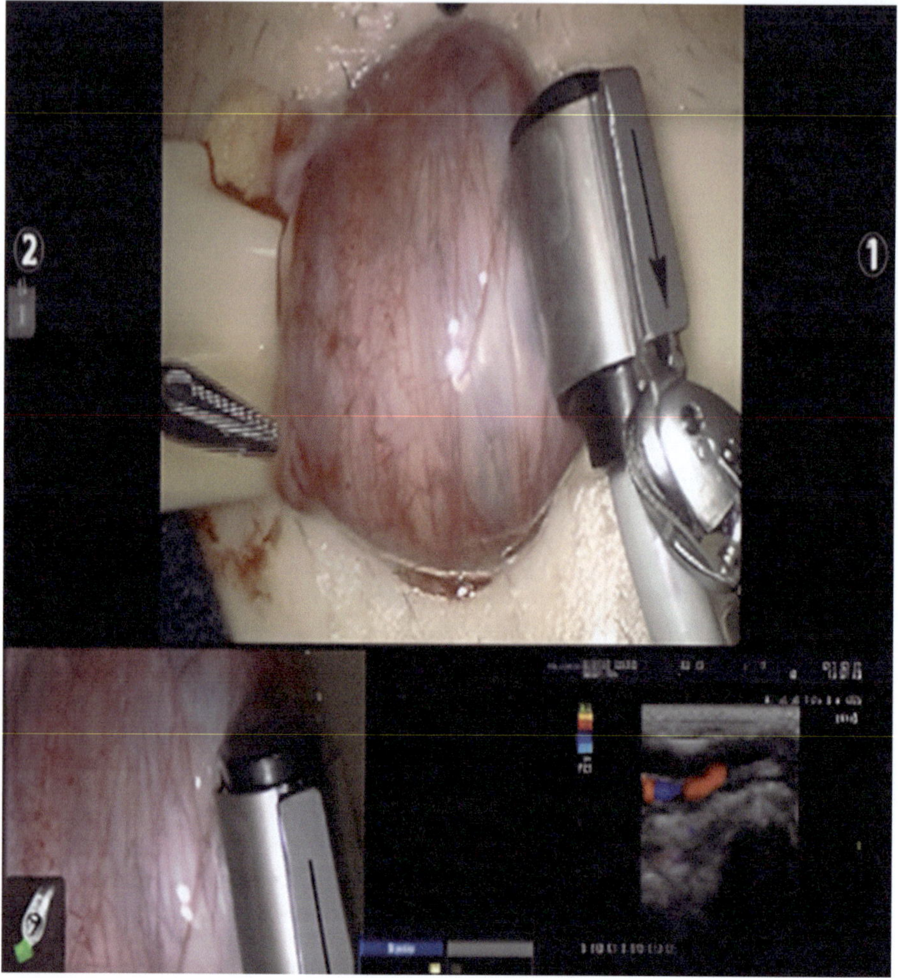

Fig. 7 Identification of the spermatic cord vessels via micro-Doppler probe

8 VeinViewer

A new biomedical advancement was made for inaccessible veins called VeinViewer. The system works on the principle of near-infrared light fluorescence. The system emits a certain wavelength of light to the patient's skin and hemoglobin in veins gets excited by this light and starts to emit another wavelength of light which is ultimately captured and processed by the device. The system automatically projects a greenlight over the skin indicating the vessels' demarcations. The system has been proved advantageous in a randomized trial on the pediatric population [20]. In urological practice, it has been found useful in defining venous structures in

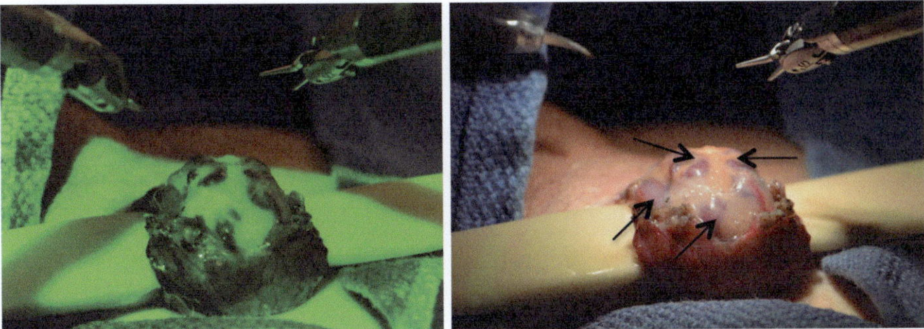

Fig. 8 VeinViewer utilization during robotic microsurgical varicocelectomy

hypospadias cases [21]. In our experience, we found the device to be beneficial for detecting varicose veins during robotic-assisted microsurgical varicocelectomy (Fig. 8). It comes in handy, especially in difficult cases where there's extensive scar tissue. Like the micro-Doppler, the device also lets us know if the vessel is a vein or artery which helps tremendously during these procedures.

9 Tools for Ligation/Ablation in Robotic Microsurgery

Microsurgery requires precise ligation and delicate dissection of the surrounding tissues. Instruments with monopolar and bipolar electrocautery technology are most commonly sufficient for this purpose; however, electrical energy tends to disperse in close proximity which may become important in microsurgical applications. Novel advancements have been made to provide easier, more precise techniques with less thermal spread.

10 Flexible Fiber Optic CO_2 Laser Probe

Carbon dioxide energy has been in use since the 1960s. Nevertheless, its use with a flexible probe was introduced in the late 2000s [22]. This technology has been used by multiple specialties of medicine [23–25] thanks to its minimal energy spread property. The laser has a long wavelength of 10.6 µm. This causes high absorption from the target tissue and water around it. High absorbance of this energy results in the conversion of the energy to heat energy in a small designated area that has been irrigated with saline, preventing damage to the surrounding structures [26]. We reported our experience with CO_2 laser technology (OmniGuide, Cambridge, MA) compared to monopolar electrocautery (ERBE Inc., Atlanta, GA) on a fresh human cadaver spermatic cord model [27]. We found remarkably decreased peripheral tissue damage caused by CO_2 energy versus standard monopolar technology. The

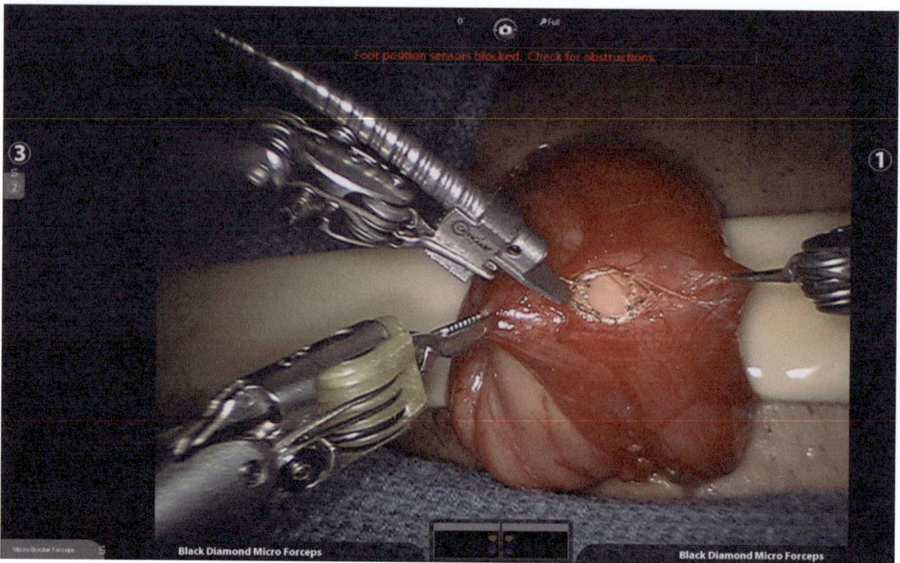

Fig. 9 Flexible fiber optic CO_2 laser probe provides highly precise dissection

Black Diamond microforceps was used to effectively maneuver the flexible probe. The tip of the CO_2 laser probe provided a blunt edge that also helped to separate tissue planes while ligation was performed. This tool can be considered for procedures with delicate anatomy requiring precise ablation and minimal thermal injury to nearby structures (Fig. 9).

10.1 Water-Jet Dissection

High-pressure water-jet dissection is done by a high-pressure stream of saline through a probe (Erbejet 2, ERBE Inc., Atlanta, GA). This technique has been applied to various procedures mostly in neurosurgery [28, 29]. Recently it has been used for ureterolysis procedures in cases with retroperitoneal fibrosis resulting in excellent dissections [30]. In our practice, we demonstrated the use of this advancement to ablate small nerve fibers on the vas deferens while preserving the blood vessels in animal models [31]. We also utilized this technology during robotic targeted microsurgical denervation of the spermatic cord to ablate residual nerve fibers in specific locations around the vas deferens that are thought to be responsible for chronic scrotal content pain (Fig. 10) [32, 33].

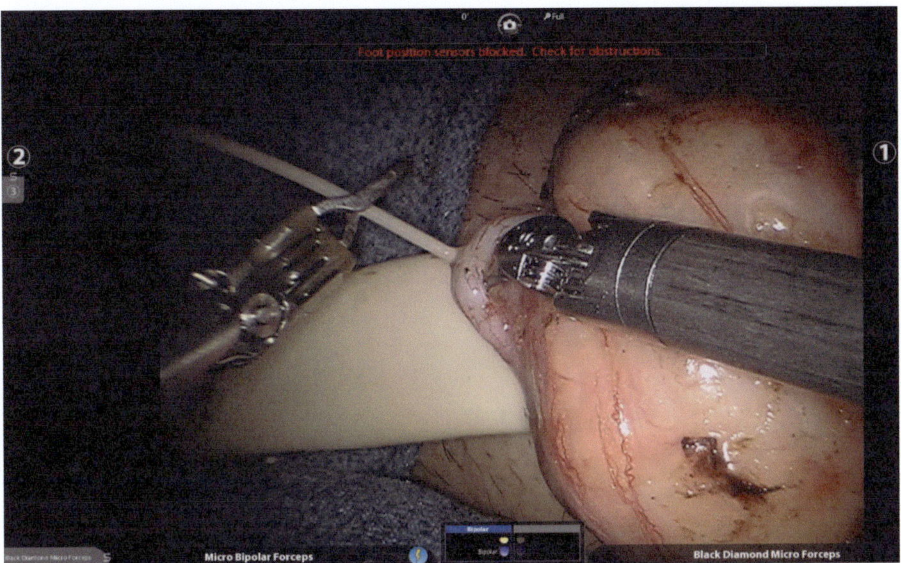

Fig. 10 High-pressure water-jet dissection for the remaining nerve fibers

11 Robotic Microsurgery: Current Urological Applications

From our standpoint on urologic robotic microsurgery, we have a large, possibly the largest, cohort of patients with chronic scrotal content pain and male infertility. We mostly utilized the robotic platform for robotic-assisted vasectomy reversals (RAVR) during the robot-assisted vasovasostomy (RAVV)/vasoepididymostomy (RAVE) stage. We have results from 264 RAVR cases (162 bilateral RAVV, 102 RAVE) with a median 12-month follow-up. Patency rates, defined as >one million sperm/ejaculate, were 91% in the RAVV group and 60% in the RAVE group. In addition, we used the robot for our varicocelectomy procedures in 588 cases. 65% of patients undergoing this procedure for oligospermia had a significant improvement in their sperm count and motility, and azoospermia converted to oligospermia in 15% of patients. 72% of patients, who underwent the procedure for scrotal pain, had a significant decrease in pain. In these two applications, our results proved the robotic approach is not only comparable to pure microsurgical approach but also very efficient for the surgeon.

Another use of the robot in our practice was in microsurgical testicular sperm extraction procedures (micro-TESE). We brought the robot in after the scrotum was delivered and kept it until the sampling was done and assessed under the microscope displayed on the surgeon's console. We also found the fourth robotic arm to be beneficial for deeper dissection when there's no viable sperm from the initial sampling stage.

Lastly, we used the robot for robotic-assisted targeted microsurgical denervation of the spermatic cord (RTMDSC), a procedure we defined and developed for chronic scrotal content pain treatment algorithm explained in detail in our previous studies [33, 34]. We used the robotic platform with the adjunctive instruments like the CO_2 laser probe, micro-Doppler, and hydro-dissection probe. We performed 1356 RTMDSC cases between 2008 and 2020. With 70 months of median follow-up, 84% of our patients encountered a significant decrease in pain by 6 months post-op. There were only 98 complications (95 of which were minor complications like hematoma at the surgical site, wound infection, etc.) and we concluded this robotic technique to be safe and feasible.

12 Robotic Microsurgery: Future Applications

As technology advances, imaging tools are expected to improve. Robotic systems bring the perfect infrastructure for the integration of such advancements. More application areas for potentially better outcomes combining these technologies should be explored with more studies.

12.1 Confocal Laser Endomicroscopy

Confocal laser endomicroscopy (Cellvizio, Mauna Kea Technologies, Paris, France) is an optical imaging method frequently used by gastroenterologists and neurosurgeons [35–37]. This technology allows the surgeon to evaluate the histology of tissues on a cellular level intraoperatively. It implements real-time in vivo images up to 1–5 μm resolution. A synchronous laser beam provides optical imaging with/without fluorescein. Figure 11 shows the utilization of this technology captured from the surgeon console (TilePro is used for real-time visualization) during a robotic microsurgical spermatic cord denervation case.

12.2 Multiphoton Microscopy

Multiphoton microscopy is an additional modality that measures nonlinear interactions between a laser photo beam and tissues of interest [38]. This technology has sharper image quality than confocal microscopy and can even show subcellular structures. This device can identify nerve fibers in tissues without any contrast-enhancing markers. Multiple studies suggesting the use of this modality for micro-surgical denervation of spermatic cord based on animal models have been made [39, 40]. In addition to the imaging properties, the device can also be used as a cellular level ablation tool when laser energy is increased accordingly.

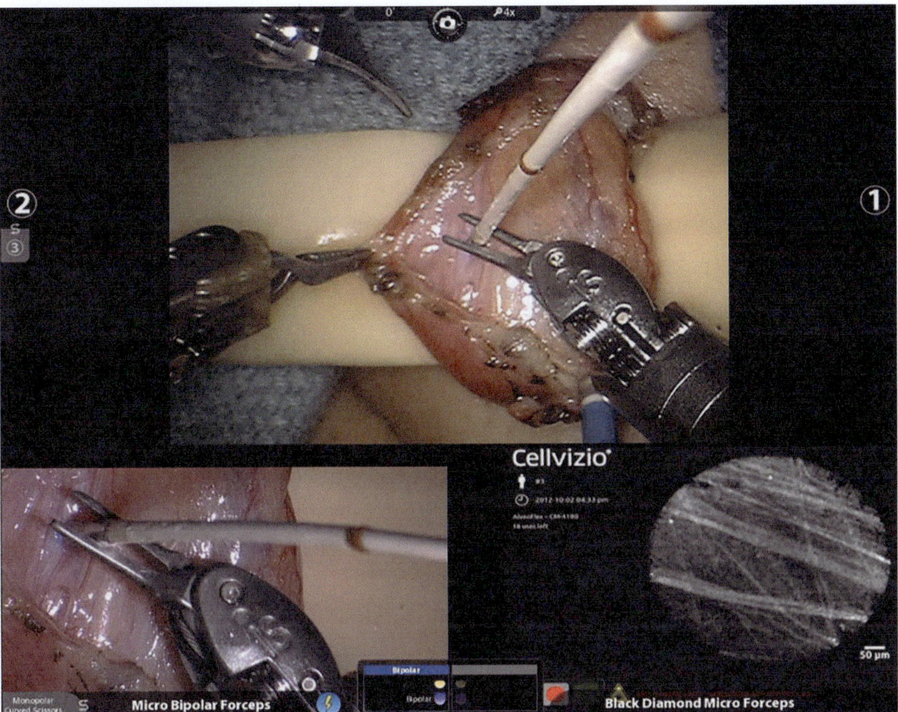

Fig. 11 Confocal laser endomicroscopy view in the surgeon console (lower right-hand side)

12.3 Prototype Platforms

Several new robotic platforms are being developed and multiple have been on the human trial stage. SPORT (Single Port Orifice Robotic Technology; Titan Medical Inc., Toronto, Ontario, Canada) is one such new platform focusing on minimal invasiveness. It has multiple abstract appearances in Europe but results with more human studies should be pursued. The same company rebranded its system to Enos robotic single-access surgical system in 2020, but more studies are yet to be published about this platform.

An interesting robotic system was named Sofie (Surgeon's Operating Force-Feedback Interface Eindhoven) and was developed at Eindhoven University of Technology in the Netherlands back in 2010. This robot was developed to be the first robotic system with tactile feedback but was never made publicly available. It is still unknown what advancements/pullbacks have been made on the project. Tactile feedback in robotic surgery might be an area of primary focus for the upcoming robotic platform developments.

13 Conclusion

Despite the superiorities of robotic platforms in microsurgery, there are limitations that have partially been explained in this chapter. High costs and lack of tactile feedback are the two major limitations of all the current platforms. For the time being, tactile feedback can be overcome with the help of the abovementioned adjunctive tools. Cost seems to be in a decreasing trend over the years inversely correlated with the number of new platforms announced. So far, we have been able to reduce the out-of-pocket costs for our patients undergoing robotic procedures by increasing surgical throughput. In order to do this, we have increased the daily number of robotic-assisted microsurgery cases which ended up covering a similar amount of time to pure microsurgical cases. This improvement resulted from surgical efficiency, higher case volumes, and decreased dependence on a skilled assistant. The authors have performed over 2000 robotic-assisted microsurgical procedures in urologic settings and continue to explore new applications in urology.

There is a growing market in the robotic field with many more competitors added every year which will likely benefit both the healthcare quality and cost in the future. Newer and cheaper robotic platforms are likely to emerge as well. We hope future surgical advancements in this area will be easier to access worldwide to improve the quality of care. Needless to say, more prospective, randomized studies on these new platforms with more patients followed up for longer periods are warranted.

Financial Disclosure The authors report no financial disclosures or sponsors for this chapter.

References

1. Kwoh YS, Hou J, Jonckheere EA, Hayati S. A robot with improved absolute positioning accuracy for CT guided stereotactic brain surgery. IEEE Trans Biomed Eng. 1988;35(2):153–60.
2. Lane T. A short history of robotic surgery. Ann R Coll Surg Engl. 2018;100(6_sup):5–7.
3. Etafy M, Gudeloglu A, Brahmbhatt JV, Parekattil SJ. Review of the role of robotic surgery in male infertility. Arab J Urol. 2018;16(1):148–56.
4. Lindenblatt N, Grünherz L, Wang A, Gousopoulos E, Barbon C, Uyulmaz S, et al. Early experience using a new robotic microsurgical system for lymphatic surgery. Plast Reconstr Surg Glob Open. 2022;10(1):e4013.
5. van Mulken TJM, Schols RM, Scharmga AMJ, Winkens B, Cau R, Schoenmakers FBF, et al. First-in-human robotic supermicrosurgery using a dedicated microsurgical robot for treating breast cancer-related lymphedema: a randomized pilot trial. Nat Commun. 2020;11(1):757.
6. van Mulken TJM, Wolfs J, Qiu SS, Scharmga AMJ, Schols RM, Spiekerman van Weezelenburg MA, et al. One-year outcomes of the first human trial on robot-assisted Lymphaticovenous anastomosis for breast cancer-related lymphedema. Plast Reconstr Surg. 2022;149(1):151–61.
7. Fan S, Dai X, Yang K, Xiong S, Xiong G, Li Z, et al. Robot-assisted pyeloplasty using a new robotic system, the KangDuo-surgical Robot-01: a prospective, single-centre, single-arm clinical study. BJU Int. 2021;128(2):162–5.

8. Wang J, Fan S, Shen C, Yang K, Li Z, Xiong S, et al. Partial nephrectomy through retroperitoneal approach with a new surgical robot system, KD-SR-01. Int J Med Robot. 2022;18(2):e2352.

9. Fan S, Zhang Z, Wang J, Xiong S, Dai X, Chen X, et al. Robot-assisted radical prostatectomy using the KangDuo surgical Robot-01 system: a prospective, single-center, single-arm clinical study. J Urol. 2022;208(1):119–27.

10. Fan S, Xiong S, Li Z, Yang K, Wang J, Han G, et al. Pyeloplasty with the Kangduo surgical robot vs. the da Vinci Si robotic system: preliminary results. J Endourol. 2022;36:1538.

11. Crew B. A closer look at a revered robot. Nature. 2020;580(7804):S5–7.

12. Gudeloglu A, Brahmbhatt JV, Parekattil SJ. Robotic-assisted microsurgery for an elective microsurgical practice. Semin Plast Surg. 2014;28(1):11–9.

13. Jourdes F, Valentin B, Allard J, Duriez C, Seeliger B. Visual haptic feedback for training of robotic suturing. Front Robot AI. 2022;9:800232.

14. Jewell EL, Huang JJ, Abu-Rustum NR, Gardner GJ, Brown CL, Sonoda Y, et al. Detection of sentinel lymph nodes in minimally invasive surgery using indocyanine green and near-infrared fluorescence imaging for uterine and cervical malignancies. Gynecol Oncol. 2014;133(2):274–7.

15. Dijkstra BM, Jeltema HJR, Kruijff S, Groen RJM. The application of fluorescence techniques in meningioma surgery—a review. Neurosurg Rev. 2019;42(4):799–809.

16. Wada H, Hirohashi K, Anayama T, Nakajima T, Kato T, Chan HH, et al. Minimally invasive electro-magnetic navigational bronchoscopy-integrated near-infrared-guided sentinel lymph node mapping in the porcine lung. PloS One. 2015;10(5):e0126945.

17. Kaplan-Marans E, Fulla J, Tomer N, Bilal K, Palese M. Indocyanine green (ICG) in urologic surgery. Urology. 2019;132:10–7.

18. Tobis S, Knopf JK, Silvers C, Messing E, Yao J, Rashid H, et al. Robot-assisted and laparoscopic partial nephrectomy with near infrared fluorescence imaging. J Endourol. 2012;26(7):797–802.

19. Simone G, Tuderti G, Anceschi U, Ferriero M, Costantini M, Minisola F, et al. "Ride the green light": Indocyanine green-marked off-clamp robotic partial nephrectomy for totally endophytic renal masses. Eur Urol. 2019;75(6):1008–14.

20. Hess HA. A biomedical device to improve pediatric vascular access success. Pediatr Nurs. 2010;36(5):259–63.

21. Gupta A, Sunil K, Singh GP, Kureel SN. Study of variations in axial pattern vessels of penile Dartos in hypospadias and implied surgical significance. Urology. 2020;146:201–6.

22. Ryan RW, Spetzler RF, Preul MC. Aura of technology and the cutting edge: a history of lasers in neurosurgery. Neurosurg Focus. 2009;27(3):E6.

23. Chen SX, Cheng J, Watchmaker J, Dover JS, Chung HJ. Review of lasers and energy-based devices for skin rejuvenation and scar treatment with histologic correlations. Dermatol Surg. 2022;48(4):441–8.

24. Wang C, Zhao Y, Li C, Song Q, Wang F. Meta-analysis of low temperature plasma radiofrequency ablation and CO(2) laser surgery on early Glottic laryngeal carcinoma. Comput Math Methods Med. 2022;2022:3417005.

25. Candiani M, Ottolina J, Tandoi I, Bartiromo L, Schimberni M, Villanacci R, et al. Fertility sparing procedure using carbon dioxide fiber laser vaporization of ovarian Endometrioma. J Vis Exp. 2022;(185).

26. Brahmbhatt JV, Gudeloglu A, Liverneaux P, Parekattil SJ. Robotic microsurgery optimization. Arch Plast Surg. 2014;41(3):225–30.

27. Gudeloglu A, Kattoor AJ, Brahmbhatt J, Parekattil S, Agarwal A. Prospective control trial: flexible CO(2) laser vs. monopolar electrocautery for robotic microsurgical denervation of the spermatic cord. Int J Impot Res. 2020;32(6):623–7.

28. Toth S, Vajda J, Pasztor E, Toth Z. Separation of the tumor and brain surface by "water jet" in cases of meningiomas. J Neurooncol. 1987;5(2):117–24.

29. Tschan CA, Tschan K, Krauss JK, Oertel J. First experimental results with a new waterjet dissector: Erbejet 2. Acta Neurochir. 2009;151(11):1473–82.

30. Abdessater M, Elias S, Boustany J, El Khoury R. Bilateral laparoscopic ureterolysis using hydrodissection in retroperitoneal fibrosis: a new application of an old technique. Res Rep Urol. 2019;11:131–5.
31. Gudeloglu A, Brahmbhatt JV, Allan R, Parekattil SJ. Hydrodissection for improved microsurgical denervation of the spermatic cord: prospective blinded randomized control trial in a rat model. Int J Impot Res. 2021;33(1):118–21.
32. Parekattil SJ, Gudeloglu A. Robotic assisted andrological surgery. Asian J Androl. 2013;15(1):67–74.
33. Parekattil SJ, Ergun O, Gudeloglu A. Management of chronic orchialgia: challenges and solutions–the current standard of care. Res Rep Urol. 2020;12:199.
34. Parekattil S, Gudeloglu A, Ergun O, Etafy M, Calixte N, Brahmbhatt J, et al. PD58-06 What is the predictive value of a spermatic cord block prior to microsurgical denervation of the spermatic cord? J Urol. 2020;203(Supplement 4):e1202.
35. Abramov I, Park MT, Gooldy TC, Xu Y, Lawton MT, Little AS, et al. Real-time intraoperative surgical telepathology using confocal laser endomicroscopy. Neurosurg Focus. 2022;52(6):E9.
36. Abramov I, Park MT, Belykh E, Dru AB, Xu Y, Gooldy TC, et al. Intraoperative confocal laser endomicroscopy: prospective in vivo feasibility study of a clinical-grade system for brain tumors. J Neurosurg. 2022;138:587–97.
37. Vaculová J, Kroupa R, Kala Z, Dolina J, Grolich T, Vlažný J, et al. The use of confocal laser endomicroscopy in diagnosing Barrett's esophagus and esophageal adenocarcinoma. Diagnostics (Basel). 2022;12(7):1616.
38. Ustione A, Piston DW. A simple introduction to multiphoton microscopy. J Microsc. 2011;243(3):221–6.
39. Sun HH, Tay KS, Jesse E, Muncey W, Loeb A, Thirumavalavan N. Microsurgical denervation of the spermatic cord: a historical perspective and recent developments. Sex Med Rev. 2022;10:791.
40. Ramasamy R, Sterling J, Li PS, Robinson BD, Parekattil S, Chen J, et al. Multiphoton imaging and laser ablation of rodent spermatic cord nerves: potential treatment for patients with chronic orchialgia. J Urol. 2012;187(2):733–8.

New Platforms in Robotic Surgery

Gustavo Cardoso Guimarães

1 Introduction

In the late twentieth century and early twenty-first century, the first steps toward a high-performance robotic system were taken.

Since the 1970s, agencies such as the US National Aeronautics and Space Administration (NASA) have been interested in the application of telesurgery for application to astronauts, with the idea that a machine equipped with surgical instruments could be remotely controlled by a surgeon in the Earth performing surgery on an astronaut on a space station. Similarly, the US Defense Advanced Research Projects Agency (DARPA) invested in developing a remote telesurgery unit that would allow for operating wounded on the battlefield. These initiatives led to advances in robotic telesurgery concepts and telecommunications technologies that enabled the 2001 Lindbergh Operation, in which French physician Jacques Marescaux and Canadian surgeon Michel Gagner performed a remote cholecystectomy from New York City on a patient in Strasbourg, France [1].

In 1978, Unimate developed the PUMA (Programmable Universal Manipulation Arm), which was later used in 1985 to perform stereotactic biopsies in neurosurgery [1].

In 1988, the Probot robot used for transurethral resection of the prostate was developed by Imperial College London. The system uses an image-guided three-dimensional model of the prostate, and the surgeon determines the area for resection. Based on these data, Probot calculates and performs the excision, and the procedure is performed by the robot autonomously, leaving the surgeon to supervise the procedure [1].

G. C. Guimarães (✉)
Surgical Oncology, Department and Robotic Surgery Program, BP—A Beneficência Portuguesa de São Paulo, Sao Paulo, Brazil

J. P. Manzano, L. M. Ferreira (eds.), *Robotic Surgery Devices in Surgical Specialties*, https://doi.org/10.1007/978-3-031-35102-0_16

In 1992, ROBODOC (Integrated Surgical Systems, Sacramento, CA, USA) was launched to assist in orthopedic hip replacement surgery, where this robotic system performs the preparation of the femoral implant cavity. It comprises a computerized preoperative planning workstation (ORTHODOC) and a five-axis robotic arm (ROBODOC). In August 2008, ROBODOC obtained FDA approval for total hip replacement. This technology was sold to Curexo Inc. in 2007, which in 2014 became THINK Surgical, Inc. [1, 2].

The first robotic system for use in laparoscopic surgery was introduced by Computer Motion (Santa Barbara, CA) in 1994. The AESOP moved your arm through voice commands from the surgeon.

In 1996 the ZEUS robot (Computer Motion), a fully integrated system, composed of arms and surgical instruments controlled by the surgeon, introduced the very concept of telepresence, in which the surgeon (master) commands the servo (robot). The ZEUS robot consisted of three arms, each independently attached to a surgical table, having an AESOP arm controlling the endoscope and two other surgical arms with four degrees of freedom [2].

The da Vinci robotic surgical system (Intuitive Surgical, Sunnyvale, CA) was introduced in Europe in 1997, and Dr. Guy Cadiere performed the first procedure, a robot-assisted laparoscopic cholecystectomy, in Brussels. The da Vinci became the first FDA-approved robotic surgical system in July 2000. In 2003, Intuitive Surgical acquired Computer Motion.

Since then, Intuitive Surgical's da Vinci system has become the most widely used robotic system in the world [1]. Its first model had only three arms but already had seven degrees of freedom and three-dimensional (3D) vision due to the binocular camera.

In the last 20 years, it has had continuous evolution and has passed with constant advances since the release of the da Vinci version and soon after the da Vinci S (Fig. 1).

The da Vinci Si model of third generation and soon after a fourth generation of robotic systems, the da Vinci X models and the da Vinci XI.

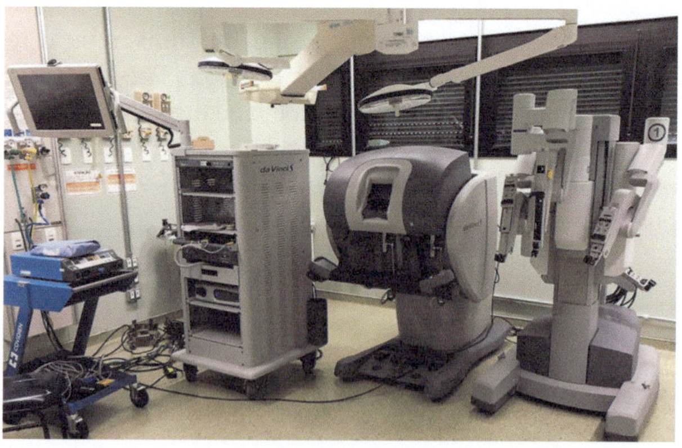

Fig. 1 da Vinci Surgical System S

Still considered a fourth generation, Intuitive Surgical launched the da Vinci SP system. This is now changing from the idea of systems with multi-ports to the single-port system, hence the nine da Vinci SP (single port).

More recently, a significant number of new robotic platforms have been launched on the market, not only for robots for use in laparoscopic procedures, such as the da Vinci by Intuitive Surgical, but also for other medical specialties.

Some of these new platforms and systems are already being commercialized in different parts of the world, other robotic platforms are in different stages of development, a fact that makes it virtually impossible to exhaust in a single chapter all the new technologies that exist and that will be launched in future years. However, the reality is that we will experience a new era in surgery in the coming years with a change in the way of performing surgeries with benefit for patients, surgical teams and the entire health system.

2   New Platforms

2.1   Platforms in Orthopedic Surgery

The ROSA Robotic Knee System (Zimmer Biomet, 2012) was approved by the FDA in 2019 with a rapid acceptance since then. The SA system was designed for total knee arthroplasty. In a 2020 study by Seidenstein and colleagues, it showed that surgeries with the ROSA system were more accurate and reproducible than with conventional instrumentation [3]. In the same way that it showed more accuracy in relation to target angles and resection thickness [4], there were fewer cases with outliers and 100% of cases within 3° of the targeted neutral alignment and lower outliers with the ROSA Knee for all angles of bone resection [3, 4].

The Mako® Total Hip 4.0 Robotic System is a robotic arm for assisted surgery, launched by Stryker in 2020 with the aim of performing robotic knee and hip arthroplasty surgery. This system uses 3D reconstruction of the region to be operated for the planning system (SmartRobotics™) [5].

The new Mako Total Hip 4.0 software is designed to enhance the user experience with region-based, approach-specific pelvic registration and allows for implant position planning, considering changes in pelvic tilt in various positions and allowing for visualization of the relationship between the femur and pelvis and their components to help detect the risk of a possible impact. Using AccuStop™ haptic technology and a patient-specific CT scan, the Mako Total Hip enables single-stage reaming and guided impactions to help promote accurate implant placement [5].

The Mazor™ X robotic system was launched in October 2021 by Medtronic for robotic-guided spinal surgery.

The Mazor platform incorporates the StealthStation™ S8 surgical navigation capabilities existing in the Mazor Core Technology robotic-assisted surgery platform. Real-time image guidance, visualization, and navigation are informed by interactive 3D planning and information systems to provide workflow predictability and procedural flexibility. This three-dimensional platform allows you to visualize the anatomy and structures of the spine in relation to each other, allowing access to plan and simulate spinal cages and screws in advance, with the aim of increasing surgical efficiency and precision. It also integrates Midas Rex™ MR8 high-speed electric drill systems that enable improved trajectory accuracy, starting with pilot hole creation and offering dissection tools and accessories designed to drill accurately at speeds up to 75,000 rpm, allowing the surgical team to use intersomatic features navigated in the Mazor system to visualize disc preparation and intersomatic placement during a robotic surgery in an orthopedic surgery procedure [6].

2.2   Cranial Robotic Guidance Platforms

Medtronic's Stealth Autoguide™ robotic cranial guidance platform is designed to provide stereotaxic positioning and trajectory guidance for neurosurgical procedures.

The Stealth Autoguide™ System is a remotely operated positioning and guidance system that is designed for any neurological condition where the use of stereotaxic surgery may be appropriate such as stereotaxic biopsy, stereotaxic electroencephalography (EEG), and laser tissue ablation. It offers continuous real-time visualization, feedback, and robot-assisted motion that allow fast and accurate alignment to surgical plans for cranial procedures. The system allows the integration of StealthStation™ with Midas Rex™ drilling technology, enabling efficient workflow with minimal operating room space [7].

The Neuromate® robot, launched in 2019 by Renishaw for stereotaxic brain procedures, provides a platform that can be used in a wide range of functional neurosurgical procedures such as electrode implantation procedures for deep brain stimulation (DBS) and stereoelectroencephalography (SEEG), as well as stereotactic applications in neuroendoscopy [8].

2.3   Robotic Platforms for Endoscopic Procedures

Monarch, Auris. In 2018 Auris Health received marketing approval for a robot for endoscopic procedures. Initially for bronchoscopy and more recently for endourological procedures, it comprises an endoscope with a telescopic design and integrated camera for continuous vision and accurate access, offering a four-way articulation and cutting-edge 3D tracking technology to support guided access. All control is done by an easy-to-use joystick [9].

Still with the same concept, Intuitive launched in 2019 the Ion (Intuitive Surgical) for performing endoscopic procedures. With an "ultrathin" design, it has advanced maneuverability allowing navigation to peripheral pulmonary branches and features a 3.5 mm outer diameter catheter with a 2.0 mm working channel allowing access to small and difficult to navigate. It also features a peripheral vision probe that allows direct vision while navigating [10].

2.4 Robots for Endovascular Procedures

Corindus CorPath GRX (Siemens Healthcare). It presents an integrated robot proposal for endovascular examinations and treatments, both for cardiac and peripheral vascular and neurovascular procedures, and features a radiation-protected workstation and a set of joysticks and touchscreen controls that translate the doctor's movements during surgery for endovascular. Robot-assisted intervention allows accurate measurement of anatomy and device positioning with the added benefit of radiation protection for the clinician and potentially reduced radiation exposure for medical staff and patients [11].

3 Robot in Ophthalmology

R2D2 – Robotic Retinal Dissection Device (Oxford University). It is a robot created for retinal eye surgery. The R2D2 is designed to eliminate tremors during instrument movement allowing for precise, millimeter-wide movement within the eye. Without using the R2D2, surgeons need to slow the pulse and make precise movements between heartbeats. With the use of R2D2, it is possible to perform high-precision procedures that cannot be done by the human hand. The robot uses 7 independent computer-controlled motors to make precise movements at a scale of 1/1000 mm. The eye surgeon uses a joystick and touchscreen to control the robot and can monitor its progress through a surgical microscope [12, 13].

3.1 New Platforms for Laparoscopic Surgery

Versius CMR Robotic System (Cambridge Medical Robotics). From an English start-up founded in 2014, it quickly developed a really light, versatile, and modular system. In 2015 it presented its prototype and in 2019 it already performed its first surgery on humans. It was introduced in India and in England in 2019. With rapid expansion, it announced its first 5000 procedures performed, in more than 50 centers spread across 13 countries, in multi-specialties, in June 2022.

It presents the concept of an open console modular robot and full HD 3D vision with the use of glasses. Unlike other systems, its control console used by the surgeon can be used both in a sitting and standing position. And all controls, both arms, camera, and power are on the handpiece, not using foot control [14].

Hugo RAS (Medtronic). It received the approval of the European Community (CE mark approved) in October 2021. This robotic system from the Medtronic company comes with the proposal to be modular, with an open console and full HD 3D vision system, and with the use of glasses. It was approved in the European Community in 2022 and its primary use in humans was in 2021 [15].

Ottava surgical robotic system (Johnson & Johnson). The Ottava system was designed with six arms to allow greater control, flexibility, and patient access during surgery; it was planned that throughout 2021, Johnson & Johnson should work on validating the Ottava system and plans to start clinical trials in 2022; however, the company announced the expected delay of 2 years due to technical and supply difficulties [16].

Senhance Surgical System (Asensus Surgical, Inc., formerly TransEnterix, Inc.). It received FDA marketing clearance in March 2021 for use in general surgery. Its system also uses the concept of modular units and an open console with glasses for full HD 3D viewing [17].

Revo-I Surgical Robotic System (Revo Surgical Solution). This robot was approved for human use in Korea in 2017 and is basically used only in this country. It has attributes and functionality like the da Vinci Si and X system [18].

Hinotori™ (Medicaroid, Japanese company). It was developed as a robotic-assisted surgery system to reproduce the surgeon's sensitive movement and founded from a joint venture formed by the partnership between Kawasaki Heavy Industry and Sysmex Corporation in 2012.

With the robotic arms coming from a raised base, it allows for an open and wide operating field. It maintains the "closed" console concept with 3D vision system without the need for additional glasses [19].

DLR MiroSurge robotic system (Institute of Robotics and Mechatronics—Germany). The MiroSurge Telesurgery DLR System includes a surgeon's console with a 3D display and two tactile input devices and three robotic arms. Two arms move the laparoscopic instruments, and the third one guides an endoscope. According to the manufacturer, it presents feedback on the force used, allowing the surgeon not only to see where the arms are moving but also to partially feel it in the haptic input devices [20].

Enos robotic single access surgical system (Titan Medical). The Enos system is a system designed to offer single-port access for robot-assisted surgery. It is composed of two components: the patient's car and a console. The company expects to receive FDA approval for 2023 [21].

4   Conclusion

It is quite clear that this is an expanding market and that it will change very quickly with new devices and companies on the market, as well as new generations of existing devices, bringing new functionality and new uses. It is to be expected that with each passing day these systems become smaller, more efficient, faster, safe, interactive, and, who knows, even with navigation systems and, why not, autonomous functions.

References

1. Britannica. Robotic surgery. 2022. https://www.britannica.com/science/robotic-surgery#ref1225036. Accessed 15 Oct 2022.
2. Atluri S, de Oliveira BNA, Parekh DJ. História da Cirurgia robótica. In: Guimaraes GC, Parehkh DJ, Távora JEF, de Oliveira BNA, Junger GM, editors. Cirurgia Robótica. Principios e Fundamentos. Minas Gerais: Editora Universitária Ciências Médicas; 2022. p. 35–9.
3. Seidenstein A, Birmingham M, Foran J, Ogden S. Better accuracy and reproducibility of a new robotically-assisted system for total knee arthroplasty compared to conventional instrumentation: a cadaveric study. Knee Surg Sports Traumatol Arthrosc. 2021;29:859–66.
4. Parratte S, et al. Instability after total knee arthroplasty. J Bone Joint Surg Am. 2008;90(1):184.
5. Stryker. Stryker releases Mako total Hip 4.0. 2020. https://www.stryker.com/kz/en/about/news/2020/stryker-releases-mako%2D%2Dtotal-hip-4-0-software-upgrade.html. Accessed 15 Oct 2022.
6. Medtronic. Medtronic Canada announces the commercial launch of Mazor™ X, the first robotics platform dedicated to spinal surgery in Canada. 2021. https://canadanews.medtronic.com/2021-10-25-Medtronic-Canada-announces-commercial-launch-of-Mazor-TM-X,-the-first-dedicated-robotic-spinal-surgery-platform-in-Canada. Accessed 15 Oct 2022.
7. Medtronic. STEALTH AUTOGUIDE™. Cranial Robotic Guidance Platform. 2019. https://www.medtronic.com/us-en/healthcare-professionals/products/neurological/cranial-robotics/stealth-autoguide.html. Accessed 15 Oct 2022.
8. Renishaw. neuromate® stereotactic robot. 2022. https://www.renishaw.com.br/pt/neuromate-stereotactic-robot%2D%2D10712. Accessed 15 Oct 2022.
9. Ethicon. Monarch Platform. 2022. https://www.aurishealth.com/monarch-platform. Accessed 15 Oct 2022.
10. Intuitive. Ion by Intuitive. 2022. https://www.intuitive.com/en-us/products-and-services/ion. Accessed 15 Oct 2022.
11. Siemens Healthineers. CorPath GRX. 2022 https://www.siemens-healthineers.com/br/angio/endovascular-robotics/corpath-grx. Accessed 15 Oct 2022.
12. Medical Design and Outsourcing. Oxford robotic surgery, advances in synthetic retina could help visually impaired. 2017. https://www.medicaldesignandoutsourcing.com/oxford-robotic-surgery-synthetic-retina-visually-impaired/. Accessed 15 Oct 2022.
13. The Engineer. Robotic surgery is easy on the eye. 2017. https://www.theengineer.co.uk/content/in-depth/robot-surgery-is-easy-on-the-eye/. Accessed 15 Oct 2022.
14. CMR Surgical. Versius—CRM Surgical. 2022. https://cmrsurgical.com/versius. Accessed 15 Oct 2022.
15. Medtronic. Hugo Ras System. 2022. https://www.medtronic.com/covidien/en-gb/robotic-assisted-surgery/hugo-ras-system.html. Accessed 15 Oct 2022.
16. Medical Device Network. Johnson & Johnson's new robotic surgical system to rival Intuitive Surgical's da Vinci. 2022. https://www.medicaldevice-network.com/analysis/ottava-robotic-johnson/. Accessed 15 Oct 2022.
17. Insights Care. Asensus Surgical announces FDA clearance in general surgery indications expand to include new procedures in large general surgery market. 2021. https://insightscare.com/asensus-surgical-announces-fda-clearance-in-general-surgery-indications-expand-to-include-new-procedures-in-large-general-surgery-market/. Accessed 15 Oct 2022.

18. Revo Surgical. Revo-I. 2022. http://revosurgical.com/#/main.html. Accessed 15 Oct 2022.
19. Medicaroid. Corporate history. 2022. https://www.medicaroid.com/en/company/history.html. Accessed 15 Oct 2022.
20. DRL Institute of Robotics and Mechatronics. 2018. https://www.dlr.de/rm/en/desktopdefault. aspx/tabid-11674#gallery/28728. Accessed 15 Oct 2022.
21. User Walls. Titan medical provides update to Enos project timeline. 2022. https://www.user-walls.news/n/titan-medical-update-enos-project-timeline-3431363/. Accessed 15 Oct 2022.

Single-Port

**Dorival Duarte Jr., Artur de Oliveira Paludo,
Leonardo Martins Caldeira de Deus, Milton Berger, João Pádua Manzano,
and André Kives Berger**

1 Introduction

Platforms for robotic surgery have undergone constant improvements and technological changes. Since its implementation, approximately two decades ago, the
quality of optics and the range of motion of instruments and software technology
have constantly evolved [1]. The global trend in robotic surgery is the development
of technologies that deliver fine and precise movements, associated with minimally
invasive surgeries, in the act of endoscopic surgeries or with minimal incisions. At
this view we have the *single-site* laparoscopic *(LESS)* [2] and, later, the da Vinci
single-port (SP) robotic system.

Hirano et al. [3] pioneered the LESS concept, using trocars and laparoscopic
forceps in a single puncture site to perform retroperitoneal adrenalectomy. Rane
et al. [4] and Desai et al. [5] described, on the other hand, the performance of
laparoscopic LESS nephrectomy. The first study used laparoscopic and optical
instruments introduced by the R-port, while the second introduced the concept of
"scarless" with the technique.

D. Duarte Jr. (✉) · A. de Oliveira Paludo · M. Berger
Moinhos de Vento Hospital, Porto Alegre, RS, Brazil

Federal University of Rio Grande do Sul, Porto Alegre, RS, Brazil

L. M. C. de Deus
Moinhos de Vento Hospital, Porto Alegre, RS, Brazil

J. P. Manzano
Department of Surgery, Universidade Federal de São Paulo, São Paulo, Brazil
e-mail: jmanzano@unifesp.br

A. K. Berger
Moinhos de Vento Hospital, Porto Alegre, RS, Brazil

University of Southern California, CA, EUA, Los Angeles, CA, USA

J. P. Manzano, L. M. Ferreira (eds.), *Robotic Surgery Devices in Surgical
Specialties*, https://doi.org/10.1007/978-3-031-35102-0_17

233

However, the poor reproducibility of LESS techniques seems to have pushed the method away from surgeons. According to Moschovas et al. [6], the acceptance of laparoscopic procedures among urologists has reduced in recent years, with the robotic approach.

Robotic surgeries performed with robotic arms at the same puncture site began to be described in 2010 by Joseph et al. [7]. The authors described the "chopstick" surgery, which consisted of crossed punctures, achieving a certain triangulation with the robotic arms with a good presentation of the surgical target. Tugcu et al. [8] and Mattevi et al. [9] also described the clinical use of a single surgical access using the arms together with a multiport robot with different diagrams of the robotic arms.

To overcome the challenges related to the *LESS* and, as part of the refinement of minimally invasive surgery, the da Vinci SP platform was created. The first use of a da Vinci SP prototype (SP999) was reported by Kaouk et al. [10] in 2014, based on 11 SP robotic prostatectomies. The progression of the prototype model was developed to what we know today as the da Vinci SP (SP1098); and its first description of clinical use took place a few years later, in the performance of two radical prostatectomies by the same authors [11]. Subsequently, other surgeries, such as pyeloplasty and radical nephrectomies, were added to the feasibility of the technology, using the GelPOINT technique to introduce the trocater SP [12, 13].

The development of the da Vinci SP model allowed a new paradigm in the concept of robotic surgery. First, the use of multiarmed robots favors, in some situations, the clashing of robotic arms in patients with little space for triangulations. The SP allows robotic arms to be integrated through a single-specific robotic trocar. The arrangement and triangulation of the robotic arms is then carried out within the cavity, either abdominal or endoscopic, and using smaller instruments measuring 6 mm [1] (Fig. 1).

2 Features

The da Vinci SP has 25 mm trocar, integrated by the scope and three robotic arms, all inside your device. The camera is articulated and has an oval shape of 12×10 mm. In turn, the robotic arms are thinner than those of the multiport model, with only 6 mm, containing two articulation centers in each arm [1]. Furthermore, each instrument occupies a position along the "clock," i.e., 3, 6, 9, and 12 h [14].

One of the most outstanding features of the da Vinci SP model is the possibility of rotating the entire camera system and arms together inside the cavity, with the relocation pedal, maintaining the surgical target. The model also allows the visualization of a three-dimensional figure with the projection of the surgical instruments for spatial orientation to the surgeon on the console.

The SP platform was initially developed to introduce a single trocar into the peritoneal cavity [15]. With the trocar inserted, a space of 10 cm from the trocar tip to the joint is required. Thus, in small spaces, such as the retrocavity, "floating docking" is often performed [15]. The trocar docking outside the cavity is performed

Fig. 1 Single-port
overview. (With permission
from the corresponding
author)

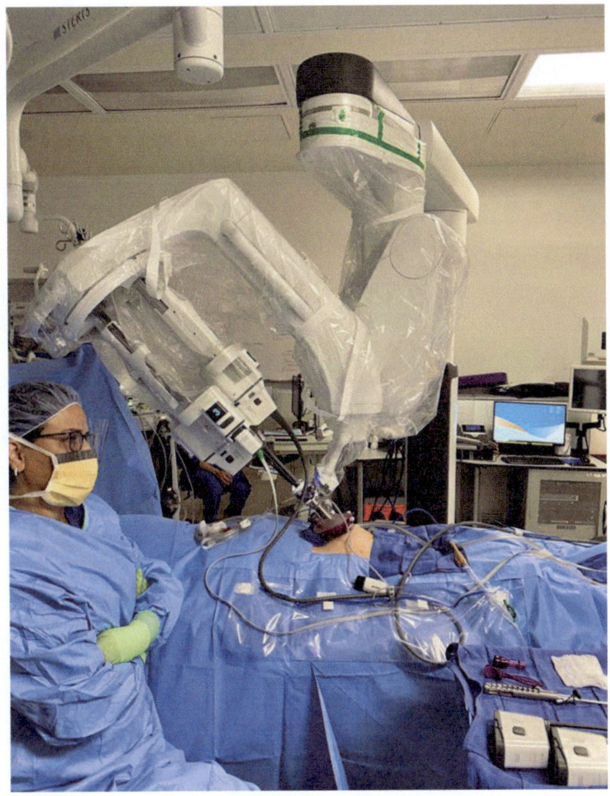

10 cm from the skin and the introduction of instruments can be done through the
GelPOINT Mini (Applied Medical) or the SP access portal (Intuitive) (Fig. 2), and
even the auxiliary trocar can be placed on the same GelPOINT.

As for docking in pelvic surgeries, the da Vinci SP trocar is placed 20 cm from
the pubis, under an incision of approximately 3 cm, introduction using the Hasson
technique, and an angulation of 26° in Trendelenburg [1]. The side docking is then
performed, contra-laterally to the side of the auxiliary portal. In pelvic surgery, different camera angles may be necessary; in radical prostatectomy, for example, def-
fating maneuver can be performed with 30° flexed down, while neurovascular
dissection can be performed with 20–30° upward [16].

3   Differences with the Xi Model

The main differences between the multiport and SP system are described in Table 1.

Fig. 2 Single-port GelPOINT docking. (With permission from the corresponding author)

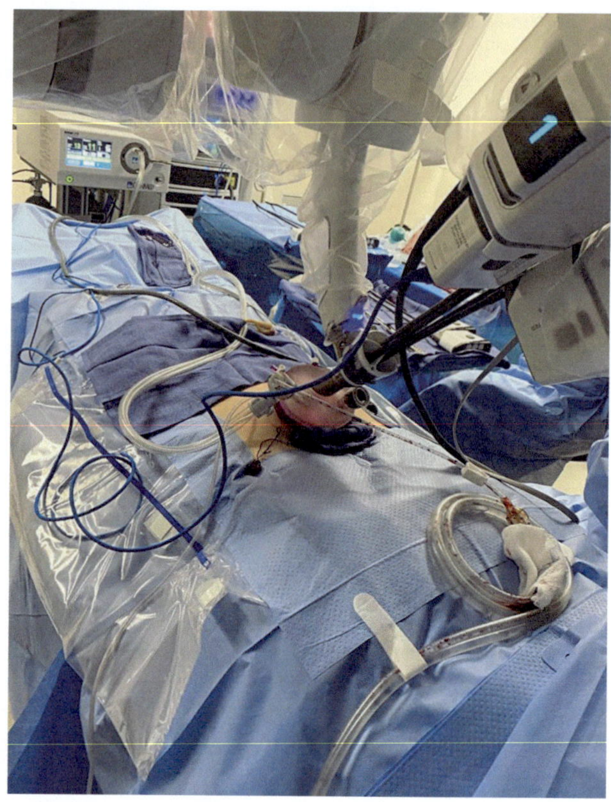

Table 1 da Vinci single-port x Da Vinci Xi (multiarmed)

Characteristic	Model Xi	Model SP
Portals	Multiport	Single-port
Arm spacing	Spaced out	Elbows are needed to spread out and triangulate inside the SP
Working distance	Closer to the target	Longer working distance
Relocation	No relocation (no relocation pedal)	Robotic system completely relocated in each quadrant of surgery
Scope	0°/30°	Flexible 3D technology
Instruments	8 mm	6 mm
Grip and dissection strength	Usual	Reduced
Sum of incisions	32 mm	25 mm

4 Single-Port and Its Applications

Moschovas et al. [17] published a systematic review of the literature involving PS and urology. The authors selected and analyzed 43 studies, with application for clinical use and in cadavers, confirming that the use of the da Vinci SP robot in urological procedures is safe and feasible. Some of the studies reported less postoperative pain and earlier discharge from robotic SP extraperitoneal surgeries compared to multiport surgeries [18, 19]. In a non-systematic review, Moschovas et al. filmed the SP radical prostatectomy urological procedures, through a 12 mm accessory port in the surgery. The footage helped to study the flexible camera movements of the SP and to understand the new technology range of motion [6].

The feasibility of the SP technology was also pointed out by Kaouk et al. [20], in a descriptive study of the first 100 cases of their center using the da Vinci SP. In their series, only 1% of the patients required surgical conversion due to intense abdominal adhesion from previous surgeries.

In different specialties, urology is the pioneer in the use of SP technology. In one of the first reviews on the topic [1], the authors described the "step by step" of SP robotic radical prostatectomies in a single high-volume service. In this study, 26 patients were selected between 2018 and 2019, with cT2 pathologies, prostate <80 g, and BMI <35 kg/m^2. Console time averaged 85.3 min (which decreased as the surgeries progressed), operating room time averaged 121.5 min, and the estimated blood loss was 50 mL. The hospital stay lasted an average of 16 h 38 min, with the removal of the urinary catheter on the fourth postoperative day. The same group of authors presented a new review, after 50 SP surgeries from June to December 2019, with 80% of patients with cT2 pathology and 20% with cT3 pathology. The average console time decreased by approximately 5.3 min and 14% had positive margins in the anatomopathological examination. Length of urinary catheterization and hospital stay was similar [21].

Agarwal et al. [22] presented a series of 49 radical prostatectomy surgeries performed by three different surgeons. Prior techniques and Retzius sparing have been described. The authors did not use GelPOINT and performed systematic intraoperative freezing for their cases. The rate of positive margins was 28% and 8% of patients had Clavien 1 complications. On the other hand, Ng et al. [23] performed a study of complications and surgical conversions in SP procedures. The results of the 20 patients showed the absence not only of Clavien 2 complications but also of surgical conversions.

In the meta-analysis by Hinojosa-Gonzalez et al. [24], which included 6 studies and 1068 patients, SP ($n = 324$) and multiport ($n = 744$) radical prostatectomy surgeries were compared, with no evidence of statistically significant differences in blood loss ($p = 0.25$), operative time ($p = 0.34$), or positive surgical margins. Length of stay was significantly shorter in SP ($p = 0.003$), with no differences in complication rates.

Also in radical prostatectomy surgery, Kaouk et al. [25] described the transvesical approach for patients with hostile abdomens and low- and moderate-risk prostate cancer, in addition to transperineal prostate surgery.

Two other reviews compared patients undergoing multiport surgery and single-port surgery: While Saidian et al. [26] showed no statistically significant differences between patients undergoing robotic radical prostatectomy with a da Vinci Xi robot and SP (47 × 48 patients), Vigneswaran et al. [27] found less pain and shorter hospital stay in their SP groups.

In the context of the treatment of benign prostatic hyperplasia, in a recent review, Khalil et al. [28] described a series of 75 patients who underwent robotic simple prostatectomy surgery, 47 of which were multiport and 28 SP. Surgical time, estimated blood loss, and length of hospital stay had no statistically significant difference between the groups. There was a higher rate of complications in the SP group, but without statistical significance (42.86% vs. 21.28%, $p = 0.09$). On the other hand, Steinberg et al. [29] reported ten cases of simple robotic SP prostatectomy without Clavien three complications. Kauk et al. [30] reported another 10 cases with a variation in surgical time of 146–203 min and estimated blood loss of 68–175 mL.

Another feasible urologic surgery with SP technology is radical cystectomy. Kaouk et al. [19] described the step by step of a series of 4 cases, in which 75% of the reconstructions were intracorporeal shunts. Zhang et al. [31] also reported 4 cases, with 100% of the surgeries with intracorporeal bypass and without records of Clavien 3 complications. Furthermore, the authors [31] reported superior cosmetic results and pain reduction when compared to the open and robotic multiport approach.

SP robotic partial nephrectomy is also cited in the literature. Key studies in the description of this type of surgery were those carried out by Kaouk et al. [32] and Valero et al. [33]. The first authors [32] reported 3 cases of partial nephrectomy, with a mean surgical time of 180 min, estimated blood loss of 180 mL, and ischemia time of 25 min. Only one case had Clavien 3 complications. The second study [33] reported the first case of partial nephrectomy and SP robotic radical prostatectomy in the same intraoperative period. The surgical time was 256 min and the estimated blood loss was 250 mL.

Surgeons have also applied SP technology in robotic pyeloplasty surgeries. Heo et al. [34] described a series of three cases using GelPOINT under the Anderson-Hynes technique.

In addition to urology, gynecology has also implemented robotic surgeries SP. Iavazzo et al. [35] mention, in a literature review, 18 case series and 8 cases of robotic SP hysterectomy, totaling 505 patients. The results showed a mean surgical time of 122 min, an estimated blood loss of 50 mL, and a hospital stay of 1.5 days. There were 0.8% intraoperative complications and surgical conversion (to multiport robotics, laparoscopy, or laparotomy) in 2.8% of cases. Acar et al. [36] reported 11 cases of SP vaginoplasty, with an operative time of 267 min and an estimated blood loss of 131 mL, with only 2 patients with Clavien 3B complications. Sacrocolpopexy SP was also described by Ganesan et al. [37], with 3 cases of operative time of 198–240 min and estimated blood loss of 10–50 mL.

The expansion of SP robotic surgery in coloproctology and general surgery has also been present in recent years. Liu et al. [38] described a review on the subject, showing the advances in colonic resections with the SP robot.

Regardless of the surgical specialty or type of surgery, it is worth remembering that the comparison between centers that perform SP surgery is difficult, as we must keep in mind that in most procedures there is no standardized surgical technique.

Likewise, different access routes for the same surgery, different docking techniques, different patient selections, and different postoperative routines are performed in SP centers, which makes comparison difficult [15].

5   Challenges and Benefits

Regarding console commands and surgical dynamics, understanding the distance between the arms, quantifying the triangulation needed to work, and correctly relocating the robotic arms are the biggest challenges at the beginning of the da Vinci SP learning curve. Likewise, working with flexible camera rotation and angulation demands training and expertise.

About training, Maschovas et al. [14] describe the experience of sequenced training in dry lab, followed by training in wet lab. The next step was the observation of 5 (five) cases with the da Vinci SP, followed by 2–3 surgeries in the proctorship phase [14]. Another challenge faced is the increase in surgical time related to the use of the reallocation pedal. Constant use of this pedal increases operative time as the entire system is slowly reallocated to a new target [39].

The real benefits of using the SP robot are still being debated [17]. The lack of large trials and series that compare the oncological and functional results of the different multiport and SP technologies is one of the future answer that should be clarified over time. It is worth mentioning that no benefits were found in the satisfaction of patients operated by multiport robots and SP in the SSQ-8 questionnaire [40]. However, patients were significantly more satisfied with the single scar of SP surgeries compared to multiple scars in multiport robotic surgeries.

We still have a lack of data in the literature comparing surgical and functional outcomes between patients operated on with multiport robotic surgery and SP. This obstacle is due, in part, not only to the few hospitals that have the SP robot (some centers in the United States and another center in Korea) but also due to the reduced number of certified and qualified surgeons to perform SP surgeries [17]. Few are the SP procedures described in some surgeries. In the case of pycloplasty, cystectomy, and ureteral reimplantation, the total number of surgeries described does not reach 15 surgeries per procedure.

6   Conclusion

As a new technology, SP surgery is feasible and requires training and caution. The learning curve of the method is not negligible and the challenges and improvements for performing surgeries using this robot must be kept in mind.

Urology is a pioneer in the use and development of the SP platform, with radical prostatectomy being the most performed procedure using this robotic system [17]. It is expected that, in a few years, there will be an increase in the number of surgeries described with SP, as well as a greater number of comparisons of these surgeries with multiport surgeries.

We believe in the subsequent evolution of technology. The da Vinci SP is a version 1.0, and as the technology of multiport robots has been refined, we believe that new models and options for SP robots will soon be available and with greater technological complexity built-in.

References

1. Moschovas MC, Bhat S, Rogers T, Onol F, Roof S, Mazzone E, Mottrie A, Patel V. Technical modifications necessary to implement the da Vinci single-port robotic system. Eur Urol. 2020;78(3):415–23.
2. Greco F, Hoda MR, Mohammed N, Springer C, Fischer K, Fornara P. Laparoendoscopic single-site and conventional laparoscopic radical nephrectomy result in equivalent surgical trauma: preliminary results of a single-Centre retrospective controlled study. Eur Urol. 2012;61:1048–53.
3. Hirano D, Minei S, Yamaguchi K, Yoshikawa T, Hachiya T, Yoshida H, Takimoto Y, Saitoh T, Kiyotani S, Okada K. Retroperitoneoscopic adrenalectomy for adrenal tumor via single large port. J Endourol. 2005;19(7):788–92.
4. Rane A, Rao P, Bonadio F, Rao P. Single port laparoscopic nephrectomy using a novel laparoscopic port (R-port) and evolution of single laparoscopic port procedure (SLIPP). J Endourol. 2007;21:A87.
5. Desai MM, Rao PP, Aron M, et al. Scarless single port transumbilical nephrectomy and pyeloplasty: first clinical report. BJU Int. 2008;101:83–8.
6. Moschovas MC, Seetharam Bhat KR, Onol FF, Rogers T, Ogaya-Pinies G, Roof S, Patel VR. Single-port technique evolution and current practice in urologic procedures. Asian J Urol. 2021;8(1):100–4.
7. Joseph RA, Salas NA, Johnson C, et al. Chopstick surgery: a novel technique enables use of the da Vinci robot to perform single-incision laparoscopic surgery [video]. Surg Endosc. 2010;24:3224.
8. Tugcu V, Simsek A, Evren I, et al. Single plus one port robotic radical prostatectomy (SPORP); initial experience. Arch Ital Urol Androl. 2017;89:178–81.
9. Mattevi D, Luciani LG, Vattovani V, Chiodini S, Puglisi M, Malossini G. First case of robotic laparoendoscopic single-site radical prostatectomy with single-site VesPa platform. J Robot Surg. 2018;12:381–5.
10. Kaouk JH, Haber GP, Autorino R, et al. A novel robotic system for single-port urologic surgery: first clinical investigation. Eur Urol. 2014;66:1033–43.
11. Kaouk J, Garisto J, Bertolo R. Robotic urologic surgical interventions performed with the single port dedicated platform: first clinical investigation. Eur Urol. 2019;75:684–91.
12. Kaouk JH, Sagalovich D, Garisto J. Robot-assisted transvesical partial prostatectomy using a purpose-built single-port robotic system. BJU Int. 2018;122(3):520–4.
13. Bertolo R, Garisto J, Gettman M, Kaouk J. Novel system for robotic single-port surgery: feasibility and state of the art in urology. Eur Urol Focus. 2018;4:669–73.
14. Checcucci E, De Cillis S, Pecoraro A, Peretti D, Volpi G, Amparore D, Piramide F, Piana A, Manfredi M, Fiori C, Autorino R, Dasgupta P, Porpiglia F, Uro-technology and SoMe working Group of the Young Academic Urologists Working Party of the European association of urology. Single-port robot-assisted radical prostatectomy: a systematic review and pooled analysis of the preliminary experiences. BJU Int. 2020;126(1):55–64.

15. Moschovas MC, Brady I, Noel J, Zeinab MA, Kaviani A, Kaouk J, Crivellaro S, Joseph J, Mottrie A, Patel V. Contemporary techniques of da Vinci SP radical prostatectomy: multicentric collaboration and expert opinion. Int Braz J Urol. 2022;48(4):696–705.

16. Moschovas MC, Bhat S, Sandri M, Rogers T, Onol F, Mazzone E, Roof S, Mottrie A, Patel V. Comparing the approach to radical prostatectomy using the Multiport da Vinci xi and da Vinci SP robots: a propensity score analysis of perioperative outcomes. Eur Urol. 2021;79(3):393–404.

17. Moschovas MC, Bhat S, Rogers T, Thiel D, Onol F, Roof S, Sighinolfi MC, Rocco B, Patel V. Applications of the da Vinci single port (SP) robotic platform in urology: a systematic literature review. Minerva Urol Nephrol. 2021;73(1):6–16.

18. Aminsharifi A, Sawczyn G, Wilson CA, Garisto J, Kaouk J. Technical advancements in robotic prostatectomy: single-port extraperitoneal robotic-assisted radical prostatectomy and single-port transperineal robotic-assisted radical prostatectomy. Transl Androl Urol. 2020;9(2):848–55.

19. Kaouk J, Garisto J, Eltemamy M, Bertolo R. Step-by-step technique for single-port robot-assisted radical cystectomy and pelvic lymph nodes dissection using the da Vinci® SPTM surgical system [published online ahead of print, 2019 mar 13]. BJU Int. 2019;124:707. https://doi.org/10.1111/bju.14744.

20. Kaouk J, Aminsharifi A, Sawczyn G, et al. Single-port robotic urological surgery using purpose-built single-port surgical system: single-institutional experience with the first 100 cases. Urology. 2020;140:77.

21. Moschovas MC, Bhat S, Onol F, Rogers T, Patel V. Early outcomes of single-port robot-assisted radical prostatectomy: lessons learned from the learning-curve experience. BJU Int. 2021;127(1):114–21.

22. Agarwal DK, Sharma V, Toussi A, Viers BR, Tollefson MK, Gettman MT, Frank I. Initial experience with da Vinci single-port robot-assisted radical prostatectomies. Eur Urol. 2020;77(3):373–9.

23. Ng CF, Teoh JY, Chiu PK, Yee CH, Chan CK, Hou SS, Kaouk J, Chan ES. Robot-assisted single-port radical prostatectomy: a phase 1 clinical study. Int J Urol. 2019;26(9):878–83.

24. Hinojosa-Gonzalez DE, Roblesgil-Medrano A, Torres-Martinez M, Alanis-Garza C, Estrada-Mendizabal RJ, Gonzalez-Bonilla EA, Flores-Villalba E, Olvera-Posada D. Single-port versus multiport robotic-assisted radical prostatectomy : a systematic review and meta-analysis on the da Vinci SP platform. Prostate. 2022;82(4):405–14.

25. Kaouk J, Beksac AT, Abou Zeinab M, Duncan A, Schwen ZR, Eltemamy M. Single port transvesical robotic radical prostatectomy: initial clinical experience and description of technique. Urology. 2021;155:130–7.

26. Saidian A, Fang AM, Hakim O, Magi-Galluzzi C, Nix JW, Rais-Bahrami S. Perioperative outcomes of single vs multi-port robotic assisted radical prostatectomy: a single institutional experience. J Urol. 2020;204(3):490–5.

27. Vigneswaran HT, Schwarzman LS, Francavilla S, Abern MR, Crivellaro S. A comparison of perioperative outcomes between single-port and multiport robot-assisted laparoscopic prostatectomy. Eur Urol. 2020;77(6):671–4.

28. Khalil MI, Chase A, Joseph JV, Ghazi A. Standard multiport vs. single-port robot-assisted simple prostatectomy: a single-center initial experience. J Endourol. 2022;36(8):1057–62.

29. Steinberg RL, Passoni N, Garbens A, Johnson BA, Gahan JC. Initial experience with extraperitoneal robotic-assisted simple prostatectomy using the da Vinci SP surgical system. J Robot Surg. 2020;14(4):601–7.

30. Kaouk J, Sawczyn G, Wilson C, Aminsharifi A, Fareed K, Garisto J, Lenfant L. Single-port percutaneous Transvesical simple prostatectomy using the SP robotic system: initial clinical experience. Urology. 2020;141:173–7.

31. Zhang M, Thomas D, Salama G, Ahmed M. Single port robotic radical cystectomy with intracorporeal urinary diversion: a case series and review. Transl Androl Urol. 2020;9(2):925–30.

32. Kaouk J, Garisto J, Eltemamy M, Bertolo R. Pure single-site robot-assisted partial nephrectomy using the SP surgical system: initial clinical experience. Urology. 2019;124:282–5.
33. Valero R, Sawczyn G, Garisto J, Yau R, Kaouk J. Concomitant multiquadrant robotic surgery for radical prostatectomy and left partial nephrectomy. Of the procedures by means of a single approach. Minutes Urol Esp. 2020;44:119–24.
34. Heo JE, Kang SK, Koh DH, Na JC, Lee YS, Han WK, Choi YD, Jang WS. Pure single-site robot-assisted pyeloplasty with the da Vinci SP surgical system: initial experience. Investig Clin Urol. 2019;60(4):326–30.
35. Iavazzo C, Minis EE, Gkegkes ID. Single-site port robotic-assisted hysterectomy: an update. J Robot Surg. 2018;12(2):201–13.
36. Acar O, Sofer L, Dobbs RW, et al. Single port and multiport approaches for robotic vaginoplasty with the Davydov technique. Urology. 2020;138:166–73.
37. Ganesan V, Goueli R, Rodriguez D, Hess D, Carmel M. Single-port robotic-assisted laparoscopic sacrocolpopexy with magnetic retraction: first experience using the SP da Vinci platform. J Robot Surg. 2020;14(5):753–8.
38. Liu H, Xu M, Liu R, Jia B, Zhao Z. The art of robotic colonic resection: a review of progress in the past 5 years. Updates Surg. 2021;73(3):1037–48.
39. Moschovas MC, Bhat S, Rogers T, Noel J, Reddy S, Patel V. Da Vinci single-port robotic radical prostatectomy. J Endourol. 2021;35(S2):S93–9.
40. Noël J, Moschovas MC, Sandri M, Bhat S, Rogers T, Reddy S, Corder C, Patel V. Patient surgical satisfaction after da Vinci® single-port and multi-port robotic-assisted radical prostatectomy: propensity score-matched analysis. J Robot Surg. 2022;16(2):473–81.

Future of Robotic Surgery

Rafael Silva de Araújo, João Pádua Manzano, and Lydia Masako Ferreira

1   Introduction

For two decades, Intuitive Surgical's da Vinci® system has maintained a monopoly on minimally invasive robotic surgical treatment. Restricted patents, well-developed marketing strategies, and high-quality products ensure the company's leading market share [1]. However, a lot of Intuitive Surgical's earliest patents will expire within the following couple of years due to nuances in US patent regulation. With this in mind, many of Intuitive Surgical's competitors (with backgrounds in medical and industrial robotics) have released robotic packages, some of which are now available [2].

More recent robotic systems have been created: ALF-X by TransEnterix [3], Single Port (single-port system) [4] and Ion Endoluminal System [5] by Intuitive Surgical, Inc., and Monarch robotic endoscopy system by Auris [6] have been accredited by the FDA. The Monarch and Ion systems compete for pulmonary use and are still in early clinical trials. PROCEPT is an FDA-approved Aquablation robotic machine advanced for the resection of benign prostate gland [7], while Revo-i (Korea) [8], Single Port Orifice Robotic Technology (SPORT) (Titan) [9], Medicaroid (Kawasaki and Sysmex) [10], Versius (Cambridge Medical Robotics) [10], and AVRA (German Aerospace Center) are being made around the world [11].

Robotic surgery is just starting to broaden. Merely due to its virtual nature, robotic systems will surely be in the middle of future innovations in liver surgical

R. S. de Araújo (✉)
Department of Plastic Surgery, Federal University of São Paulo, São Paulo, SP, Brazil

J. P. Manzano
Department of Surgery, Universidade Federal de São Paulo, São Paulo, Brazil
e-mail: jmanzano@unifesp.br

L. M. Ferreira
Plastic Surgery Department, Universidade Federal de São Paulo, São Paulo, Brazil

                243
J. P. Manzano, L. M. Ferreira (eds.), *Robotic Surgery Devices in Surgical Specialties*, https://doi.org/10.1007/978-3-031-35102-0_18

procedure. Completion further drives technological progress as intellectual property regulations recede and new groups input the marketplace [12]. We can expect better single-incision robotic surgery systems that can be combined with natural body hole sampling [13]. In addition, advances in parenchymal anatomical decoys consisting of the Cavitron Ultrasonic Surgical Aspirator (CUSA) for robotic systems are especially predicted. But we are also on the verge of a technological revolution, including "smart instruments," big data, emerging integrated sensors, and deep-learning techniques [12].

2   The General Future of Surgical Robotic Surgery

Harnessing its true potential, we are fast approaching an era of robotic surgery where a robot could either perform preprogrammed tasks or learn from its own experience through a feedback pipeline of good and not-so-good outcomes (reinforcement learning) [14]. In these robots, the automation would be driven by deep-learning models (DLM) that are designed, defined, and continuously evolved by the application of artificial neural networks (ANN). ANNs are the digital equivalent to the biological nervous system. DLM built with ANN are the intermediate stage for building autonomous robots. An intelligent robot will recognize organs, tissues, and surgical targets to execute a task that is either supervised by a surgeon or robot automatically, thereby complementing human performance.

To build DLM, large amounts of high-quality annotated data would be required; ideally, these data would be sourced from multiple centers following uniform standards. It has been observed that DLM, when deployed for clinical use, learn on their own and learn much faster than the human brain can ever do. DLM have a voracious appetite for data before their performance starts plateauing when the law of diminishing returns comes into force. A driverless car continuously captures and processes data through multiple sources and, thereby, constantly improves its own performance. Similarly, it is feasible to collect surgical data through intraoperative sensors and external and internal videos and as a direct feed from machines used for monitoring the patient during anesthesia [15]. These sensors could also potentially highlight blood vessels, nerve cells, tumor margins, or other important structures that could be hard to visualize [16].

The massive data obtained through relevant sources is profoundly rich and its immense potential to underline the indicators of surgical performance. DLM built with this big data would be able to preempt unexpected events and, correspondingly, lend an opportunity to the surgeon to preempt, intervene, and prevent potential complications. The futuristic robotic systems would be able to recognize the presence of a specific surgeon sitting at the console and provide him/her the instant access to one's own analyzed performance data in the backdrop of the global data relevant to the procedure displayed in real time for an instant and smarter surgical decision-making. With the advent of cloud services, low latency, and 5G Internet, it has been possible to instantly exchange information between machine–machine, machine–human, and human–human [17].

The large image repository of big data and the libraries of past case information along with the experience of the master surgeons are rich ingredients of building robust DLM. At the simplest level, a surgeon could view the data, animation, videos, and simulation for real-time interaction and, accordingly, would harness its immense potential in much improved surgical decision-making [18]. Validated DLM would be stored in the cloud to access on demand. It would not only overlay clearly laid blood vessels in relation to a tumor but also provide "pearls of wisdom" on how an expert surgeon would negotiate tricky bends in troubled waters. Furthermore, intelligent robots would be capable of selecting appropriate instruments and provide high-quality support in decision-making of the surgeon. "Digital Surgery," a health technology start-up company based in London, launched the first dynamic artificial intelligence system as a live-operating tool [19].

The reference tool helps to support surgical teams through complex medical procedures that are described akin to "Google Map for surgery." Digital surgery system aims at five billion people around the world who do not have access to well-tolerated surgical care. The platform leverages cameras and computer vision to recognize what is happening during surgery while cross-referencing a vast library of surgical guides and, thereupon, helps in predicting difficult situations to choose a correct approach. Surgical teams get real-time analysis and feedback via audio and visual cues, and thereby, they can guide using a wireless pedal. This is a true intersection of technology and surgery. Verb Surgical (Verb Surgical Inc., J&J/Alphabet, Mountain View, CA, USA) is a digitally enabled surgical platform with advanced instrumentation, low-latency connectivity, data analytics, advanced robotics, advanced visualization, simulation, and machine learning. The company is projecting its goal to democratize surgery and increase information to the surgeon given during a procedure [14].

Recently, Intuitive Surgical, Inc. obtained the FDA 510(k) approval for IRIS 1.0 System which processes medical images and delivers personalized segmented image studies (3D anatomical models) to the surgeons as a roadmap to the surgery of the patient. The surgeon would be able to manipulate the labeled multiplanar reconstructions on their iOS device to develop a surgical plan. It would also be possible for the da Vinci surgical system TilePro input to display 3D models and high-resolution stereo viewer via hardwire connection from the iOS device. This tool will allow image processing, review, analysis, communication, and media interchange of multidimensional digital images acquired from CT images [20].

3   Autonomous Robots

The primary prerequisite for developing autonomous robots is the availability of reliable, relevant, and robust data. It is from here that additional building blocks, generally reliant upon computer vision, may be laid. Computer vision is a deep-learning technique to understand image data and deal with tasks such as object detection, classification, and segmentation. Convolutional neural networks are a type of deep-learning algorithm designed to process data that exhibits natural spatial invariance (images whose meaning does not change under translation). Object detection and segmentation algorithms identify specific parts of an image corresponding to objects. Currently, some of these tools required to build autonomous robots are thought to be 2D surgical scene segmentation, depth-map reconstruction, surgical skill evaluation [21], and surgical simulation and planning [22]. Owing to the limited availability of high-quality data, many of these building blocks are being built from data from a select few competitions. In our excitement at the public release of data, we competed in two separate competitions [21, 22]; one for 3D segmentation and the other for 2D segmentation. The prior competition is geared toward presurgical planning and diagnostics, and the latter is oriented toward real-time object detection.

4 Big-Data Capture and Data Sharing

Healthcare is expected to generate 2314 exabytes (one billion gigabytes) of data by 2020 in the USA that is growing 48% annually (Stanford report), but it is also true that most of the data remain uncaptured or unutilized. Currently, we have unstructured, heterogeneous data available in silos not ready to be used meaningfully. Organizing and cleaning data are labor-intensive, immensely costly, and time-consuming tasks [14].

In the current medicolegal climate and data-conscious society, organizing such a repository is an endeavor of astronomical complexity and cost. As the balance between investment for scientific innovation and keeping it business-wise is often difficult to achieve, even for technology companies with deep pockets, it is difficult to build such repositories that are integral to building autonomous surgical robots. Gaining the consent of patients (current and past) would be an uphill task that has potential to be a legal and ethical minefield. As a corollary to this, the world-class artificial intelligence researchers have extremely limited access to high-quality surgical data for their research, which is a huge missed opportunity for the growth of autonomous robotic surgery. It is worth highlighting that the legal agreements between hospitals and the companies investing in innovations have been challenged by the regulatory bodies guarding the interest of patients, for example, Google and the University of Chicago Medical Center data sharing agreement has been challenged legally raising privacy concerns [23].

5 Nanosurgery

The smallest and most interesting leap for minimally invasive surgery is nanotechnology, because it would harness many potent facets of biotechnology: robotics, natural orifice surgery, and genetic/protein level cellular rearrangements of an illness. Researchers at the Hospital of the University of Pennsylvania are working on ways to use nanotechnology to treat acute respiratory distress syndrome with liposomes targeted to the pulmonary endothelium. They are approximately 100 nm in size and function as drug carriers coated with antibodies that bind to the inflamed pulmonary capillary endothelium [24].

6 Soft Robots

Equally impressive, but more on a macro scale, the origami robot is an ingested robot that unfolds within the visceral lumen and is magnetically controlled extracorporeally to image/diagnose or repair damaged organs [25]. Soft robotics may offer the greatest integration with the quickest timeline of current technology and surgical principles at hand by incorporating minimally invasive access and human control. Through soft robotics, the near future of robotics seems most attainable. Harvard University's Octobot is the first fully soft robot that is controlled by a microfluidic logic system rather than a rigid chip and fueled by hydrogen peroxide cells. In addition, it potentially offers the potential of controlled or autonomous intra-abdominal surgery and imaging [26].

7 Conclusion

With so many amazing new and overlapping technologies, surgeons are on the verge of a robotic surgery explosion that will yield dozens of unique robotic fusions. How can human surgeons remain competitive and at least semiautonomous? Basically, the answer lies with the surgeon: surgeons must view the development of robotics in surgery as a meaningful journey of discovery to gain more knowledge for the benefit of our patients. As robotic surgeons, we are committed to pursuing a safer and less invasive platform that, combined with the dual interaction between surgeon and robot, will enable us to achieve greater outcomes for patients while ensuring that we have holistic identity in their care.

References

1. Rassweiler JJ, Autorino R, Klein J, et al. Future of robotic surgery in urology. BJU Int. 2017;120:822–41.
2. Brodie A, Vasdev N. The future of robotic surgery. Ann R Coll Surg Engl. 2018;100(Suppl 7):4–13.
3. Samalavicius NE, Janusonis V, Siaulys R, et al. Robotic surgery using Senhance® robotic platform: single center experience with first 100 cases. J Robot Surg. 2020;14:371. https://doi. org/10.1007/s11701-019-01000-6.
4. Chan JY, Tsang RK, Holsinger FC, et al. Prospective clinical trial to evaluate safety and feasibility of using a single port flexible robotic system for transoral head and neck surgery. Oral Oncol. 2019;94:101–5; https://linkinghub.elsevier.com/retrieve/pii/S1368837519301654.
5. Ion lung biopsy system from Intuitive Surgical wins FDA approval. https://www.therobotreport. com/ion-lung-biopsy-intuitive-surgical-fda/.
6. J&J's Auris touts Monarch robotic bronchoscopy feasibility study: MassDevice. https://www. massdevice.com/jjs-auris-touts-monarchrobotic-bronchoscopy-feasibility-study/.
7. Misrai V, Rijo E, Zorn KC, et al. Waterjet ablation therapy for treating benign prostatic obstruction in patients with small- to medium-size glands: 12-month results of the first French Aquablation clinical registry. Eur Urol. 2019;76:667. https://linkinghub.elsevier.com/retrieve/pii/S0302283819305147.
8. Kang CM, Chong JU, Lim JH, et al. Robotic cholecystectomy using the newly developed Korean robotic surgical system, Revo-I: a preclinical experiment in a porcine model. Yonsei Med J. 2017;58:1075. https://doi.org/10.3349/ymj.2017.58.5.1075.
9. Seeliger B, Diana M, Ruurda JP, et al. Enabling single-site laparoscopy: the SPORT platform. Surg Endosc. 2019;33:3696–703. https://doi.org/10.1007/s00464-018-06658-x.
10. Rassweiler JJ, Autorino R, Klein J, et al. Future of robotic surgery in urology. BJU Int. 2017;120:822–41. https://doi.org/10.1111/bju.13851.
11. Home-AVRA Medical Robotics. https://www.avramedicalrobotics.com/.
12. Kinross JM, Mason SE, Mylonas G, et al. Next-generation robotics in gastrointestinal surgery. Nat Rev Gastroenterol Hepatol. 2020;17:430–40.
13. Kim W, Choi Y, Cho JY, et al. Robot single incision left lateral sectionectomy via da Vinci(R) xi single site & vaginal extraction of the specimen. Surg Oncol. 2020;33:254–5.
14. Peters BS, Armijo PR, Krause C, et al. Review of emerging surgical robotic technology. Surg Endosc. 2018;32:1636–55. https://doi.org/10.1007/s00464-018-6079-2.
15. Chand M, Ramachandran N, Stoyanov D, Lovat L. Robotics, artificial intelligence and distributed ledgers in surgery: data is key! Tech Coloproctol. 2018;22:645–8.
16. Rai S. Cognitive computing and artificial intelligence systems market in healthcare. BCC research report.
17. Kim SS, Dohler M, Dasgupta P. The Internet of Skills: use of fifth-generation telecommunications, haptics and artificial intelligence in robotic surgery. BJU Int. 2018;122:356–8. This article highlights the futuristic technological advances such as low-latency fifth generation network (5G), Internet of Things (ultrasensitive miniaturized sensors needed for real.
18. How robots and AI are creating the 21st-century surgeon: robotics business review. https://www.roboticsbusinessreview.com/healthmedical/how-robots-and-ai-are-creating-the-21st-century-surgeon/.
19. Digital Surgery's AI Platform guides surgical teams through complex procedures VentureBeat. https://venturebeat.com/2018/07/16/digital-surgerys-ai-platform-guides-surgical-teams-through-complex-procedures/. This article highlights the current use of machine learning in surgery.
20. Intuitive's IRIS 1.0 Medical Image Processing Software. http://surgrob.blogspot.com/2019/04/intuitives-iris-10-medical-image.html.
21. EndoVisSub2019-SCARED: Home. https://endovissub2019-scared.grand-challenge.org/.
22. KiTS19: Home. https://kits19.grand-challenge.org/.

23. Google and the University of Chicago are sued over data sharing. The New York Times. https://www.nytimes.com/2019/06/26/technology/googleuniversity-chicago-data-sharing-lawsuit.html.
24. Brenner JS. Nanomedicine for the treatment of acute respiratory distress syndrome. Ann Am Thorac Soc. 2017;14:561–4.
25. Walcutt L. Ingestible origami surgeon could be coming 'soon' to a pill near you. Forbes Mag. May 24, 2017.
26. Burrows L. The first autonomous, entirely soft robot. Harvard Gazette. August 24, 2016.

Index